Care of the Long-Stay Elderly Patient

Care of the Long-Stay Elderly Patient

SECOND EDITION

Edited by
Michael J. Denham

Consultant Geriatrician
Northwick Park Hospital

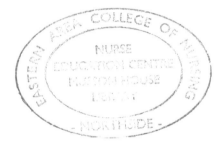

CHAPMAN AND HALL

LONDON • NEW YORK • TOKYO • MELBOURNE • MADRAS

UK	Chapman and Hall, 2–6 Boundary Row, London SE1 8HN
USA	Chapman and Hall, 29 West 35th Street, New York NY10001
JAPAN	Chapman and Hall Japan, Thomson Publishing Japan, Hirakawacho Nemoto Building, 7F, 1–7–11 Hirakawa-cho, Chiyoda-ku, Tokyo 102
AUSTRALIA	Chapman and Hall Australia, Thomas Nelson Australia, 102 Dodds Street, South Melbourne, Victoria 3205
INDIA	Chapman and Hall India, R. Seshadri, 32 Second Main Road, CIT East, Madras 600 035

Second edition 1991

© 1991 Chapman and Hall

Typeset in 10½ on 12pt Palatino by
Mews Photosetting, Beckenham, Kent

Printed in Great Britain by
St Edmundsbury Press, Bury St Edmunds, Suffolk

ISBN 0 412 34770 9

British Library Cataloguing in Publication Data

Care of the long-stay elderly patient. – 2nd ed.
   1. Residential institutions. Long-stay patients : Old persons. Care
   I. Denham, Michael J. (Michael John), *1935*–
362.16
ISBN 0–412–34770– 9

Library of Congress Cataloging-in-Publication Data

Care of the long-stay elderly patient / [edited by] Michael J. Denham.
   — 2nd ed.
   p cm.
   Includes bibliographical references.
   Includes index.
   ISBN 0–412–34770–9
   1. Aged—Long term care—Great Britain. I. Denham, Michael J. (Michael John)
   [DNLM: 1. Long Term Care—in old age. 2. Long Term Care—methods.
WT 30 C2715]
RA998.G7C37   1990
362.1′6—dc20
DNLM/DLC
for Library of Congress

Contents

Contributors

Juliette Alvin, FGSM   Founder of the British Society for Music Therapy

Pam Brereton, SRD   District Dietitian, Harrow Health Authority, Northwick Park Hospital, Harrow

M.J. Clarke-Williams, MA, MB, FRCP   Formerly Consultant Physician in Geriatric Medicine, Queen Alexandra Hospital, Cosham, Portsmouth

M. Cathy Conroy, Occupational Therapist, Moorgreen Hospital, Southampton

Tim Dartington, BA   Author, Head of the National Organisations Management Unit, London

M.J. Denham, MD, FRCP   Consultant Physician in Geriatric Medicine, Northwick Park Hospital, Harrow

E. Sonia Glossop, MCSP, SRP   Formerly District Physiotherapist, Harrow Health Authority, Northwick Park Hospital, Harrow

S. Haywood, Health Services Management Centre, Park House, Edgbaston, Birmingham

Pam Hibbs, OBE, BA, RCN, RHV   Chief Nursing Officer, St Bartholomew's Hospital, West Smithfield, London

Sandra Holley,   Formerly Speech Therapist, Northwick Park Hospital, Harrow

S. Jones, BA, PhD, ABPsS   Independent Consultant in Education, London

D.M. Langley,   Drama Therapist, Exeter

G.E. Langley, MB, FRCP, FRC Psych, DPM   Formerly Consultant Psychiatrist, Exe Vale Hospital, Exminster, Exeter

H. McGregor, RCN   Formerly Nurse Manager, Harrow Health Authority, Northwick Park Hospital, Harrow

Margaret Meikle, LCST, MCST   District Speech Therapist, Portsmouth and South East Hampshire Health Authority, Portsmouth

Sylvia Poulden, NDD   Author and Lecturer on Attitudes to Ageing – Intergenerational Communication, Department of Adult Education, University of Southampton

Ruth Sander, RCN   Head of Home, Jubilee House, Cosham, Portsmouth

Contributors

Barbara J. Sutcliffe, MCSP, SRP, Physiotherapy Consultant, London

C. Twining, MA, MSc, PhD, Top Grade Clinical Psychologist, Whitchurch Hospital, Whitchurch, Cardiff

Preface to the second edition

Since the first edition of this book was published there have been considerable changes in continuing care. NHS nursing homes have been created, enthusiasts have developed new initiatives, and attempts have been made to improve attitudes. The recent White Paper on Community Care is likely to accelerate the transfer of large numbers of elderly patients from long-stay hospital beds to private-sector accommodation: a move often accompanied by much anxiety about standards of care. Although Health Authorities visit private nursing homes and apply the National Association of Health Authorities' standards to them, anxieties continue. Unfortunately for the patients who remain in hospital, many Health Authorities seem reluctant to apply these same standards to their own long-stay departments, since many would fail abysmally. The 1987 annual report of the Health Advisory Service (see Chapter 3) presents a damning indictment of the care given to old people:

> A recent review of twelve consecutive HAS Reports on services for older people in hospitals shows that long-stay wards consistently offered environments which were unable to offer privacy, homely surroundings, personal space and possessions or adequate furniture. In the twelve districts there was not one comprehensive personalised clothing service. Half of the reports commented on the lack of effective management of continence. Catering was often provided according to the needs of the institution rather than those of the resident patients. Privacy was widely neglected . . . Impersonal ward routines for bed-times, waking times, and evening visiting times . . . The contribution of disciplines other than nursing was meagre . . . The level of medical participation was minimal and infrequent . . .

Good quality continuing care requires the integrated, imaginative input of many professions and professionals combined with alert, perceptive, strong leadership. This leadership means motivating all those in the unit to achieve the agreed aims. It may come from doctors, administrators or members of the rehabilitation professions, but perhaps, most appropriately, from the nursing profession. This is because nurses have such a strong, close working relationship with the patients – and without good nursing care all else fails. That leader should have a proven track record of recognizing patients' social and physical needs, and must persuade those closely involved with the patients to adopt a more open, questioning, flexible and self-critical approach to care. Custodial styles of care, with a suffocating emphasis on 'safety at all costs', must be avoided since they induce total dependency by effectively smothering any form of independence. It should be possible to define a philosophy of care which improves standards of practice and methods of working. Change can be achieved as the contributors, and the case studies show.

Preface to the first edition

Considerable attention, interest and enthusiasm are now focused on the acute medical and psychiatric problems of the elderly. Much has been achieved and many patients are enabled to return to the community. However, a number of patients will, unfortunately, be unable to do this and will need to remain in hospital for the rest of their lives. It was usual to speak of 'long-stay patients' or 'long-term care' in this situation, although there is now a tendency to adopt the description 'continuing care' which has more positive connotations. Until relatively recently, the needs of this group of patients have been somewhat neglected or ignored, but now more attention is being directed towards improving quality of life.

The writers in this book describe various ways in which this aim can be achieved. All make clear the important factor of the attitude of caring staff towards their clients. I hope that those who are keen to improve the quality of life for residents or patients will find the contents helpful, valuable and thought-provoking.

Michael J. Denham

Institutionalization and the elderly

The fifty elderly psychiatric patients were living on a ward in a totally protected environment with intensive nursing attention. The patients were allowed to do almost nothing for themselves for fear they might fall and hurt themselves. During the day they sat . . . staring into space, mumbling to themselves, ignoring everything that went on around them, expecting and getting total care and having no responsibility other than to breath, swallow and excrete . . .

The employees of the hospital shunned this ward and had to be forced to accept tours of duties when vacancies occurred (Folsom, 1968, see references in Chapter 1).

Part One

PREVENTING INSTITUTIONALIZATION: POLICY ISSUES

Chapter 1

The elderly in continuing-care units

INTRODUCTION

Elderly patient medicine had its origins some 50 years ago, when dedicated doctors, initially working independently in poor law infirmaries, in ortho-paedic departments and in the community, took an interest in the medical care of the elderly. It was soon realized that much could be done to improve the quality of care by instituting medical treatment, by com-mencing rehabilitation procedures, and by vigorous up-grading of the ward environment. Dr Marjory Warren, for example, who was appointed to the West Middlesex Hospital in England, found that when elderly patients with strokes were admitted, they were often put straight to bed and kept there. This rapidly led to institutionalization. She developed a radical approach to their treatment, introducing remedial exercises to encourage remobilization. Together with the assistance of facilities pro-vided by the social services departments, she found that she could discharge a high proportion of her patients. Thus it was that elderly patient medicine began, with a strong emphasis on rehabilitation. Later, elderly patient departments developed their expertise still further by combining a rehabilitation function with the admission, investigation and treatment of acutely ill elderly patients (Hodkinson and Jefferys, 1972; Bagnall et al., (1977).

Interest in the psychiatric care of the mentally ill old person developed mainly after the Second World War. As was the case with elderly patient medicine, it was found that much could be done to help not only the patient but also the relatives. Community support was increased, for example, by the use of intermittent or total day care, the help of psychiatric nurses working outside the hospital setting, and intermittent hospital admission for short or long-stay periods. The development of new drugs assisted the situation still further. Liaison between geriatricians and psychiatrists increased and improved and, in places, joint assessment units have been established. Indeed, just how far services for the elderly mentally ill have developed over the years can be assessed by reading 'The Rising Tide' (1982). It is unfortunate, however, that it is still necessary to record that the number of senior training posts for doctors interested in the speciality remains quite small and limits the creation of new consultant 'psychogeriatric' posts.

Unfortunately, even today, some very old elderly may still fear admission to elderly patient departments because they equate them with the gaunt, inhospitable-looking buildings of the old workhouses, so well described by Townsend (1962), and rather expect that once they are admitted they will not come out alive. They may be unaware that many admission units are now in newer accommodation which forms part of the district general hospital. However, their fears may be well founded in respect of continuing-care units where the elderly are often housed in older buildings, frequently 'handed-down' from other specialities which no longer need them and which are entirely unsuited for their new function – indeed, sometimes retaining some of the worst features of the workhouse. In spite of upgrading, these wards can still look depressing, lacking both privacy and personal space for the patient (Health Advisory Service Annual Report, 1987). The patients may be dressed in clothing which is not their own, and sit in rows along the wall, staring vacantly into space and doing nothing (Brocklehurst, 1977). In such an establishment, where the staff may consider there is nothing further to be done, institutionalization will rapidly develop.

INSTITUTIONS AND INSTITUTIONALIZATION

In recent years several authors have attempted to define the characteristics of institutions and their effects on inmates. When these factors are understood it will be easier to plan how best to reverse at least some of the features of institutionalization.

Types and characteristics

Goffman (1960), in his important contribution, considered that there are five types of institution:

1. Those established to care for persons thought to be incapable and harmless and who need protecting from the environment, e.g., homes for the aged.
2. Those places caring for persons incapable of looking after themselves, or who are a threat to the community, e.g., TB sanatoria or mental hospitals.
3. Those established to pursue some technical task, e.g., army barracks or boarding schools.
4. Those organized to protect the community against potential dangers to it, e.g., jails and prisoner-of-war camps.
5. Those designated as retreats from the world, e.g., convents.

In many institutions the activities of daily life, such as sleep, work and play are carried out under one roof, governed by one authority. Each phase of a person's daily routine is rigidly fixed and is carried out in the company of others, who are all treated alike. The enforced activities are part of the overall plan designed to fulfil the official aims of that institution. The inmates, who have restricted access to the world outside, are, on admission, stripped of 'wonted supports', such as personal possessions, and 'self' is systematically, if unintentionally, mortified. The inmate is often introduced to a privilege system where there are house rules, and a system of rewards or punishment. He may react to this by withdrawing from events except those around him, and may adopt a rebellious line, or become converted to the status required of him in order to stay out of trouble. Those inmates most likely to survive are the 'tough' ones (Turner, Tobin and Lieberman, 1972).

King and Raynes (1968) described four main factors which can produce institutionalization:

1. Depersonalization – where inmates have limited personal possessions and privacy.
2. Social distance – where staff live away from the inmates and do not join in with socially orientated activities.
3. Block treatment – where everyone is dealt with as a group. The inmates have to wait in a queue until all have been dealt with before the next activity starts.
4. Lack of variation in daily routine – inmates are treated the same way, no matter how much they differ from each other.

Pincus (1968), who studied homes for the aged, considered that there are four dimensions related to the institutional environment:

1. Public/private – that is, the ability of the resident to have a private domain which is not open to public view or use, and which the institution will not transgress.
2. Structured/unstructured – the degree to which the resident is expected to conform to rules and discipline, and his ability to make decisions or to have a choice.
3. Resource sparse/resource rich – this assesses the degree of the resident to be able to engage in work or lesser activities.
4. Isolated/integrated – which assesses the opportunity for communication and reaction with the world outside the home. This point is made clearly by Martin (1984) in a review of official inquiries into maltreatment of patients and poor management in some long-stay psychiatric hospitals.

Physical features

The institutional environment is influenced by a number of physical and psychological factors. Among these are the size and structure of the accommodation, the furnishings and the ward atmosphere, as well as human factors of the personality and attitudes of both staff and residents. There seems to be no general agreement about the size of the ideal long-stay unit. Townsend (1962), when considering old people's homes, suggested that size correlated with quality of care, that the smaller establishments, often run by voluntary organizations, having better staffing, toiletting facilities and freedom of choice for the resident, and therefore gave better care than the larger units. Greenwald and Linn (1971) who studied nursing homes in America and rated them according to bed usage, staff ratios, services available, administrative policies and general physical characteristics, came to similar conclusions.

There is increasing concern that the design of long-stay units should reduce the barriers to patient movement and communication, and improve privacy. There is more emphasis on smaller bedroom units, and supplying clues for the patient to identify a room, area or toilet facility by the use of varying colour schemes. Where there is reasonable privacy, e.g., single bedrooms, there is a greater tendency for patients to have a neutral attitude towards the communal rooms, and less tendency for them to develop territorial attitudes towards certain positions or furniture in these rooms. However, a possessive attitude towards seating positions is a complex problem. There is increasing emphasis on the need for accommodation and facilities to allow the patient to undertake various diversional activities which will foster an active role and reduce institutionalization (discussed further in Chapters 10, 11, 12 and 13). The lack of such facilities can produce a passive role, social withdrawal, a complaining attitude, or just sitting and watching (Lawton, 1970).

The Department of Health and Social Security has issued a series of excellent building notes. Number 37, 'Hospital Accommodation for Elderly People', covers the requirements for District General Hospitals and Community and Day Hospitals. It does not apply to elderly patients with mental illness (see Building Note No. 35). The note gives sound advice, is comprehensive, and considers many factors involved in ward design – including fire precautions, lighting, noise, critical dimensions, heating, ventilation, fittings, decorations, design features, colour schemes, bed space, etc. It is to be recommended to all those involved in the design of new ward accommodation or with up-grading existing wards. It should be read in conjunction with Common Activity Spaces, Volume 1 (Building Note No. 40).

The atmosphere of a ward can clearly influence a patient, and it relates to the degree of institutionalization. Bennett (1963) has attempted to measure this by constructing a ten-item index of totality. An institution received a high score if, for example, it was designed as a permanent residence; all activities were arranged sequentially for the entire group of inmates; there was continual observation by the staff of the inmates, who were not allowed to make decisions regarding their time or property, most of which had been removed; and where congregate living was required as the usual pattern of accommodation. Bennett found that mental hospitals tended to have high totality and public homes low totality.

Personality and physical status

The personality of people in institutions has been much studied, particularly to assess the effects of admission. Lieberman (1969), in a review, has listed the psychological characteristics of inmates which includes poor adjustment to the new environment, depression, intellectual inefficiency, negative self-image, a view of themselves as old and a feeling of insignificance. Lieberman, Prock and Tobin (1968) have attempted to find out whether these features were present before admission, or were the result of it, by comparing subjects at home and waiting admission with those who have actually been admitted. Seven areas of psychological functioning were studied, including cognitive functioning, personality traits, self-image, time perception and relationships with other people. It was concluded that some factors such as despair and psychological distance from others were present before admission, but that other features developed later. They suggested that institutionalization was a complex process which begins when a person first considers entering a home and continues throughout the time a person is there. However, people with certain types of personality seem most likely to apply for admission, i.e., there is a degree of self-selection into homes. Those who survive best in institutions were those: (1) who accepted and conformed to the system and organization of the homes; (2) who wanted to be admitted; and (3) whose physical arrangements in the home were better than in their own home. On the other hand, Turner and colleagues (1972) concluded that aggressive characteristics helped survival in homes. Lieberman (1969) pointed out that people who enter institutions find it increasingly difficult to re-enter the community, presumably due to the factors mentioned above.

Several workers have attempted to assess both physical and social factors which predict the need for admission to an institution. Liberakis (1981) found that institutionalization tended to be associated with biological and social handicaps which affect communication and the activity of the patient. Wingard *et al.* (1987), in their critical review of a large number of studies of those in institutional care, concluded that four factors were repeatedly identified as predictors of the need for care. These were: increasing old age, especially if the person was very old; being female; lack of care-givers and social support; and poor mental and physical health associated with the need for assistance with the activities of daily living. However, differing philosophies or styles of care can also influence the type of institution chosen. Cross *et al.* (1983) found that elderly confused patients in London were more likely to be in residential care, whereas in New York they were more likely to be in nursing homes. Overall, admission to a home appears to be most beneficial for those whose existence in the community is most at risk.

The effects of the institution on the patient

A number of attempts have been made to measure the effect of the institutional environment on the inmates by devising scales or inventories. King and Raynes (1968) developed a 16-item Inmate Management Scale as a method of discriminating between institutions with different patterns of managing their inmates. The scale is designed for the management of children, but has some relevance to the elderly. Four parameters of function were measured – rigidity of the regime, treatment of the inmates, depersonalization of inmates, and social distance between staff and inmates. King and Rayner found that the rigidity of care of the children appeared to be dependent on management attitudes rather than on the degree of dependency of the inmates. Houts and Moos (1969) devised a Ward Initiative Scale which measured patient and staff perception of the behaviours expected and supported on the wards. Seven subscales were measured, including involvement on the ward, aggression, submission to staff, and revealing self to others. The scale is considered useful in allowing wards to be compared when assessing the effect of treatment. Raynes, Pratt and Roses (1979) have attempted to measure the quality of communication between staff and residents by measuring the frequency of different types of speech – whether informative, controlling, any other kind of speech, or no speech. Wing and Brown (1970) described a Ward Restrictiveness Scale, for use in mental hospitals, which assessed, for example, the freedom of the patient to move about the ward and hospital, bathing and toiletting arrangements and clothing availability. Spiegel and Younger (1972) devised a Ward Climate Inventory of 23 items, which consists of three main factors – concern of the personnel for patients, concern of the patients for the patients, and ward morale. McReynolds (1968) describes the Hospital Adjustment Scale which is, however, more related to measuring the patient's level of functioning in spite of psychiatric symptoms rather than the effect of the environment of the patient.

The attitude of the staff, both caring and administrative, can have a considerable effect on institutional life. Thus, homes which induce conformity by a system of authority, adhering to well-established patterns of caring without question, discouraging complaining, introducing disciplinary procedures with privilege and sanction systems, are likely to produce severe institutionalization, and the index of totality is marked (Bennett, 1963). In addition, not all staff are trained to cope with the social, psychological, psychiatric and physical problems of the patient. Indeed, the difficulties experienced in trying to cope with such patients can easily induce stress in the staff, which in turn can make them less receptive to ideas and concepts of changes in care. Finally, the general environment of the unit can make them less attractive places to work in and it may be difficult to attract staff – leading to high turnover with loss of drive, initiative and morale (Folsom, 1968).

PREVENTING INSTITUTIONALIZATION

The dangers and effects of institutionalization have been detailed, but preventing them is not easy since there are a number of problems. Firstly, the consultant physician or psychiatrist may take the view that everything that can be done for the patient has already been done, and since their time is limited, it should be spent on those patients who are most likely to benefit and be discharged home. Other caring staff may take a similar attitude. Secondly, the ward accommodation is often unsuitable for long-stay patients, both from a nursing point of view and as a site for diversional activities. Bathing and toileting facilities may be unsuitable, badly sited and lacking privacy. Access to ward areas may be difficult, thus restricting movement of patients, and making the management of incontinence more difficult. The physical outlook may be depressing, while bedding, chairs and other equipment may be old and unsuitable for the elderly infirm. Diversional activity areas may be limited. Thirdly, the organization of the patient's day may be arranged to fit the nursing schedules rather than the patient's benefit. Patients may still be woken up at 5 a.m. and put to bed at 2 p.m. In addition, they may not have their own clothing or may be provided with obvious institutional clothes. Privacy, particularly for toileting may be restricted. The ability of the patient to make even the smallest decision is taken away. On the other hand, an enlightened, enthusiastic attitude among caring staff can lead to considerable improvement in the care of patients in long-stay accommodation (Folsom 1969, Wing and Brown 1970, Loew and Silverstone 1971, Gottesman 1973, Savage 1974, McIver 1978, HAS Annual Report 1986/7). Recently, advice and guidelines for improving care of the elderly in hospital have been published by the Royal College of Nursing (1987). Fourthly, carers may fail to consider the patient's previous intellectual capacities and illnesses but if interest is taken in past hobbies and jobs, it may be possible to 'light–up' the mind. The subsequent chapters in this book show in greater detail what can be achieved.

One of the pleasures of being a consultant physician or psychiatrist in charge of the elderly is the immense job satisfaction to be obtained not only from treating the acutely ill person, but also by improving the quality of life for patients in long-stay accommodation. It *is* possible to get away from the situation of patients sitting around walls staring vacantly into space. Much can be done to help patients use their minds actively.

Nursing a long-stay patient requires its own special attributes and attitude of mind. The nurse must be aware of the effects and risks of institutionalization and dependency. Case conferences are important when all the caring staff meet to discuss patient care. The remedial and nursing staff, together with volunteers, should all be closely involved in the diversional activities. It can be helpful to invite patients to join nursing/management committees to comment on the organization of the patients' day. Questionnaires of all caring staff, patients and relatives (Raphael and Mandeville, 1979) can be very revealing about the quality of care being given. To the sceptical, diversional activities may still seem a waste of time. However, case examples in the last section of the book show what can be achieved.

CONCLUSION

Some people fear the onset of old age, visualizing deteriorating memory and intellect, incontinence, and loss of independence leading to an institutional existence. Some have even committed suicide to avoid the situation. This is very sad since the reality can be quite different. However, much can be done – and still has to be done – to improve the quality of life in continuing-care wards.

REFERENCES

Bagnall, W.E., Dalta, S.R., Knox, J. and Horrocks, P. (1977) Geriatric medicine in Hull – a comprehensive service. *Brit. Med. J.*, **2**, 102–4.

Bennett, R. (1963) The meaning of institutional life. *Gerontologist*, **3**, 117–25.

Brocklehurst, J.C. (1977) The quality of life in long-stay geriatric units in *Quality of Life of the Elderly in Residential Homes and Hospitals – a Report of a Seminar held by the Department of Adult Education, University of Keele*. Beth Jonson Foundation.

Cross, P.S., Gurland, B.J. and Mann, A.H. (1983) Long-term institutional care of demented elderly peple in New York City and London. *Bull, N.Y. Acad. Med.* **59**, 267–75.

DHSS (Department of Health and Social Security) (1973) Department of Psychiatry (Mental Illness) for a District General Hospital. Hospital Building Note 35, HMSO, London.

DHSS (1986) Hospital Accommodation for Elderly People. Building Note 37, HMSO London.

DHSS (1986) Common Activity Spaces, Vol. 1. Building Note 40, HMSO, London.

Folsom, J.C. (1968) Reality orientation for the elderly mental patient *Geriatr. Psychiatry,* **1**, 291–306.

Goffman, E. (1960) Characteristics of total institutions, in *Identity and Anxiety* (eds Stein, M.R., Vidick, A.J. and White, D.M.), Free Press of Glencoe, Illinois.

Gottesman, L.E. (1973) Milieu treatment of the aged in institutions. *Gerontologist,* **13**, 23–6.

Greenwald, S.R. and Linn, M.W. (1971) Intercorrelation of data on nursing homes. *Gerontologist,* **11**, 337–40.

Health Advisory Service.Annual Reports, 1986, 1987. NHS Health Advisory Service, Sutherland House, 29–37 Brighton Road, Sutton, Surrey SM2 5AN, England.

Hodkinson, H.M. and Jefferys, P.M. (1972) Making hospital geriatrics work. *Brit. Med. J.,* **4**, 536–9.

Houts, P.S. and Moos, R.H. (1969) The Development of a ward initiative scale for patients. *J. Clin. Psychiatry,* **25**, 319–24.

King, R.D. and Raynes, N.V. (1968) An operational measure of inmate management in residential institutes. *Soc. Sci Med.,* **2**, 41–53.

Lawton, M.P. (1970) Assessment, integration and environments for older people. *Gerontologist,* **10**, 38–46.

Liberakis, E.A. (1981) Factors predisposing to institutionalisation. *Acta Psychiatrica Scan.,* **63**, 356–66.

Lieberman, M.A. (1969) Institutionalisation of the aged: effects on behaviour. *J. Gerontology,* **24**, 330–40.

Lieberman, M.A., Prock, V.N. and Tobin, S.S. (1968) Psychological effects of institutionalisation *J. Gerontology,* **23**, 343–53.

Loew, C.A. and Silverstone, B.M. (1971) A programme of intensified stimulation and response facilitation for the senile aged. *Gerontologist,* **11**, 341–7.

MacIver, V. (1978) Freedom to be. *Can. Nurse,* **74**, 19–26.

Martin, J.P. (1984) *Hospitals in Trouble,* Blackwell, Oxford.

McReynolds, P. (1968) The Hospital adjustment scale 3. *Psychol. Rep.* **23**, 823–35.

Pincus, A. (1968) The definition and measurement of the institutional environment in homes for the aged. *Gerontologist,* **8**, 207–10.

Raphael, W. and Mandeville, J. (1979) Old People in Hospital. King Edward's Hospital Fund for London, London.

Raynes, N.V., Pratt, M.V. and Roses, S. (1979) *Organisational Structure and the Care of the Mentally Retarded,* Croom Helm, London, and Praeger, New York.

Royal College of Nursing (1987) *Improving Care of the Elderly in Hospital.* The Royal College of Nursing in collaboration with the British Geriatrics Society and the Royal College of Psychiatrists. Royal College of Nursing, London.

Savage, B. (1974) Rethinking psychogeriatric nursing care. *Nursing Times,* **70**, 282–4.

Spiegal, D. and Younger, J.B. (1972) Ward climate and community stay of psychiatric patients. *J. Consult. Clin. Psychol.* **39**, 62–9.

The Rising Tide (1982) Developing Services for Mental Illness in Old Age. NHS Health Advisory Service, Sutherland House, 24–37 Brighton Road, Sutton, Surrey SM2 5AN, England.

Townsend, P. (1962) *The Last Refuge,* Routledge and Kegan Paul, London.

Turner, B.F., Tobin, S.F. and Lieberman, M.A. (1972) Personality traits as predictors of institutional adaptation among the aged. *J. Gerontology,* **27**, 61–8.

Wing, J.K. and Brown, G.W. (1970) *Institutionalisation and Schizophrenia,* Cambridge University Press, Cambridge.

Wingard, D.L., Jones, D.W. and Kaplan, R.M. (1987) Institutional care utilisation by the elderly: a critical review. *Gerontologist,* **27**, 156–63.

Chapter 2

Standards of institutional care for the elderly

This chapter considers two aspects of standard setting: the content and nature of standards and the process of monitoring them. Both are problematic. Concern about standards of care for elderly patients in institutions rightly persist, shared by leaders of NHS professional groups: '' . . . while there has been considerable progress, inhumanity and inadequate care have not been eradicated from every ward where old people are treated'' (Royal College of Nursing, 1987). Arrangements for monitoring public and private provision also have many critics, partly because they have not rooted out poor standards. They have proved inadequate for the task.

Day and Klein (1987) impishly suggest that ''the only sure way of avoiding scandals in institutions is to close them down''. However, the increasing numbers of the very old and frail, combined with professional aspirations to care and treat, preclude such a development. They will continue to be major users of acute hospital and community health services, with a sizeable number spending their last years of life in institutions. Even when deterrents to admission were introduced in the 19th century, elderly people found their way into workhouses.

Indeed, there is every likelihood of an increase in institutional care. In some countries a higher proportion of the elderly than in the United Kingdom live in institutions (Laing, 1987), so there is no reason to think that the trend will inevitably be downwards. Recently, the trend has been upwards because of the growth of the private sector, which provided an additional 20 000 nursing home beds in England between 1985 and 1987. The effect has been to increase the likelihood of an elderly person being in residential care. Laing estimated that it was 13% higher in March 1986 than it had been in 1981. While ''this age standardized index of provision fell back slightly in 1987 (it) remained 12% higher . . than in 1981'' (Laing, 1987, p. 175). So, the issue of standards in institutions will remain an important factor in the quality of life of the elderly.

There is no sign of the surge in private provision tailing off, or of it going into reverse. It is now as important as the NHS in the provision of long-term institutional care. In 1987 there were 110 000 beds for the elderly in nursing homes and NHS elderly patient facilities in England (Table 2.1). Over 50% were in the private nursing home sector.

Table 2.1 Beds for the elderly: England, 1987

Region	*Number of beds**	
	NHS elderly patient	Private nursing homes
Northern	3 949	2 039
Yorkshire	4 827	5 562
Trent	5 263	5 550
East Anglia	2 499	1 524
North-west Thames	3 564	1 048
North-east Thames	4 662	1 729
South-east Thames	3 829	6 252
South-west Thames	2 877	6 038
Wessex	3 433	5 065
Oxford	1 822	2 371
South-western	3 773	7 324
West Midlands	6 072	4 507
Mersey	3 042	3 157
North-West	5 163	4 563
Total	54 775	56 729

*Figures for NHS elderly patient beds are for 1986 (data supplied by the Unit for Inter-authority comparisons, University of Birmingham). Figures for private nursing homes are for December, 1987 (survey conducted by the Health Services Management Centre, University of Birmingham)

The regional data, of course, obscure wide variations between district health authorities (DHAs), although there are now few without a significant private sector. The number of DHAs with 20 or more private nursing home beds per 1000 resident population aged 75 years or over increased from 30 to 67 between 1985 and 1987. In some places private provision is very large with 30 or more beds for each 1000 resident population aged 75 or more (Figure 2.1). So a discussion of the quality of institutional care should give at least equal prominence to private suppliers.

STANDARDS: PUBLIC AND PRIVATE

The Royal College of Nursing reports progress in the NHS (1987, para 1.16), and Day and Klein (1987, p. 384) feel that standards in the private sectors have also been improving. However, few observers would deny a concern with general standards. NHS professionals and the media frequently direct attention to the failings of the private nursing homes. Some have been closed. Similarly, the final report of the outgoing Director

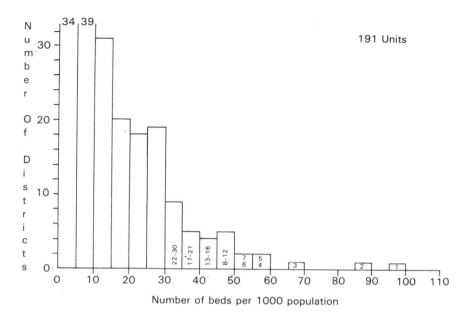

Figure 2.1 Number of nursing home beds per 1000 resident population aged 75+ in England, 1987.

of the Health Advisory Service (HAS) was equally worrying about NHS standards (Health Advisory Service, 1987): 'The quality of long-term care offered to elderly people in hospital is still generally very poor. There is a growing contrast with the individual personal care offered in many local authority homes to elderly people with degrees of disability not significantly different from those seen in hospital. . . . in the hospitals "traditional" care is still prevalent. One recurrent issue is the unnecessary use of restraint . . . (The) reasons include staff shortages . . . and suffocating emphasis on "safety at all costs" which operates at the expense of rehabilitation and self respect for elderly people' (Health Advisory Service, 1987, pp. 14–15).

Improvements in the quality of life for elderly people in institutions require dramatic improvements on past performance. The literature abounds with pleas for higher standards and more effective arrangements to reinforce them. However, exhortation is easy, and the history of the NHS is littered with similar sentiments. There are clearly no magic formulae, quick fixes or quality assurance systems which could solve the problems 'at a stroke'. It will be a hard, long slog. However, improvements are possible through more general application (rather than rhetoric) of increasingly accepted wisdoms. Quality is improved by more attention to the outcomes of care, in which patient preferences are accorded centre-stage.

STANDARDS

What standards?

The debate on existing standards is not very well informed; there is no set of standards of good practice to which all would subscribe or data on which to base general judgements. DHSS statistics on nursing homes are confined to capacity: the number of hospitals and homes, facilities and beds. Performance indicators for NHS elderly patient services focus mainly on the adequacy of inputs and the efficiency with which facilities are used, rather than quality of care. This is well illustrated by the DHSS booklet explaining performance indicators. It picks out 'key indicators . . . to give a broad view of health service activity in the country as a whole . . . ' and suggests questions for attention (DHSS, 1988, p. 6). The questions for services for elderly people are: 'How long do elderly people stay in hospital? How many people spend very long periods in hospital? To what extent do districts make use of day care for the elderly? How adequate are district nursing services?' (ibid, p. 51). None of these questions addresses the issue of standards of care except indirectly: a shorter length of stay, ample day-care provision and district nursing services are presumed to limit the need for, and exposure to, institutions. Also, while shorter lengths of stay may be a useful proxy of good practice for rehabilitation they tell us nothing about the quality of care for those in institutions for the remainder of their life. For them, the booklet refers to the aim of providing continuing care in 'small, homely units' (p. 51) on which there is little information.

Structure, process and outcome

The difficulties in standard setting still stem from legitimately different perceptions of what is good quality care and the facts that should inform judgements. Unacceptable standards may be relatively easy to identify (but even then only when they have been subject to an enquiry, e.g., the Nye Bevan Lodge Part III Home inquiry) but most residents are hopefully living out their time in hospitals and homes much better than this. For them there is no agreement on whether the plethora of norms and guidelines cover and give due weight to the most important aspects of care.

One way of imposing some discipline on ideas about the content and measurement of quality is the one suggested by Donabedian (1980). His methodology has been a familiar feature on training courses for many years. He distinguishes between structure (number and calibre of personnel, quality of buildings, equipment etc.); process (the way the resources are used); and outcomes (the benefits to the patient). Standards of good practice should include aspects of all three elements.

The NHS remains preoccupied with structure and process considerations in quality, in spite of acknowledgements of the importance of outcome measures. There are few outcome measures in DHSS performance indicators or the guidelines on the registration and inspection of nursing homes, prepared by the National Association of Health Authorities (NAHA). Comments of registration officers on training programmes for registration officers at the Health Services Management Centre (HSMC), University of Birmingham, make it clear that this 'neglect' extends to practice in inspections of private nursing homes. Attention focusses on staffing issues and accommodation requirements. It is likely that this reflects NHS practice since most inspectors are drawn from its management. The effect of this preoccupation with structure and process is well illustrated by a comparison of the National Association of Health Authorities guidelines (1985, 1988) with the booklet 'Home Life'. The guidelines were produced by a working party sponsored by the Department of Health and Social Security (1984) for residential homes.

The booklet 'Home Life'

The booklet (Avebury, 1984) opens with a statement on the principles of care, referring to the 'conviction' which underlies the recommendations and requirements set out in the code: 'those who live in residential care should do so with dignity; that they should have the respect of those who support them; should live with no reduction of their rights as citizens . . . and should be entitled to live as full and active a life as their physical and mental condition will allow' (para 1.1).

Personal fulfilment, dignity, autonomy, individuality, esteem, quality of experience, emotional needs and risk and choice are covered in a discussion of residents' rights.

This opening sets the scene for sections on social care, physical features, approach to different client groups, staff and the role of the inspection authority. General guidance is offered, often calling for qualitative judgements. For example, in the section on staff there are 31 recommendations. Four of these concern staff numbers with a suggested approach to a calculation of the number of care hours per resident. The others concern personal qualities and skills, appointment procedures, training, and the importance of management. There are references to the importance of 'shared aims', 'personal warmth', 'patience', 'responsiveness' and 'respect for the needs of the individual' (p. 49).

The section on physical features refers to official guidance which is followed by discussion of suitable locations, size, accommodation and space and arrangements for own rooms. The latter is intended to re-inforce the general message of individuality and respect: 'special reasons will be expected where there are more than two people to a room'. People should be able to bring their own furniture to bedsitting rooms, and private wash basins should ensure 'privacy . . . for personal care considered private' (pp. 33–34).

NAHA guidelines

The NAHA guidelines have two sections. One offers advice to health authorities; the second suggests model guidelines which follow these suggestions closely. The tone is quite different to Home Life, even allowing for the wider remit of the guidelines: they also cover private acute hospitals. While there are brief references to the 'importance of flexibility and individual care' and 'sensitivity to the changing needs' of the elderly and a recommendation of regular occupational and leisure activities (para 1.3) there is no equivalent to Home Life's statement of philosophy. Rather, the NAHA publication in its own words – 'continually refers to legislation and associated regulations concerned with the physical standards of nursing homes and the qualifications and suitability of staff. The working party has emphasised statutory requirements as it considers that a good understanding and compliance with these requirements together with vigilance on the part of registering authorities will lead to higher standards of care' (para 1.2).

The advice on staffing provides a good illustration of the effect of different perspectives on quality. Home Life concentrates on personal qualities and experience. In contrast, the NAHA guidelines discuss legal requirements, qualifications, delegation, notice of absence, nursing levels, staffing ratios, records, medical advice and staffing, and arrangements for services for other types of staff (pp. 63–79). NAHA guidelines on accommodation similarly reflect administrative rather than patient pre-occupations. They discuss location of premises, construction, sanitary facilities, heating, lighting and ventilation, telephones, emergency electrical supplies, the nature and adequacy of accommodation for patients and regard for the provisions of the Health and Safety at Work Act (pp. 70–75).

A supplement to the handbook (September, 1988) moves NAHA guidance a little in the direction taken by Home Life. There is a discussion of qualitative factors in sections on the patient relationship, including the right to privacy and full information and relations between staff and patients (pp. 2–5). However, most of the supplement is taken up with other topics which reflect an administrative/professional concern with inputs rather than quality of life. Discussions of management and staffing issues (pp. 6–11) remain pre-occupied with qualifications and staffing ratios. The remainder of the supplement is concerned with sanctions (pp. 12–22) and arrangements for the control, supply, storage and administration of drugs and medicines (pp. 23–27).

What is lost by this relative neglect of outcome considerations, true of most health services? It could be argued that the systems ensure adequate premises, space, staff, qualifications, high-standard nursing and medical practices and pre-requisites of quality. Maybe, but not all the soul-less and joyless units described in HAS reports were so deprived. Something else was missing which might have been captured by a concern with outcomes. Also, structural and process standards reflect professional judgements which are not necessarily synonomous with priorities of patients and their families.

Making outcomes matter more

The absence or neglect of outcome considerations in assessing quality is unsurprising: there are many gaps in our knowledge of the impact of therapeutic and caring interventions on recipients. However, the problem has deeper roots than the lack of information. The absence of information was no bar to drawing up a list of subject headings related to all three elements in a training manual for health authority members (National Health Service Training Authority, 1988). Possible indicators, for each of the areas in which standards could be set, were also identified (Table 2.2).

One explanation for the continuing NHS preoccupation with inputs and process considerations is not ignorance, but that it reflects NHS beliefs. The aim is to have more professionals and facilities available. From this viewpoint, provision of services is an end in itself, evident in a concern to ensure equal access and commitment to retention of hospital beds. Nor is this imbalance automatically corrected by implementing one of the many quality assurance schemes now on offer.

Table 2.2 Long-term care for the elderly: inputs, process, outcomes*

Measuring input and structure – possible indicators

nurse staffing (number, mix)
access to physiotherapy, chiropody, dentistry, OT, speech therapy
medical cover
staff training opportunities
record system
physical environment
use of voluntary help
resident's personal environment (e.g. personal clothes, memorabilia, etc.)

Measuring process – possible indicators

nursing procedures
flexibility in the resident's day
variability/choice in food
range of patient/resident activities
access to visitors
frequency of trips and outings

Measuring outcome – possible indicators

mobility
self care
physical condition
incontinence
mental condition
independence
social integration

*From: Manual for Health Authority Chairmen and Members (NHSTA, 1988)

Energies are sometimes directed to choice and implementation of systems rather than outcome measures and appropriate standards. Also it is not evident that they will necessarily tilt attention from professional assessments of the adequacy of resources allocated to them to outcome measures (which are more threatening to professional interests).

Outcomes: consumer preferences

HSMC programmes for registration officers have tried to cut through these problems by focussing on a central tenet of the NHS to which all subscribe. The choice of outcome measures is largely determined by whether they accord with the priorities, wishes and aspirations of patients and perhaps relatives.

Consumerism has the slight disadvantage of being 'in fashion' and understandably annoying to those who see the many years of their previous professional life having been devoted to the care of patients. Nevertheless, consumer preferences as a starting point for assessments of quality and how to improve it are useful. They provide an antidote to an obsession with the adequacy of staffing and accommodation. Consumerism also has the advantage of consistency with the self-image of NHS personnel and is less threatening, since the outcomes of professional procedures will not be subjected to rigorous scrutiny.

The more obvious disadvantage is finding a practical way of ensuring that patients' wishes are given priority in assessing quality of care. For example, who are the consumers, and how does one measure quality for the mentally confused? Also, a basic ingredient of satisfaction is missing for the many elderly people who did not want to go into a home or hospital in the first place.

One way around these problems is to require providers to think about the specifics of how they would like to be treated. In HSMC programmes, registration and inspection officers are invited to undertake an exercise 'to judge services against the standards society holds for the people it values, rather than the living situations which services typically make available to elderly people with physical or mental infirmities' (ESCATA, 1984, p. 2). It requires them to allocate each of a number of statements about particular aspects of life (for example, being talked to loudly even though you're not deaf) to one of three categories: (i) things they do not value for myself or friend; (ii) don't mind; (iii) things I value for myself or friend. The intention is to: (i) clarify personal values and attitudes towards a range of personal options and social situations; (ii) reflect on – and more closely identify with – lifestyles and opportunities made available to elderly people, including those with mental infirmity, in the light of values we express for ourselves and our peers; (iii) focus on possibilities for positive change in personal behaviour and in the services provided for elderly people (ESCATA, 1984, p. 1).

The exercise is based on the principle of 'normalization', maximizing choice and control over aspects of life such as physical settings, activities, and the use of time, relationships, language labels and images. The outcome remains challenging for most registration officers since comparisons of existing practice (NHS and private) with things that are valued for themselves produce a sigificant deficit. Many valued aspects of life are not captured by existing guidelines or NHS concerns with staffing and accommodation. The exercise flags up values related to personal dignity as a prime source of outcome measures, rather than input and process considerations. They provide powerful measures (although qualitative) to assess performance and the effectiveness of professional activities such as the nursing process.

Patients' rights

A variant of this approach is to start from the notion of a charter of rights for patients. The protection and enhancement of patients' rights and values is central to assessments of the quality of outcomes: they are the things that matter most to the beneficiary. It is not merely an 'add-on' to input and process considerations: it transforms them, directing attention to different considerations when standard setting for care.

Table 2.3 is a charter of rights used by a social services department in registering residential homes. Figure 2.2 illustrates the impact of such an approach on practice. It contrasts the starting points for an assessment

Table 2.3   A patient's charter of rights

Patients in a private home shall have the right:

1. to retain their personal dignity and independence irrespective of the severity of their physical or mental infirmity.
2. to have skilled sensitive care to enable them to achieve the highest possible quality of life.
3. to have their social, emotional, religious, cultural, political and sexual needs accepted and respected.
4. to have their personal privacy respected.
5. to be consulted about daily living arrangements in the home, and to participate in discussions about any proposed changes to those arrangements.
6. to be fully involved in and fully informed about their individual assessment of need.
7. to make informed choices about their future personal care plans.
8. to have a regular review of their individual circumstances, at which they have the right to be present.
9. to be fully informed about the services provided by the home and the department.
10. to choose their own medical practitioner and dentist, and to consult them in private.
11. to be responsible for their own medication and to make decisions about their medical treatment, whenever possible.
12. to manage their own financial and personal affairs.
13. to have the same access to facilities and services in the community as any other citizen.
14. to not be moved without consultation.
15. to have access to a formal complaints procedure, and to be represented by a friend and adviser if they so wish.

The only restrictions are those legal ones necessary to provide the level of care the resident needs, and those necessary to protect the health and safety of the resident and other residents.

The NAHA guidelines (who? where? what?)

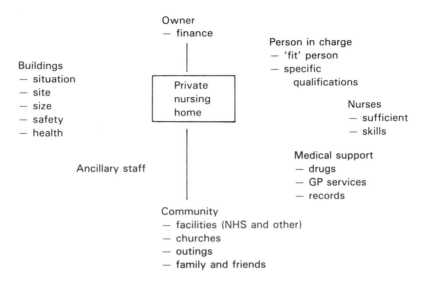

Policy/management guidelines (how?)

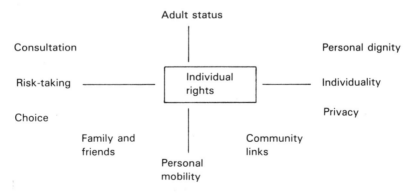

Figure 2.2 Guidelines for home-owners. (From Davis, 1986, with permission).

of quality of care using the NAHA guidelines and those prompted by a statement of patients' rights. The first puts the building and services centre stage. The second puts the emphasis on policy and management issues.

Negative outcomes

Another useful antidote to structural and process thinking is assessments which take 'negative outcomes' into account. Day and Klein (1987) have reported on such an arrangement in New York. 'Negative' outcomes are 'those . . . that should be avoidable given adequate quality of care. . '. It is based on a comparison of the number of 'sentinel incidents' such as bedsores, control of behaviour by restraints and drugs, grooming. Homes with a very high or low incidence of such indicators, for which the information is obtained from regular assessments of patients, are investigated (ibid, p. 387).

Standards: structure and process

The emphasis in this chapter has been on giving practical expression to a widespread wish to give more weight to outcome considerations in assessments of quality of service. The purpose is not to deny the importance of structural and process considerations but to put them into context. However, they are not unaffected by the argument on the over-riding importance of patient preferences and rights. For example, there is a conflict, recognized in Home Life, between them and taking every safeguard against injury and freedom of choice: 'Responsible risk-taking should be regarded as normal, and residents should not be discouraged from undertaking certain activities solely on the grounds that there is an element of risk. Excessive paternalism and concern with safety may lead to infringement of personal rights. Those who are competent to judge the risk to themselves should be free to make their own decisions so long as they do not threaten the safety of others' (ibid. para 2.8).

Another test is whether structural and process standards do justice to changes in general expectations about the balance between the institution and the individual. Williamson's (1987) summary of trends in standards of non-clinical care provides a useful checklist of acceptable standards for the 1990s (Table 2.4). While not all the examples are appropriate to institutional care for the elderly, their drift is relevant and it helps to widen the range of considerations to be taken into account. Reminders are very necessary. The Royal Commission on the National Health Service commented on the continuing early wakening times for many patients 18 years after a national report urging delay (1979, para 10.37). Considerations of staff convenience continued to determine practice.

Structure, process and outcome: a balance

Measures and standard setting for outcomes must not merely be added to those on structure and process: that route leads to overload,

Table 2.4 Changing trends in standards of non-clinical care

Environmental provision

From:	To:
Public	Private (bathing and toilet facilities, single rooms)
Large-scale	Small-scale (normal houses for mentally handicapped group homes)
Utilitarian	Comfortable (flowers, carpets)
Fostering dependence	Fostering independence (facilities for ambulant patients to make their own tea and coffee)

Institutional routines

From:	To:
Rigid	Flexible (patients are not woken up at a set time)
Imposed conditions	Negotiated conditions (patient given choice of times for out-patient appointments, in-patient admission)
Batch	Individual (staggered appointments system for out-patients)
Closed care	Open care (access to partner or friend in childbirth. Open access/overnight arrangements for parents of sick children)

Staff–patient interaction

From:	To:
Impersonal	Personal (continuing care from same practitioner in pregnancy)
Autocratic	Consultative (e.g. patient participation in drawing up care plans with nursing staff)
Inducing dependency	Supporting autonomy (e.g. fostering self responsibility in treatment, taking own blood pressure, or medication)

bureacratic procedures to cope with the information, and ineffectiveness. They should replace some measures of structure and process, with selection influenced by their likely contribution to valued outcomes.

MONITORING

The development of appropriate standards is only the first step in the process in improving the quality of care in institutions. The next step is producing the conditions which encourage and sustain their application.

Current arrangements for external monitoring of performance have not precluded scandals or poor services; nor have the normal processes of supervision. For example, health authority personnel did visit Stanley

Royd hospital, where conditions led to the death of some patients. 'It is obviously difficult to assess the quality of a hospital . . . members of health authorities do make formal visits . . . but, as has been pointed out in other inquiries, these are "unsurprisingly uncritical" and speak "almost uniformly of the usual high standard of hygiene and physical care . . . (when) there was adverse comment . . . assurances of improvement appear to have been accepted and more recent reports are uncritical, appearing to concentrate more on praising the good than criticising defects . . . ' (DHSS, 1986, para 17).

There are two elements in more effective monitoring: the tools to do the job and the promotion and reinforcement of high standards. The technology for effective monitoring is increasingly available in the surfeit of 'systems' (official, home-grown and commercial) used to evaluate services. Managerial responsibility for quality has also been given a higher profile since the advent of general management in the NHS: most DHAs now have a director with a specific responsibility for quality of services and/or customer relations. There is also a training programme for officers responsible for the registration and inspection of nursing homes. Attempts to improve the effectiveness of monitoring should focus on the refinement of these and other developments, rather than radical innovations.

Monitoring: tools of the trade

The test of the effectiveness of current systems for assessing quality is not confined to whether they give sufficient weight to outcome considerations. Also important are criteria for assessment which allow scores (more or less), and therefore more discrimination between shades of performance rather than absolutes (yes or no).

Another consideration is the level of performance expected. It is not always clear whether the (implicit) standards are based on minimum requirements, informed by professional or planning norms: what could reasonably be expected given the performance of others, or what is required for an optimal service? It is an important issue for nursing-home inspectors who sometimes require standards higher than those achieved in the elderly patient hospitals of the DHA which employs them. There is no categorical answer about the level on which expectations should be based. What is required is more clarity about the level of assessment.

The most important issue is selectivity, if monitoring is to be more effective and meaningful. Attention has to focus on key elements which also give a good indication of the general quality of the institutional care. Otherwise there is always the danger of assessments becoming a compendium of information requiring a laborious form-filling process.

The City and Hackney Health Authority's arrangements for monitoring meet many of these points; they specify a manageable number and achievable standards for services to the elderly patient (King Edward's Hospital Fund for London, 1987). The report includes rating scales for each standard and guidelines on considerations to inform assessments. The standards cover:

1. physical environment of wards or nursing homes (22 for aspects of structure, living conditions and equipment);
2. personal services (12 for social activities, personal grooming, ancillary personal services, religious and cultural beliefs, language);
3. nutrition (12 for nutritional requirements, choice of food, presentation of food, meal times as a social activity, provision of alcohol/special drinks);
4. nursing services (21 for objectives of care, staffing ratios, care plans, incontinence, pressure sores, freedom of movement, personal hygiene, eliciting views of patients and relatives);
5. para-medical and therapeutic services (nine standards);
6. medical services (three on specialist medical care and provision of medical services);
7. social work (nine standards).

The monitors

There is a need to quicken the pace of improvement. The 1987 'review of twelve consecutive HAS reports . . . showed that long-stay wards consistently offered environments . . . unable to provide privacy, homely surroundings, personal space and possessions or adequate furniture. In the twelve districts there was not one comprehensive personalized clothing service' (Health Advisory Service, 1987, p. 15). Increased awareness of unacceptable standards, coupled with professional commitment and the basic human kindness of those who work in the service would still seem insufficient to effect the necessary changes.

The problem is not the availability of people to review and check standards. In addition to managers, who have this responsibility, there are already a number of external agencies with an interest in quality of care. Professional associations are involved when approving training posts, and the HAS has been around for over a decade. Similarly, in the private sector there are registration and inspection officers and reviews by representatives of nursing home associations on applications for membership.

The problem is the limited impact of the monitors, which raises questions about the appropriateness of the institutions and ways of working. There are no ready-made solutions. A report on the operation of the HAS does not commend it as a model for reviews of acute hospital and primary health care services. This is partly because the HAS has its origins in a different 'culture' and environment. However, the text makes it plain that the effectiveness of HAS within its present remit cannot be assumed. The environment may have changed but HAS 'has not adapted fully'. Rather than expanding its remit, 'HAS should be developing and improving its capacity to do what it already does' (Health Advisory Service, 1987, p. 52).

There may be a case for expanding the remit of registration and inspection officers to cover NHS long-stay units for the elderly, but this would require an independent organization to ensure even-handedness. More important is the preparation of these officers for their responsibilities. The early months of the HSMC programme brought to light a number of cases where relatively junior personnel were allocated the responsibility at short notice (one/two weeks) with no systematic preparation. The job requires knowledge and a different range of skills to those developed within the NHS. Examples include familiarity with the law on registration, an appreciation of financial viability of small businesses, and communicating across organizational boundaries. Better preparation and reviews of performance would do much to improve the effectiveness of registration and inspection officers.

FINAL COMMENTS

Institutions will remain a significant element in services for the elderly. Community care, even if effectively implemented, will not eliminate the need for shelter for the very frail, and some of this shelter will be found in nursing-home-type provision in both public and private sectors.

This chapter started from the premise that standards need to improve. In so doing, it assumed that there is no magic solution. The problem is how to generalize what the good are already doing and turn good intentions into practice. This is no easy thing to accomplish. Otherwise, the HAS would have found less reason to criticize standards in the NHS and there would be less concern about nursing homes.

Perhaps one of the obstacles to quicker progress is a pre-occupation with quality of service, rather than quality of life. This chapter has underlined the pre-occupation of many with ensuring there were sufficient inputs and the process of care was up to standard. A counter-balance is needed with more practice, reinforced by effective review, centred on human values and patients' rights. Both provide a reminder that quality of life, from the vantage point of the individual, is the crucial factor in quality.

This chapter has outlined ways in which this aim could be more nearly realized. There are tools available to facilitate the necessary changes. The problem of unacceptable standards for the elderly in institutions is therefore not one of poor systems and information. It is a problem amenable to the sustained application of what is already known.

REFERENCES

Avebury, Lady K. (1984) *Home Life. A Code of Practice for Residential Care*. Report of a Working Party. Centre for Policy on Aging, London.

Davis, A. (1986) *Managing to Care in the Regulation of Private Nursing Homes*, Patten Press, Hayle, Cornwall.

Day, P. and Klein, R. (1987) Quality of institutional care and the elderly: policy issues and options. *Brit. Med. J.*, **294**, 384.

DHSS (1988) Comparing health authorities. Health service indicators 1983–86, DHSS, London, March.

DHSS (1986) Committee of inquiry into an outbreak of food poisoning at Stanley Royd Hospital. Report, HMSO, London, Cmnd 9716.

Donabedian, A. (1980) *The Definition of Quality and Approaches to its Assessment*, Health Administration Press, Ann Arbor, Michigan, USA.

ESCATA (1984) Lifestyles. A staff training exercise based on normalisation principles. Brighton.

Health Advisory Service (1987) Annual Report, Health Advisory Service, London.

King Edward's Hospital Fund for London. (1987) Achievable Standards of Care for the Elderly Patient. Project Paper. King Edward's Hospital Fund For London.

Laing, W. (1987) *Review of Private Health Care*. Laing and Buisson Publications, London.

National Association of Health Authorities (1985) Registration and Inspection of Nursing Homes. NAHA, Birmingham.

National Association of Health Authorities (1988) Supplement. NAHA, Birmingham.

National Health Service Training Authority (1988) A Manual for Health Authority Chairmen and Members. NHSTA.

Royal College of Nursing (RCN), in collaboration with the British Geriatric Society and Royal College of Psychiatrists. (1987) *Improving the Care of Elderly People in Hospital*, RCN, London.

Royal Commission on the National Health Service (1979) Report. Cmnd. 7615, HMSO, London.

Williamson, C. (1987) Reviewing the Quality of Care in the NHS. NAHA, Birmingham.

Chapter 3

The physician and the continuing-care patient

The pace of devolving continuing care from hospital wards to private accommodation, NHS nursing homes or facilities managed by voluntary or charitable organizations is accelerating. Increasing numbers of consultants are finding that they have few, if any, continuing-care patients. It is almost as if the speciality of elderly patient medicine is losing its *raison d'etre*, since it began in the days when consultants such as Marjory Warren took over continuing care wards. However, there will still be consultants in elderly patient medicine who will retain direct clinical care of long-stay patients, and it is to them that this chapter is particularly directed.

Physicians in elderly patient medicine are trained to work in a multidisciplinary manner. They lead the multidisciplinary team in the acute and rehabilitation departments of the elderly patient unit. However, they are less likely to have this leadership role within the continuing-care unit, where it may be taken by the Nurse Manager. This is not to imply that medical input is now unimportant, or is to be abrogated or withdrawn.

The consultant with continuing-care patients must continue to take an active interest in them for four reasons. Firstly, the consultant is responsible for the clinical management of patients, unless they are in nursing unit beds, where medical responsibility is rather different (Punton, 1989), or in NHS nursing homes, which are not consultant-led. Furthermore, the consultant needs to supervise, to a variable degree, the doctor who provides the day-to-day medical cover. He/she is usually a general practitioner or clinical assistant who hopefully will have been trained in elderly patient medicine and will have the Diploma of Geriatric Medicine. Secondly, the consultant may be involved when difficult ethical decisions have to be taken about the giving or withholding of treatment. Evans (1987) has pointed out that doctors are recruited, trained and expected to take such decisions and to accept responsibility for the outcome. No other caring professions have a similar function. Ethical dilemmas can also develop when research in the elderly in continuing care is being considered. Thirdly, the consultant should be involved in discussions of any changes in the pattern, style or model of continuing care which are to be developed. Fourthly, it is only by visiting the wards that the consultant will be able to assess general standards of care as well as the morale and attitudes of staff. Lack of senior medical input can irritate staff and impair morale, since it can be interpreted as a lack of interest or concern – which may unfortunately be true. These points are developed below.

ETHICAL DILEMMAS OF TREATMENT VERSUS NON-TREATMENT

The aim of continuing care must be to add life to years, not years to life, i.e., to make the patient's life as dignified, pleasant and interesting as he/she wishes. Ethical dilemmas relating to treatment or the witholding of it seldom occur when it is clear that the elderly patient will benefit from proposed therapy which has few, if any, important risks. However, debate can occur about the most appropriate form of treatment for the very frail, dependent, or terminally ill aged people, who, in spite of their disabilities, are not a homogeneous group (Berg *et al*, 1988). The question which may have to be faced is whether the individual has a life of sufficient or acceptable quality that it should be maintained at all costs (Fox, 1987; McNicholl, 1987). It may be that permitting the patient a natural painless death from water deficiency is preferable to prolonged pain and discomfort by intravenous infusions or tube feeding (Norberg *et al*, 1980; Lynn and Childress, 1983). Death should not necessarily be looked upon as defeat, and caring staff may need to be reconciled with this view (Chapter 17).

All aspects of the patient's health and wishes need to be considered by the members of the multidisciplinary caring team when taking ethical decisions regarding the witholding or giving of treatment. These include the patient's quality of life, the nature of the patient's illness, the nature of the treatment of that condition with its risks and benefits, the presence of other diseases, and the risks and benefits of the treatment of those illnesses, the wishes of the patients and relatives, the patient's morale, mental state and age. Adequate information about these factors is mandatory. When there is doubt or lack of information, the patient should be treated. These factors are now considered in detail.

Quality of life

It is important to assess the patient's perception of his/her quality of life; unfortunately many members of the caring staff are not trained to do this. To make matters worse, quality of life can mean different things to different patients in the same situation. It can be measured objectively by assessing tangible assets, such as possessions or financial status, but this is largely irrelevant for continuing-care patients. Alternatively, subjective assessments can be made by measuring satisfaction with life or state of health, but again these features are not wholly applicable to the long-stay patient. A useful measure, however, is that of assessing morale: good morale is to do with being happy now and looking forward with interest and optimism to the future. Alternatively, the patient's symptoms can be assessed and related to the ability or otherwise to carry out the activities of daily living (Holmes and Dickerson, 1987; Davis and Lee, 1987; Davies, 1988/9). This can apply to both the physically frail but mentally alert person as well as to the quite confused patient. A very frail elderly lady with extensive rheumatoid arthritis could do virtually nothing for herself but very much enjoyed her daily sessions in the Activity Centre. Poetry readings were her particular interest. This pleasure in life was a factor in the decision to treat her frequent chest infections. The situation becomes more difficult when patients are severely demented, are not able to care for themselves in any way, are immobile and incontinent – the pre-death state (Isaacs and colleagues, 1971). What is their quality of life? They may or may not be able to indicate what their feelings are and therefore it falls to the caring staff to make a subjective judgement. Has the patient a life of sufficient acceptable quality that it should be sustained at all costs (Fox, 1987)?

The potential for good quality of life after treatment must also be considered. A very demented man with extensive carcinoma of the bladder was treated surgically and had both ureters re-sited in an ileal conduit. This was covered by a plastic bag. The patient failed to understand the need for this bag and frequently removed it, making him 'incontinent'. His wife was unable to manage him and he therefore stayed in hospital for the rest of his days.

The nature of the illness

It is axiomatic that medical staff should understand the natural history of the patient's disease if it is left untreated, and the effects of intervention. A breast tumour in a 90-year-old lady can often be managed conservatively, since these tumours are very slow growing and therefore have a good prognosis. However, a continuing-care patient developing a hyperosmolar diabetic coma will certainly require rapid and vigorous treatment if there is to be any chance of preventing death.

Knowledge of the patient's disease assumes that the diagnosis has been established. Sometimes it is not possible to be absolutely certain of the diagnosis, and the tests required to establish that diagnosis beyond doubt are invasive, physically exhausting or distressing to the patient. Only when a definitive management decision cannot be made without this knowledge should exhausting or invasive tests be carried out.

The nature of the illness: risks versus benefit

The benefit of treatment must be balanced against possible risks. Medical intervention in old age is frequently very effective, and there is no problem when the benefit is great and the risks are minimal, as treating a pernicious anaemia patient with vitamin B_{12}. However, some medical interventions are associated with increasing risks. It is well known that adverse drug reactions increase with age – an effect probably due to altered pharmacokinetics and pharmacodynamics as well as problems with compliance rather than age itself (Denham, 1990). Furthermore, surgery is not without its risk in the elderly. Post-operative mortality rises with age, especially in those with co-existing medical conditions (Palmberg and Hirsjarvi, 1979; Farrow *et al.*, 1982). Emergency surgery carries greater risks than elective procedures.

Anaesthesia, too, is not without its problems. Bedford (1955) found that 7% of elderly people developed severe dementia after operations/anaesthesia. However, Simpson *et al.* (1961) found no evidence that anaesthesia had any effect on physical activity, mental ability or personality of the patient. These findings may be due to the fact that the Simpson study included elective patients only and the pre-operative care and anaesthetic techniques had all improved between the two studies.

Anaesthetic deaths have been studied by the Association of Anaesthetists of Great Britain and Ireland (Lunn and Mushin, 1982). Although the report has been criticized, it does show that 50% of deaths attributable to anaesthesia occur in those over the age of 70 years, and that half of the deaths occurred in elective surgical cases where any adverse risk factors should have been identified, corrected or minimized. However, pre-existing disease, such as chronic obstructive airways disease, may contribute to these deaths in the old.

The presence of other diseases

It is well known that the elderly frequently have multiple pathology. The presence of these disorders, their natural history, their effects on life expectancy, quality of life, their treatment with risks and benefits, can have a considerable impact on the primary condition. A severely demented 90-year-old lady, who was totally dependent on others for all forms of care, developed large bowel obstruction, thought to be due to carcinoma. Although her quality of life was thought poor, it was considered correct to operate to relieve the obstruction since conservative management would probably have resulted in an unpleasant death.

The patient's wishes and mental state; relatives' wishes

The patient's wishes must be given great weight in the management policy decision to treat or to withhold treatment. All of us have the right to decide whether or not we wish to be treated – a point emphasized by Angell (1984) and Wagner (1984). When a patient refuses treatment but is clearly sensible, there is no problem. In this latter situation, the reasons for refusal should be identified, since some factor may have been misunderstood. If the patient still refuses, then his/her wishes clearly must be respected (Fox, 1987).

Ethical dilemmas can occur when patients are mentally unable, either due to a toxic confusional state or dementia, to give a clear indication of willingness or otherwise to have the suggested treatment. The burden of decision making should not be placed on relatives unless they have been given all the relevant facts.

A particular problem develops in those patients with advanced dementia who reject food or allow it to stay in their mouths for long periods of time or spit it out. This can be viewed as the final loss the patient is suffering before he/she dies. Fox (1987) believes that such patients are close to death at this stage and doubts the value served by providing calories and/or fluid by tube feeding, which itself is not without risks and problems. Such procedures may lengthen the days the body survives, and by so doing delude care workers and relatives, but it is unlikely to have a significant impact on quality of life and it can seriously disturb patient–carer relationships (Norberg *et al.*, 1980). Patients should certainly have the opportunity of being allowed to die with dignity (Miller, 1987). Fortunately, experience in the United Kingdom does not emulate that in the United States of America, where court decisions are required before a naso-gastric tube can be removed from a patient in the pre-death state (Lynn, 1984).

Relatives may express views about the proposed treatment of an elderly person. Where these accord with the patient's wishes, there is no problem, but difficulties arise when they are at variance. In this situation the doctor's responsibility must be to the patient, rather than to the relatives.

The patient's age

Many patients in continuing care are elderly. However, their age plays little part in the decision to give treatment or to withhold it. Age *per se* is not a bar, for example, to the insertion of pacemakers. Elderly people in the state of some dependency must not be denied the benefits of modern medicine because of their age (Fox, 1987).

Conclusion

The decision to treat or withhold treatment must be based on an unhurried, thoughtful, responsible, sensitive judgement made after considering all the relevant information obtained by members of the multidisciplinary team. Hasty decisions – and especially those based on age alone – must not be taken. No decision should be considered irrevocable: changes in circumstances or new information may warrant reconsideration. When there is a lack of information the patient should always be treated.

ETHICS OF RESEARCH IN THE CONTINUING-CARE PATIENT

Why should the elderly, and the continuing-care patient in particular, be the subject of research? It is becoming generally accepted that research on older people is needed if there is to be a reasonably rapid increase in the knowledge of the ageing process, of the diseases of old age, the changes in pharmacokinetics and pharmacodynamics with age, and the organization and delivery of care to this client group. Only well-designed research will ensure that elderly patients are given appropriate doses of drugs which do not cause adverse drug reactions while maintaining therapeutic efficiency. Furthermore, it would be unethical to start any new untried form of treatment or management of elderly patients unless it is submitted to a formal trial and subsequently shown to be of benefit. Thus, recently, the evaluation of NHS nursing homes has been reported (Bond *et al.*, 1989). The elderly in continuing care can therefore be a potentially valuable asset to the medical research worker, since they form a relatively large but, most importantly, static group of subjects with a wide range of diseases, disabilities and disorders which can be studied (Reich, 1978). However, the very fact that these patients require to be in continuing care makes them a vulnerable group since they are dependent and often 'institutionalized'. They may acquiesce to a research project without having a clear understanding of its implications. The normal ageing process, often coupled with disease of the central nervous system, makes elderly persons less able to comprehend the nature and the risks of research studies (Bernstein and Nelson, 1975). Indeed, some patients may consent to research as a *quid pro quo* – 'you have helped me, therefore I will help you'. They may also agree to participate because the activity of the project brings them into contact with different people and therefore adds interest to their lives. Such features, particularly the 'wealth of patient material', were partly the cause of the Jewish Chronic Disease Hospital case (Katz, 1972), where a number of elderly people were injected with cancerous material without their clear consent. An additional but important problem in research in this group of elderly people is that they do not tolerate change or disturbance as well as do younger people, and they find invasive procedures much more upsetting. Therefore, indirect forms of measurement are to be preferred (Royal College of Physicians, 1990).

If it be accepted that there is a need for research on the elderly, then the consultant of the continuing-care unit must consider the following factors:

Standards of research

Standards of research in the elderly must be as high as research in any other group. Just because the patient is old is no excuse for slipshod techniques. The research project must have a clearly defined, reasonably obtainable objective with its design and methods tailored to fit that study. Badly designed research should not be allowed to proceed because it may cause disturbance to patients or discomfort without benefit. Indeed, such research is unlikely to be passed by the local ethics committee.

Consent

In general, elderly patients should be assumed to be competent to give their consent unless there is evidence to the contrary. It should not be thought that, because of their age, they need to know any less about the intended research than would a younger patient. The way in which research is described to elderly patients may need to take into account special problems such as deafness, impaired vision and expectations of behaviour, which may derive from an earlier age (Royal College of Physicians, 1990). Research workers therefore need to take great care when obtaining consent from the elderly to ensure that the research proposals, either simple or complex, are understood. Not to do so will put the patient's good will, and cooperation at risk.

There seems to be little doubt, however, that excessive detail about a research project can cause confusion. Epstein and Lasagna (1969) showed that as the amount of detailed information was increased, so there was a decrease in the understanding of what was involved. Research workers, therefore, must steer a course between excessive detail and none at all. They must be considerate, understanding, patient and thoughtful in their approach to the patient or volunteer, and they must be willing to explain the project several times, answer questions and allow time for thought. Pressure to consent must not be applied under any circumstances.

Dementia research

The need to research the cause of, and to produce treatment for, dementia hardly needs reiterating, since it is medically, psychologically and financially a devastating illness. However, research into its causation presents special problems. Subjects need to be investigated at an earlier stage of the disease than perhaps is the case with other disorders. Unfortunately, there are considerable difficulties in establishing an early accurate diagnosis and, of course, there are no suitable animal models. Then again, there can be problems of obtaining consent. Not surprisingly, therefore, there is, as yet, no ethical concensus on how best to carry out research into this disorder (Ratzan, 1980).

Mental capacity

It needs to be remembered that there is a very high incidence of mental deterioration of some degree above the age of 65 years. Thus, while many of the older patients may be able to cope with routine financial matters, they may have problems in understanding unusual concepts or proposals in a research project. However, mild mental deterioration should not prevent a patient from making a competent choice. It is probably best to use a two-stage consent procedure. Initially the patient is given written details of the study, which will give the purpose of that study, the procedures involved, the risks, the benefits, and the freedom to withdraw and to ask questions. Nowadays statements are usually included about indemnity in case of accidents due to the research. At this stage the research proposal can be discussed by the patients with friends and relatives. The second part is an interview, preferably in the presence of an independent witness. It can be combined with a questionnaire to assess how well the patient has understood the information on the form (Muss *et al.*, 1979). After discussion, consent or otherwise can be obtained. This technique has much to recommend it since it gives time for discussion with relatives, but it can produce logistical problems for the investigator and can result in refusal to participate (Ratsen, 1981). It should be pointed out that the arrangements for asking relatives to consent on behalf of confused patients is illegal in the United Kingdom – only guardians can give consent to research, and then only for research that leads to potential benefits for the patient (Pryce, 1978).

Risk/benefit

Risk refers to the possibility of harm resulting from an activity and to its magnitude. For example, 'low risk' is taken to mean a low probability of a very serious harm, or, alternatively, a higher probability of a minor harm. Furthermore, 'risk' often stands for the combined probabilities and magnitudes of several potential harms. In some procedures, studies or experiments the risk is so small that it can be ignored. This can be equated to the level of risk accepted in everyday life. Examples could be the measurement of height and weight, the collection of a urine sample, the giving of a single venous blood sample by an adult (Royal College of Physicians, 1990). Research involving procedures which carry risk which is more than minimal should be permitted only in exceptional circumstances.

Benefit refers to any sort of favourable outcome of the research, which may be for the patient in particular, or for the population in general. Studies are sometimes categorized as 'therapeutic research' or 'non-therapeutic research', according to whether or not it is considered that the individual patient may obtain some benefit from participation.

Despite a lack of precision inherent in a risk/benefit analysis, it is often a straightforward matter for an ethics committee to reach a conclusion that risk is or is not reasonable in a particular case. At one end of the spectrum the committee might be prepared to consent to a procedure carrying substantial risk because the potential benefits are so great. At the other end of the spectrum it might refuse to sanction a procedure which carries no risk because the aims are trivial and the intrusion is unwarranted.

Avoiding harm

Ethics committees have a duty to protect patients or volunteers from harm, manipulation or unapproved procedure. They therefore should monitor the progress of procedures for potential problems of consent and of changes in research procedures or protocols. The ideal method of achieving this has yet to be devised. A variety of methods have been used, including the very formalized Institutional Review Board system found in the United States, ward rounds by members of the ethical committee, and annual project review forms. It is clear that both those carrying out research and those monitoring it have a responsibility to see that harm does not occur to the patient. The Medical Research Council put it clearly (1962–3) 'progress of medical knowledge has depended and will continue to depend in no small measure upon the confidence which the public has in those who carry out investigations on human subjects, be they healthy or sick . . . . . . Mistakes or misunderstandings can do incalculable harm to medical progress. It is our collective duty to see that this does not happen and so continue to deserve the confidence we now enjoy'.

Conclusion

The need for research on the elderly is being increasingly recognized. However, those in continuing care are potentially vulnerable to exploitation by research workers. Great care needs to be taken to ensure that this does not happen.

DIFFERING MODELS OF CONTINUING CARE AND THEIR MEDICAL INPUT

The consultant physician should be involved in any discussion which aims to alter the style or model of continuing care. There is now a range of models with the classical hospital approach at one end and the domestic or home style of unit at the other.

The hospital model, on the one hand, is still the most common, with the traditional wards in old buildings often handed on by other departments who no longer want them. They are often associated with very limited personal possessions for patients, and with inflexibility of staffing, which is frequently combined with problems of attitudes and resistance to change (Day *et al.*, 1988). In favour of such open wards, it has been pointed out that they can act as small communities providing sensory and psycho-social stimulation, thus making the patients less lonely and improving companionship, which can outweigh the loss of privacy (Kayser-Jones, 1986).

The domestic model, on the other hand, aims to produce an environment similar to that which the patient would find living in his/her own home. There is single accommodation and very much increased privacy, space for personal possessions, flexibility in the activity of daily living, such as getting up times and mealtimes. Flexibility in staffing ratios and duty times with elimination of rigid adherence to job specifications are frequently found. Staff may be dressed casually rather than in uniform. In this way patients are more likely to be treated as individuals, be more satisfied with their surroundings, and feel less isolated and apathetic (MacDonald *et al.*, 1988). This move towards the home style of care has clearly gathered momentum, particularly with voluntary organizations such as Anchor Housing or Abbeyfield Extra Care (Abbeyfield, 1989). It is important to remember that whichever style or model is used, caring staff should be particularly aware of the needs and requirements of ethnic minorities, who are increasingly likely to be found in continuing care. Management and staff need to be able to assess these needs and manage them accordingly (Henley, 1979).

Medical input into the new styles of care can be quite different. The consultant who visits the traditional unit regularly will be able to assess the clinical care of the patients and the ward environment as well as the morale and attitudes of the staff. He will thus have the knowledge to work with the nurse-manager for the elderly to ensure that good standards of care are maintained or improved. This may be achieved by using staff/patient questionnaires to assess job satisfaction (Raphael and Mandeville, 1979; Green, 1988), assessing and using achievable standards (Davies, 1986; King's Fund Project Paper No. 72, 1987), introducing primary nursing (Wilson and Dawson, 1989), ensuring that nurses with appropriate skills are employed on continuing-care units (Hill *et al.*, 1987), and following the guidelines for Improving the Care of Elderly people in Hospital (Royal College of Nursing, 1987).

Medical input into the domestic model is likely to be different, and will not be consultant-led. The regular medical attendant, usually a general practitioner, will generally visit several times a week as he/she would to any fragile elderly person living at home. However, logically, were the patient at home, then he/she would be expected to choose his/her own general practitioner. This seldom happens since the Health Authority usually prefers one doctor to give clinical care. In this model, the consultant should, in theory, visit only at the request of the caring staff. However, it then becomes difficult for him/her to assess standards of care as well as staff attitudes. This is an important defect, since a major factor in standards of care of the long-stay patient is the morale of the staff whose close, caring, and often long-term personal relationships with patients will deeply influence the elderly person's well-being and lifestyle.

Doctors operating in either model of care may need to support nurse management when risk to patients is debated. Junior nursing staff may be afraid to take any risks with patients in case of falls resulting in injury and accusations of negligence (Health Advisory Service, 1987). For example, physical restraints or tilt-chairs may be used to prevent falls, but these limit a patient's quality of life and should not be allowed except in very special circumstances. If they have to be used, the restraints should be removed at least every two hours when range of movement, skin care and change of position are provided (Wells and Adolphus, 1987). The use of cot sides at night for continuing care patients is another classical example of the intent to limit risk. If patients want to get out of bed, they will climb out and fall further from the cot side than if they fell from a bed in its lowest position.

Conclusion

Medical input into continuing-care units is usually less intense compared with the acute and rehabilitation departments, and will vary somewhat with the style of the organization of that unit. A doctor is less likely to be the leader of the multidisciplinary team. However, the medical role is still important, especially when considering treatment, research, staff attitudes and morale.

REFERENCES

Abbeyfield (1989) The Guide to Abbeyfield Extra Care. Abbeyfield Society 186–192 Darkes Lane, Potters Bar, Herts, EN6 1AB, England.

Angell, M. (1984) Respecting the autonomy of competent patients. *N. Engl. J. Med.*, **310**, 1115–6.

Bedford, P.D. (1955) Adverse cerebral effects of anaesthesia in old people. *Lancet*, **2**, 259–63.

Berg, S., Branch, L.G., Doyle, A.E. and Sundstrom, G. (1988) Institutional and home-based long-term care alternatives: the 1965–85 Swedish experience. *Gerontologist*, **28**, 825–8.

Bernstein, J.E. and Nelson, E.K. (1975) Medical experimentation in the elderly. *J. Am. Geriatr. Soc.*, **23**, 327–9.

Bond, J., Gregson, B.A. and Atkinson, A. (1989) Measurement of outcomes within a multicentre randomised controlled trial in the evaluation of experimental NHS nursing homes. *Age Ageing*, **18**, 292–302.

Davies, B. (1986) American lessons for British policy and research on long-term care of the elderly. *Q.J. Social Affairs*, **2**, 321–55.

Davies L. (1988/9) Assessing the quality of residential care for people with mental handicap. *J. Management Med.*, **3**, 216–28.

Davis, B.A. and Lee, P.L. (1987) Standards of gerontological long-term care nursing practices. Quarterly Review Bulletin **13**, 377–9.

Day, P., Klein, R. and Tipping, G. (1988) *Inspecting for Quality*. Centre for the Analysis of Social Policy, University of Bath.

Denham, M.J. (1990) Adverse drug reactions, in Drugs and the Elderly: New Perspectives (eds M.J. Denham and C.F. George), British Medical Bulletin, Churchill Livingstone, Edinburgh.

Epstein, L.C. and Lasagna, L. (1969) Obtaining informed consent: form or substance. *Arch. Int. Med.*, **123**, 682–8.

Evans, J. G. (1987) The sanctity of life, in *Medical Ethics and Elderly People* (ed. R.J. Elford). Churchill Livingstone, Edinburgh.

Farrow, S.C., Fowkes, F.G.R., Lunn, J.N. *et al.* (1982) Epidemiology in anaesthesia. II. Factors affecting mortality in hospital. *Br. J. Anaesth.*, **54**, 811–7.

Fox, R.A. (1987) Palliative care and aggressive therapy, in *Medical Ethics and Elderly People* (ed. R.J. Elford). Churchill Livingstone, Edinburgh.

Green, J. (1988) On the receiving end. *Health Service J.*, 4th August, 880–1.

Health Advisory Service (1987) Annual Report of NHS Health Advisory Service, Sutherland House, 29–37, Brighton Road, Sutton, Surrey, SM2 5AN, England.

Health Service Commissioner (1988/9) Second report to Parliament – epitomes of selected cases for period November 1988 – March 1989. Department of Health, London.

Henley, A. (1979) Asian patients in Hospital and at home. King Edward's Hospital Fund for London, London.

Hill, S.N., Milnes, J.P., Rowe, J. *et al.* (1987) Nursing the immobile: a preliminary study. *Int. J. Nurs. Stud.*, **24**, 123–8.

Holmes, S. and Dickerson, J. (1987) The quality of life: design and evaluation of a self assessment instrument for use with cancer patients. *Int. J. Nurs. Stud.*, **24**, 15–24.

Isaacs, B., Gunn, J., McKeckan, A. *et al.* (1971) The concept of pre-death, *Lancet* **i**, 1115–9.

Katz, J. (1972) Jewish chronic disease hospital cases, in Experimentation with Human Beings, pp. 9–65, Russell Sage Foundation, New York.

Kayser-Jones, J.S. (1986) Open ward accommodation in a long-term facility: the elderly's point of view. *Gerontologist*, **16**, 63–9.

King's Fund Project paper No. 72 (1987) Achievable standards of care for the elderly patients cared for in the acute assessment wards, continuing-care wards, nursing homes or day hospitals within the City with Hackney Health Authority, Kings Fund Centre, London.

Lunn, J.N. and Mushin, W.W. (1982) Mortality associated with anaesthesia. Association of Anaesthetists of Great Britain and Ireland. Nuffield Hospital Provincial Trust.

Lynn, J. (1984) Brief and Appendix for AMICUS Curiae. *J. Am. Geriatr. Ser.*, **32**, 915–22.

Lynn, J. and Childress, J.F. (1983) Must patients always be given food and water? *Hastings Centre Rep.* **13**, 17–21.

MacDonald, L., Subbald, B. and Hoare, C. (1988) Patient satisfaction in a long stay hospital. *International Journal of Social Psychiatry* **34**, 292–304.

MacNicholl, A.M. (1987) Models of long term care: ethical issues. *HLN Publ.*, July, 53–6.

Medical Research Council (1962/3) Responsibility in investigation on human subjects. HMSO, Cmnd 2382, London.

Miller, P.J. (1987) Death with dignity and the right to die: sometimes doctors have a duty to hasten death. *J. Med. Ethics*, **13**, 81–5.

Muss, H.B., White, D.R., Michielutte, R. *et al.* (1979) Written informed consent in patients with breast cancer. *Cancer*, **43**, 1549–56.

Norberg, A., Norberg, B., Gippert, H. and Bexele, G. (1980) Ethical conflicts in long-term care of the aged: nutritional problems and the patient-care worker relationship. *Br. Med. J.*, **1**, 377–9.

Palmberg, S. and Hirsjarvi, K. (1979) Mortality in geriatric surgery with special reference to the type of surgery anaesthesia, complicating diseases and prophylaxis of thrombosis. *Gerontology*, **25**, 103–12.

Pryce, I.G. (1978) Clinical research upon mentally ill subjects who cannot give informed consent. *Br. J. Psychiatry*, **32**, 366–9.

Punton, S. (1989) The nursing unit in a project to evaluate 'nursing beds' as an effective service provision within a DGH. *Care of the elderly*, **1**, 89.

Raphael, W. (1977) Psychiatric hospitals viewed by their patients. King Edward's Hospital Fund for London, London.

Raphael, W. and Mandeville, W. (1979) Old people in hospital. Ibid.

Ratsen, R.M. (1981) The experiment that wasn't in case report in clinical genetic research. *Gerontologist*, **21**, 297–302.

Ratzan, R.M. (1980) Being old makes you different: the ethics of research with elderly subjects. *Hastings Center Rep.* **10**, 32–42.

Reich, W.T. (1978) Ethical issues related to research involving elderly subjects. *Gerontologist*, **18**, 326–37.

Royal College of Nursing, in collaboration with the British Geriatrics Society and the Royal College of Psychiatrists (1987). *Improving Care of the Elderly in Hospital*, Royal College of Nursing, London.

Royal College of Physicians (1990) *Research Involving Patients*, Royal College of Physicians, London.

Simpson, B.R., Williams, M., Scott, J.F. and Smith, A.C. (1961) The effect of anaesthesia or elective surgery on elderly people. *Lancet* **ii**, 887–93.

Wagner, A. (1984) Cardiopulmonary resuscitation in the aged. *N. Engl. J. Med.*, **310**, 1129–30.

Wells, D.L. and Adolphus, P.D. (1987) Evaluating the care provided to long-stay patients. *Dimensions Health Serv.*, **64**, 20–2.

Wilson, N.M. and Dawson, P. (1989) A comparison of primary nursing and team nursing care in a geriatric long-term care setting. *Int. J. Nurs. Stud.*, **26**, 1–13.

Part Two

GENERAL AND SPECIFIC ASPECTS OF CARE

Chapter 4

Quality of life: assessment and improvement

INTRODUCTION

Those providing long-term care would no doubt agree that the aim is to give the patients or residents the best possible quality of life. However, just as there will be universal agreement as to this general goal, there will be a thousand and more views on just what this means and how it should be achieved. In this chapter I shall attempt to answer four questions: why measure quality of life, how can this be defined, how can this be measured, and how can such measures be applied to the evaluation of long-term care?

THE NEED FOR MEASUREMENT

It is an unfortunate paradox that the more successful we are in raising standards, the more difficult it becomes to demonstrate that what we are doing is effective. If our standards of care are so appalling that we fail to feed people adequately then we can measure any improvement in terms of basic physiological parameters. We can, for example, use mortality rates just as we might when examining the treatment of a potentially fatal illness. However, if we assume that we are already meeting the patients' basic bodily needs so that, for example, they are not dying of starvation, measuring outcome solely in terms of mortality is unlikely to be appropriate. We know that there is more to good care than this but how do we define and measure this?

In measuring the outcome of acute care, we can judge our success in terms of measures such as the average length of stay or the number of patients treated. The better our care, the shorter the stay or the more patients receiving treatment. Quite the opposite trend will be true of long-term care. The better our care, the longer will people live, and the fewer are the numbers receiving care in that particular ward or home. In the care of long-stay patients our outcome measures must be much more wide-ranging and are necessarily a little more difficult to construct.

We cannot use these difficulties as an excuse for not assessing the efficacy of long-term care. There is no universally held concept of what constitutes 'high quality care' or what steps should be taken to achieve this. It is no good simply assuming that other people will agree with us in what we think is an effective method for improving care. Even if most of our contemporaries do share some such view, later generations may show us all to be wrong. The history of care in general, and medicine in particular, is littered with outmoded treatments that were once thought to be effective.

The scientific progress which has achieved so much in acute care depends at its core on evaluating different treatments and altering our management accordingly. This is important both to see that the treatment works and to see that it does no harm. In the case of long-term care, the side effects of a change in pattern of care are unlikely to be serious, at least in terms of mortality, though even here there may be exceptions. However it is just as important that we ensure that we do no harm in other respects such as emotional well-being.

Perhaps even more importantly, the needs of long-term patients are always to be met from the finite resources available. If we are successfully to argue that resources should be devoted to some new form of care, or just to more of an existing type of care, we must justify the effort and expense. The cool breeze of evaluation grows ever stronger and it is no longer enough for an 'expert' to say 'We need more money for . . . .' for resources to be made available. It is necessary to show what the outcome is and how effective is a particular method in achieving this.

It is also widely recognized that the measurement of efficacy is a considerable problem in health care. This is true for many different types of care but none more so than that which concerns us here. Perhaps because of this the parameters that have been used to evaluate care depend at least as much on how easy they are to measure as on their relevance to outcome.

Indeed, health care as a whole has not very often been described in terms of outcome at all. More often it has been described in terms of the input of resources and the process of care. This is more easily understood if we draw a comparison with the evaluation of a manufacturing business. Let us suppose that instead of providing long-term care we were running a factory making teapots. In this case we have a clear aim in mind, namely to maximize our profit. This we can do by selling as many teapots as possibble at as high a price as we can. We need to balance the price against sales but at least we know that if we are successful the bottom line, net profit, will increase. Contrast this with long-term care. We are often in possession of only a vague idea what we are producing. I would suggest that a good quality of life might be one way of describing this. However this is difficult to measure so we look for other ways of measuring what we do. We may look at the number of staff we employ, the cost of the food or some other measure of input. This describes our service but no more so than would detailing the amount of clay or electricity we use in making our teapots each year.

We may look then at the number of times we bath people or the time we spend talking to patients. These tell us about the process of care, but again, this is only like counting the number of teapots we decorate each year or how many enquiries we get from customers. It does not tell us directly any effect on outcome. If we are making lots of teapots and then simply storing them in a big warehouse we will not be making much profit.

The answer in the end must be to measure outcome, though not simply in terms of the number of patients treated, for this is not the right measure for long-term care. We must decide on a definition of what it is that we are really trying to do and to measure this.

THE AIM OF LONG-TERM CARE

The ultimate aim of nearly all care for older people is quality rather than quantity of life. In practice there is rarely any conflict between these two goals, though when this does arise it is quite usual for people to assert that it is quality which is the more important. Thus if we are to evaluate the efficacy of our interventions we must look for improved quality of life as one, if not the most important, yardstick.

As is all too often the case, the thing that seems to be most important as a measure of outcome is also that which it is most difficult to define, let alone measure. However this should not deter us because how we approach these issues can reveal much of what we hold at the centre of our philosophy of care. To try to duck the issue, for example to measure only the process of care rather than its outcome, can be a particularly dangerous failing. We may have a set of procedures, a pattern of care which is in its individual elements excellent but which, as a whole, quite fails to achieve its overall aim.

WHAT IS QUALITY OF LIFE?

Asserting the importance of this as an outcome measure rather begs the question, 'What is it?'. We all have some notion of what it is but might find it hard to put this into words. The sort of words that are used to define quality of life include independence, privacy, choice, dignity and freedom of action. A life which is short of all or any of these is not seen to be very good. In evaluating the quality of life of those receiving medical care we also need to include things such as freedom from pain and disability.

Just as we may find it easier to measure inputs and processes rather than outcome, so many of the attempts to define quality of life include parameters which are thought to be related to quality of life rather than being direct measures of this construct. Adams (1969) defined the construct as the degree of satisfaction or dissatisfaction felt by individuals about various aspects of their lives. Such a subjective element is surely crucial to any definition of quality of life. Likewise, Ziller (1974) saw self-esteem as central, and Andrews (1974) related quality of life to the extent to which pleasure and satisfaction characterized peoples' lives.

Havighurst (1963) took a slightly broader view, including both inner factors concerning the individual's subjective view of life and external factors such as the nature and extent of behaviours such as social contact and other activities. We do know, however, that mood and activity are by no means simply related. Low levels of activity do not, for example, necessarily imply depressed mood (Simpson *et al.*, 1981).

The measure of subjective experience is always difficult, and quality of life is no exception. There are problems of response bias, where there can be a tendency to use only certain points on a rating scale, typically the mid-point or the extremes. Likewise, there may be demand characteristics whereby the subject tells the interviewer what he or she thinks the interviewer wants to hear. Responses to questions aimed at assessing a presumably fairly stable construct such as quality of life may be influenced by short-term variables such as mood-state.

In addition to all of these problems there can be cross-cultural, including socio-economic, differences in how individuals view quality of

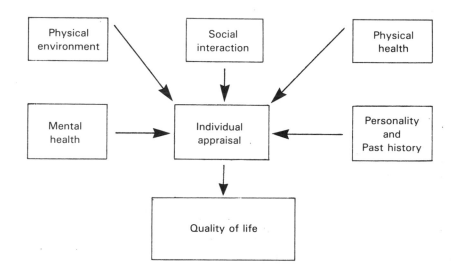

Figure 4.1 Factors which influence quality of life: a casual model.

life. A question which works well for retired North Americans may mean something quite different to older British men and women.

None of these however are reasons for abandoning any attempt to measure quality of life. Rather, they suggest ways in which we must be fastidious in both developing and applying measures. This is of course true of all measurement, be it psychological or physiological.

Despite all these difficulties we can identify a number of factors which influence quality of life. These are each important and can be represented in a causal model as shown in Figure 4.1.

This model includes several known determinants of life satisfaction, such as physical health, and allows for the influence of personal and mental health factors on individual appraisal. The assumption being made here is that quality of life depends ultimately on how each individual perceives his or her own life. Thus it can only ever be this perception, and the factors influencing this, which we can hope to measure.

MEASURES OF QUALITY OF LIFE

It will come as no great surprise to find that there have been many and varied attempts to measure this elusive concept. Some have been designed to measure the concept itself; others, perhaps the majority, have focussed on those parameters which are thought, or known, to be related to it.

Health measures

It is well known that one of the best predictors of well-being in later life is health status. It is at least as important, for example, as money in predicting how people feel. Thus many workers have chosen to look at measures of health as appropriate to measuring quality of life. This is particularly relevant to the care of long-stay patients who, almost by definition, have suffered some major deterioration in their physical or mental health.

Mortality and survival

At the high reliability end of the measurement spectrum must surely be the binary measure 'dead or alive'. It has, despite its obvious inelegance, many virtues to recommend it. In particular it consists of data which are generally easy to collect and there is little or no disagreement about which is the desired outcome value.

On the negative side, it is not always clear whether length of life is necessarily compatible with quality. This is particularly the case in the evaluation of treatments such as those for cancer (Clark and Fallowfield,

1986). On the other hand, there is some evidence that psychometric variables, particularly those relating to cognitive function, are related to time until death in older people (Botwinick, West and Storandt, 1978). Similarly, it is well-recognized that the early mortality following admission to institutional care may be very high. This is in part, of course, because those who have to be so admitted are among the frailest of those in the population. However, there can also be demonstrated effects of the institution following such a move. The topic of relocation and its effects on mortality in older people has been the subject of considerable study, often using survival data as the most important measure. Early studies seemed to show almost universal bad effects from relocation and lead some to conclude that this should be avoided whenever possible.

Later studies have however shed more light on this phenomenon, and a more balanced view would seem to be appropriate (Nirenberg, 1983). In particular, it seems that relocation may have either good or bad effects. It depends on such things as whether the individual makes the move out of his or her personal choice, and on the benefits of the receiving environment. Having to move to a deprived environment without preparation can be very bad. Good preparation and, just as important, attention to improving the environment, can have positive benefits including increased survival.

Perceived health

As with quality of life, one's own perception of one's health is at least as important in determining well-being as objectively defined medical status. Several studies have shown, for example, that such perception of one's own health is a significant predictor of life satisfaction (Palmore and Luikart, 1972; Spreitzer and Schnyder, 1974), the measurement of which I will consider in more detail later.

Furthermore, it appears that self-assessed health is especially important in settings where there is less choice and individual autonomy (Wolk and Telleen, 1976). It seems therefore reasonable to suppose that good health, or more accurately, thinking you are in good health, is an important determinant to one's quality of life.

There are several scales which have been developed to measure general health status, though in some cases this has been for quite different purposes. Both the Cornell Medical Index (Brodman *et al.*, 1951) and the General Health Questionnaire (GHQ) (Goldberg, 1978) have been concerned with perceived health as an initial measure of personal well-being. One aim has been to screen people for psychiatric morbidity. In so far as this tends to pick up psychological distress as well as frank mental illness, such measures may seem to have relevance to measuring quality of life. This is probably a fair assumption, but the higher prevalence of physical dysfunction in older people, or indeed any in long-stay care, can rather invalidate the usual norms and cut-offs. Thus, for example, the first factor on the GHQ relates to somatic complaints. In a general population of younger people living at home this may be a good way of screening for distress. In older and frailer groups it may simply reflect concurrent illness.

Whilst chronic physical illness is related to risk of depression (Murphy, 1982) not even the majority of those with such illness are depressed. Just because you have some physical symptoms does not mean that you have a poor quality of life. Nonetheless, it is true to say that assessing physical health is a very important dimension in evaluating any care pro-gramme and has been included in such studies (Kane and Kane, 1981). Improving someone's overall physical health is likely to be perceived as increasing their quality of life.

Of course, such health assessments are not necessarily self-ratings. For example, whereas the Guttman Health Scale (Rosow and Breslau, 1966) assesses health in relation to day-to-day functional activities by means of a self-administered questionnaire, the Stockton Geriatric Rating Scale (Meer and Baker, 1966) relies on ratings made by others such as nurses. The latter has been modified and combined with some simple measures of cognitive function to provide a general picture of dependency (Pattie and Gilleard, 1979). The Clifton Assessment Procedures for the Elderly have been validated on a wide range of older people. The results show both differences between groups in various settings, for example at home, in residential care or in hospital and considerable overlap between them. Again, however, it seems reasonable to suppose that a lower level of dependence allows more autonomy, and that achieving this should be part of improving quality of life.

The items on the Stockton Geriatric Rating Scale and its derivative relate to basic tasks such as bathing, dressing and eating, to the presence of disturbed behaviour such as wandering or withdrawal, and to cognitive difficulties – for example, those affecting communication. As such they give rather a coarse measure of overall function better suited to the description of groups of people rather than to the evaluation of individual ability. Moreover, the factors on the shortened scale seem to be different from those of the original (Twining and Allen, 1981).

For individuals, the use of a more detailed assessment of the activities of daily living (ADL) and mental state is much more likely to be appropriate. This is included in many sets of procedures such as the OARS (Duke University Center for the Study of Ageing and Human Development; 1978), CAMDEX (Roth *et al*, 1988) and others (Lawton, 1971). In all of these procedures there is an attempt not simply to assess an individual's basic physical abilities but also their application to the ordinary everyday activities which enable each of us to function independently. These include physical activities such as walking, bathing and dressing, together with other skills such as cooking, handling money and using public transport. It can been seen that, in respect of quality of life, these abilities are permissive, that is to say that they define the limits of independence. Of course, the individual's ability to make choices, which is central to most ideas of a high quality of life, depends not simply on his or her physical capacity but also on the availability of prosthetic aids and the person's ability to use these. Thus, someone who is physically unable to walk may, given the correct aids and environment, be able to get around very well with minimal help. Someone with less of a physical limitation may have poorer functional ability because of mental or environmental factors. If you need someone there to prompt you to make a cup of tea, you may be just as dependent as someone who needs physical help to do this.

How the measurement is carried out can make quite a lot of difference to the results. Occupational therapists take great care to match the surroundings to the individual's personal circumstances. It is no good expecting a frail older person to perform at his or her best with a gas cooker when that person has always used an electric one. Home assessment has much to commend it, and by 'home' we may mean the nursing home, residential home or hospital ward.

Mental health

Besides physical capacities and environment, the individual's mental state is a very important determinant of their activities and their own perception of their quality of life. It has already been noted that how we feel about our own health can be used as a screening tool for mental health problems. The two most common mental health difficulties for older people are of course depression and dementia. These have at once similar and very different implications. Depression is generally the more common, especially in younger old people, for example those aged under 75. It could in many ways be seen as a fairly direct measure of quality of life since we would be unlikely to say that someone with marked dysphoria has a good quality of life. Even if all the other variables are positive, their depressed mood will be reflected in their seeing things differently. In marked depression they may seek to end their life because they feel it is no longer worth living.

There are several ways that depression can be identified, ranging from an extensive structured assessment of mental state such as the Geriatric Mental Status Schedule (Copeland *et al.*, 1976), through specially designed screening scales (Yesavage *et al.*, 1983) and severity ratings (Hamilton, 1960) to checklists aimed at assessing mood which may or may not be a part of formal depressive illness (Beck *et al.*, 1961; Zung,

1965). There has even been an attempt formally to measure happiness (Kozma and Stones, 1980). Given that we are concerned here with general well-being, and not just with mental illness, the latter would seem to offer more use as ways of measuring whether we are achieving a good quality of life for our clients. Put simply, if we offer people a better quality of life we would expect them on the whole to feel happier.

Of course, the most common reason for this not happening is the other major mental illness of late life, namely dementia. Again, there are very many ways of assessing the severity of cognitive impairment varying from a lengthy research tool such as the CAMDEX (Roth *et al.*, 1988) to brief questionnaires examining mainly orientation and memory. For a brief, but slightly wider ranging, assessment there are procedures such as the CAPE (Pattie and Gilleard, 1979) and the Mini Mental Status test (Folstein *et al.*, 1975).

The real problem with dementia is of course that it affects the individual's appraisal of their situation, which is of course crucial to that person's understanding of their quality of life. Not only does this make it difficult to use self-report measures, it can produce all kinds of discrepancies between what that person thinks of their life and the way that others view things. Thus a person suffering from dementia may be distraught even when well cared for in his or her own home because he or she no longer recognizes it as such. Conversely, someone who, before developing dementia, was fiercely independent and solitary may show a 'personality change' and appear quite contented sitting doing nothing on a crowded, run-down hospital ward. It can be very hard to know how we are to define what that individual sees as a good quality of life in such cases.

Not surprisingly we tend to come to some sort of compromise and to apply those standards which, dementia notwithstanding, we think lead to a better quality of life. However we need to be flexible and to recognize that not only is each dementia sufferer an individual but that his or her needs can and most likely will change over time. We need to be sensitive to each individual's right to choose, even if that means that he or she does not join in the wonderful activity which we have so carefully designed to improve his or her quality of life. Even the inarticulate need to be allowed to vote with their feet.

ENGAGEMENT

Although it may seem obvious that someone can be happy without doing things, it is by no means always perceived to be so. Studies of frail older people and others, such as persons suffering from a mental handicap, have shown that, in institutions, there is very little going on. This is seen as a bad thing and, on the whole, such a generalization seems reasonable.

Most of us find our lives more satisfying if we are doing things. Certainly, depressed people tend to do less than people who are not depressed.

As far as institutions for frail older people are concerned, the lack of activity should not surprise us. When people are in their own homes the greater proportion of their time is taken up by sleeping and 'obligated time', that is cooking, cleaning, bathing and so on. When one takes away the need to do these latter tasks, doing nothing and sleeping are what tend to remain.

If inactivity is bad, then activity must be good. Following such logic seems to have left some workers determined to demonstrate that frail older people can do things if given the opportunity to do so. There have been careful attempts to measure the extent to which people do things, including talking to other people, and such measures are generally referred to as measurements of 'engagement'.

However much of this work originates from studies of those with a mental handicap, and the translation to older people is not always appropriate. Although it may be quite possible to show that, given the opportunity and encouragement, older people in a residential home will do things like polish coins (Jenkins *et al.*, 1977), it is not clear whether they feel better for this. Such a suspicion is confirmed by work showing that engagement and depression are not inversely correlated in such residents (Simpson *et al.*, 1981). Some people are quite happy to spend a lot of time simply sitting and thinking. The lesson here must be that if we are to use non-verbal activity measures to assess quality of life, we must complement this by measuring such things as covert reminiscence.

LIFE SATISFACTION

There is good reason to believe that how people feel about their past life relates to how they feel now. Although not all old people spend a lot of time reminiscing, many do, and for many of these people it is a pleasurable activity (Coleman, 1986). Certainly, the comparison with how things used to be is a useful way of judging how you feel about life now. The other way of judging things now is how one's own life compares with others of the same age.

Both these comparisons figure strongly in the most well-known measures of life satisfaction in old age. Neugarten, Havighurst and Tobin (1961) published two approaches to the measurement of perceived quality of life which have been strongly influential in very many subsequent studies. The measures they developed, the Life Satisfaction Indices (LSI) consisted of a series of self ratings and a set of ratings made by an interviewer on the basis of a structured interview. Both of these measures were designed to assess five areas of life satisfaction, namely:

1. Zest for life
2. Resolution and fortitude
3. Congruence between desired and achieved goals
4. Level of self esteem
5. Happy, optimistic mood

The self-assessment questionnaire has been the more widely used, and several authors have suggested amendments. Bigot (1974) reported that a shorter eight-item questionnaire was sufficient, and that this seemed to measure two components: acceptance/contentment and achievement/fulfilment.

It is worth noting here that another study (Wood *et al.*, 1969) has indicated that there may be marked age and gender differences in the validity of LSIs. These authors correlated the results from the questionnaire with ratings made by trained observers following a lengthy interview. There was a much higher correlation between the two types of measures for those aged over 70 years and for men. The authors were using the ratings to assess the validity of the questionnaires, and these results do pose some interesting questions. Why should it be that interviews disagree more with the self-ratings of women and the younger elderly? It is of course legitimate to argue that the self-ratings may be 'correct' and that all this shows is how useless are trained interviewers. However, this does little to help solve the knotty problem of validity.

One other problem with the original measures, for British workers at least, is that they are written in American rather than in English. Luker (1969) made some amendments for use with a British population but concluded that further refinement might be justified. These differences in language may be of more than passing interest. Some studies have suggested, for example, that British samples tend to show higher levels of life satisfaction than do North American ones. It is very hard to judge the significance of this, however, when correctly adjusted forms have not been used.

Lohmann (1977) compared the results of using no less than seven different measures of life satisfaction, some being the familiar questionnaires, some being measures of morale (e.g. Kutner *et al.*, 1956), and one being a simple global self-rating (How satisfied are you with your life now?). There was at best only a modest correlation between this rating and the other measures. The size of this correlation varied according to the number of items in the questionnaire. This may indicate that, as Neugarten *et al.* and subsequent authors have found, life satisfaction is multi-dimensional, and that to reduce it to a single number is to simplify beyond utility.

Studies originating in Britain (Abrams, 1973; Andrews and Withey, 1974; Hall, 1976) have also started from a large pool of items and identified a much smaller number relating more directly to life satisfaction. The most common areas relating to life satisfaction were family, home life, marriage and health. The longer the interval since the last visit to the doctor, the higher was the life satisfaction.

Retirement perhaps has less impact on life satisfaction than we might imagine, though obviously the amount of income for those on a pension is a significant factor. Indeed, only about 10% of those who are retired have significant problems in adjusting to this transition (Braithwaite and Gibson, 1987). Similarly, overall, the effects of housing and leisure activities seem to be lower down the priority order in determining how older people feel. Of course, some of these may be cohort effects, that is, how you feel now depends on when you were born, how you were brought up, and what you have been used to. This could, for example, explain partly the findings in relation to LSIs and interview ratings to which I referred earlier. The views of the younger old people may, by virtue of their experience, be closer to those of the interviewers. Such an hypothesis does not bode well for the future. It suggests that as we achieve ever higher standards of material well-being, we may become progressively more reluctant to put up with material deprivation in later life. Such a shift, the logical conclusion of ageing and consumerism, could have at least as strong an effect on the demand for resources as any change in the numbers of very elderly people.

The environment

Studies of older people in hospital have shown that the greatest causes of dissastisfaction tend to be with interpersonal rather than physical aspects of the environment. Thus, Raphael and Mandeville (1979) found that the furniture, ward and sanitary accommodation were rated by elderly patients as being the most satisfactory, while diversional activity, noise and nurses' care gave most cause for complaint or irritation. The one exception to this general rule was that day-space was also rated as a source of dissatisfaction, though even this may reflect problems in terms of the social effects of inadequate day-space. In this study, staff were also asked to give their views of the satisfaction, or otewise, of aspects of hospital life. Interestingly, there was no correlation between the rank ordering of topics by staff and patients. This does not bode well for staff trying to act as the patients' advocate.

Certainly the physical environment is important, not only for its direct effect on residents but indirectly via its influence on staff. The direct influence on residents social interaction has been demonstrated in terms of the arrangement of furniture (Peterson *et al.*, 1977) and the layout of day-space (Harris *et al.*, 1977). The latter study showed that the arrangement of space influenced the interaction of residents of old people's homes and that residents themselves are, as we always knew, a powerful force. In particular, their work demonstrated the vulnerability of the mentally frail elderly. The prime space, that is, the day-space's nearest to day-to-day activity, was dominated by mentally alert residents who effectively segregated themselves from the confused. The latter were confined to day areas away from the main stream of activity, thus compounding their handicap. However, as we might expect, whatever the design of the home, the attitudes and policies of the staff were of crucial importance.

Indirectly, the environment affects residents by way of its influence on staff behaviour, recruitment and morale. Knapp and Harrissis (1981) have shown that the likelihood of there being vacancies among the supervisory staff in a home is related to the size of the home, the amenities it offers, and its contact with the rest of the community. A small home with plenty of amenities and an adequate supply of toilets, and which provides meals-on-wheels for the surrounding community, is less likely to have problems in recruiting senior staff.

Of course, there may need to be a balance struck between the philosophy of 'small is beautiful' and the economies of scale. An Israeli study (Weihl, 1981) showed that the 'functionally independent elderly' tended to be more satisfied if they lived in homes with more than 90 places. To take one example, the author suggests that the greater level of satisfaction with personal friendships found in the larger homes may be because the residents have a larger pool of persons from whom to find a kindred spirit. The difficulties to be found in maintaining good personal relationships in some small group homes would tend to confirm that this could be a valid point.

Nonetheless, there are many arguments in favour of smaller units – perhaps not least because of the influence this has on staff behaviour and attitudes. In a small unit, staff are going to find it much easier to see each person as an individual rather than as an anonymous member of a large group. This may not matter much for the functionally independent, but it is very important for the very frail. They must depend to a much greater extent on others for their preservation of individuality and the opportunity to exercise choice and control.

It should be clear by now that 'the environment' for long-stay elderly patients must include both the physical surroundings and the social milieu of both fellow patients and staff. Of these three areas there is no doubt that it is a lot easier to measure the first rather than the second and third. Very few people are not familiar with how to use a tape measure and a thermometer. Conversely, many would have trouble knowing how to begin measuring social climate or staff policy. It may be this which has led to much greater emphasis being given to the physical aspects of care. Nonetheless, attempts have been made to take a broader approach and these deserve to be more widely applied.

In Britain, the significant expansion in private sector residential and nursing homes has meant that much more attention has been paid to the registration and monitoring of such homes. Detailed guidance has been given as to how local authorities should assess residential homes (Centre for Policy on Ageing, 1984) and how health authorities should assess nursing homes (National Association of Health Authorities, 1985).

The code of practice for residential care, 'Home Life', includes a checklist of 218 items covering five topics: social care, physical features, client groups, staff and registration. The first of these, social care, actually includes a third of all the items in the checklist and over double the number covering physical features. This seems a reasonable balance in view of what we already know of the importance of interpersonal interaction to residents' well-being. This checklist is not, of course, a measurement instrument in its own right. It cannot be compared with a tape measure or a thermometer. However, it does provide a most useful guide to checking on an institution whether this is for the formal purpose of legal registration or for other reasons.

If we are looking to measure the environment of elderly people there is one instrument available which does offer more than a checklist of features. The Multiphasic Environmental Assessment Procedures (MEAP) (Moos and Lemke, 1984a and b) have been developed from studies of older people in institutional care, and they provide both a conceptual framework for the evaluation of these environments (Moos, 1980) and a set of measuring instruments. The scales comprising the instruments cover five topics. The first four are measures of the institutions based on the reports of residents and staff, and the fifth is a set of ratings for use by an outside observer covering the same areas. The four dimensions measured by the scales are physical features, policy and program factors, resident and staff characteristics and social climate. There have been many studies using these scales on North American groups, and these studies have demonstrated good discrimination between different homes and they allow for the design of appropriate intervention programmes (e.g. Lemke and Moos, 1980; Moos and Igra, 1980; Brennan *et al.*, 1988). Because the scales consist of parallel forms for completion by residents, with help where necessary, and by staff, it is possible to compare and contrast these different views of each setting. In addition, the social climate scale has separate forms for the residents to rate the real (what is this home like now?), the ideal (what would an ideal home be like?) and the expected (what do I think it will be like when I move to this home?). This enables major discrepancies to be identified and a prospective resident to express his or her expectations of the intended home.

Social climate is an important area of care. When frail older people ask for advice on choosing a home it is rarely in terms of judging whether it looks pleasant or is adequately heated. These things they can generally judge fairly quickly for themselves on the basis of a brief visit. What is much more helpful to them is some indication of how warm and friendly is the atmosphere. Because this is usually based on loose subjective impression, this is just the sort of information which professionals are reluctant to impart. The use of this kind of structured measurement could help a great deal.

Similar approaches have been used to look at the problems of those with long-term psychiatric disability (Wing and Brown, 1970). Of course, by no means all of these people are elderly, but the problems of achieving a good quality of life are in many ways similar. Provided ideas are chosen carefully with the client group in mind they may come from a wide variety of sources.

It is also easy to see how these kinds of techniques can be used to evaluate care and suggest change. Quality of life for residents and patients is the most relevant outcome measure for long-term care. How do we bring about positive change?

IMPLEMENTATION AND EVALUATION

We saw earlier on (Figure 4.1) how a number of factors may be seen to influence quality of life. These are not neatly independent in practice, but considering them separately does help us to consider the options in a manageable way. Thus it is also useful to take the same structure and examine some of the ways in which improvement can be brought about.

Before turning in detail to each area, however, it is worth pausing to remind ourselves of some of the general principles of change which are relevant. Psychology can help us not only to understand how clients change but also how to bring about changes in what staff do. First we must remember that change is more noticeable than the status quo. Our nervous systems are built to detect change, be it movement, sound, touch or taste. We rapidly adapt to the world around us and focus our attention on what changes – not what stays the same. This habituation to things which stay the same is very important in helping us to cope with the great complexity of the world. It helps us to keep things manageable and stops us coming to harm. However, in the context of long-term care it can be a mixed blessing. We can rapidly become unaware of problems, inadequacies or even bad practice when we stay a long time in one place. Most of us can remember what impression a large old hospital made the first time we walked through the door. The sights, the noise and the smell may well have moved us greatly, and probably not for the better. We find this kind of experience stressful and may have difficulty sifting the important information from the irrelevant detail.

Unfortunately, if we work in that setting we rapidly adjust to the situation. Even things that should give us cause for concern no longer attract our attention. What really *is* a grubby wall in need of a coat of paint can fade into the background. But for those who are coming into that setting for the first time, be they new staff, patients or relatives, the impression will be much closer to that which we first had and then have forgotten. Somehow we have to try and keep that sensitivity alive and turn it to our advantage.

Similarly, many of the abilities and even the clinical condition of patients in long-term care change only slowly. It may be very hard to pick out a threshold which can alert us to someone needing extra help until the change, whether it be positive or negative is quite pronounced.

Conversely, if we are trying to change some way of doing things then that change will stand out a mile, however minor the thing we seek to change. For example, even re-arranging the chairs so as to facilitate social interaction may be resisted both by residents and by staff. This resistance may arise not because the change is for the worse but just because it is change. We have to think actively about how to bring about change and how to maintain it.

Change is therefore unsettling. Indeed, in the case of the enforced relocation of frail older people there is some evidence to suggest that it may, if handled badly, be fatal. Change can be threatening, especially if it is seen as being imposed from outside. We all need to feel that we are in control of at least a substantial portion of our lives. If we find that constantly we are out of control we may become increasingly helpless or indeed frankly depressed. People who believe that they make things happen generally feel much better that those who feel the outside world determines what happens to them. These general principles apply both to staff and to residents or patients. Both are powerful groups who play a crucial role in what happens in long-term care. Those who are not with change are against, and few innovators can achieve much if there are many who are opposed. Bearing these principles in mind, we can now consider the various factors, some internal, some external, which influence quality of life and what can be done to improve these.

The physical environment

From the examples that have already been given it is clear that the physical environment is both easy to measure and yet difficult to change. Certainly, in terms of instruments there are plenty available, and it is at least possible to set standards and to determine whether these are being achieved. We have explicit guidance available both in the form of the kinds of checklists mentioned earlier and in the building note and regulations published by bodies such as the Department of Health (DHSS, 1980).

Of course, whereas such notes tend to ensure that buildings do not fall down or are otherwise actively dangerous, they do not in themselves ensure a homely environment which supports appropriate individual and social behaviour. Such guidance is rather more complex but nonetheless can be achieved (DHSS, 1976). That these matters ought to be considered carefully need hardly be emphasized. Buildings are important and remarkably enduring. Could the Victorian Britons who designed and built so many workhouses and asylums have forseen just how many elderly peoples' lives their work would dominate and for how long? However many times you change the wallpaper, and however many sanitary annexes you build on, a ward in a lunatic asylum still looks like a series of large rooms at the end of an even longer corridor. There are some situations where the right agents for meaningful change must be the bulldozer and the pneumatic drill.

In designing and evaluating environments we must ensure that the needs of the particular client group are properly considered. Those with physical frailty may need compact accessible facilities, while those with mental frailty may need plenty of room to wander. It may be impossible to achieve both, and priorities must be decided. If we do not know what we are trying to achieve we are unlikely to be successful.

Physical health

In the case of physical health there are likewise well-established techniques for measuring outcome. In the case of long-term care, however, it is important to be aware of potentially conflicting priorities. A simple literature search of medical publications yields a very respectable number of studies which are explicitly considering the concept of 'quality of life'. However, closer examination reveals that many, indeed possibly the majority, of these papers are looking at terminal care, especially the care of those suffering from cancer. At first this may seem a little disappointing, since the issues in the care of older people are very much broader than just the management of terminal care. However, these studies do address one of the recurring questions, namely, how to balance the benefits of applying treatment – for example, the relief of pain or the prolonging of life – against possible adverse effects (such as unpleasant side-effects or pain arising from invasive procedures).

The evaluation of the outcome of physical health care in long-term settings must include the measurement of phenomena such as pressure areas and contractures and whether there is an appropriate balance between quality and quantity of life. Of course, this begs the question: who is to decide? Here, the answer is not simple, and indeed no one person, not even the physican, can decide alone on the best course of action for each and every patient. Nurses, relatives and, most importantly, the patient himself or herself have a contribution to make. Perhaps the only thing that can be definitely stated is that care which gives good quality of life must include opportunities for these difficult issues to be considered. Nobody involved, including the patient and family, should feel either excluded or left to decide such matters alone.

Social interaction

Mention has already been made of how important this is in promoting well-being. It is a fairly simple matter to measure what is, or is not, going on in a long-term care setting. This may take the form of simply noting what is the programme of activity which might give opportunity for interaction or, in much more detail, using behavioural methods such as event or time sampling. One word of caution here is that low levels of interaction are the norm, and one must not be too ambitious in trying to achieve change. It is very easy to carry out such measurement and produce a report highly critical of staff, managers and even patients. Staff are very often all too well aware of what is lacking. What they need is help to put things right.

The other important points to remember are that the lack of observable activity is, as we have already seen, no indication of individual client dissatisfaction, and activity should be meaningful – especially if it is designed to promote social interaction.

The remaining influences on quality of life may be broadly described as being more internal rather than external. They relate particularly to psychological processes and, therefore, psychological approaches are of particular relevance (Twining, 1988).

Mental health

Improving the mental health of older people means mostly alleviating depression and minimizing the effects of dementia. Of these two, the more intractable is undoubtedly dementia – although there is good evidence that depression often goes unrecognized in both the physically frail in hospital (Lim and Ebrahim, 1983; Robinson and Price, 1982) and among older people in the community (Murphy, 1982).

Approaches to dementia have tended to concentrate on the development of reality orientation programmes which have become very popular in recent years (Holden and Woods, 1988). There are some question marks over the efficacy of this in overcoming the deficits of dementia (Powell-Procter and Miller, 1982), though there may be some gains to be made in the attitudes and behaviour of staff. Much the same could be said of other interventions for the severely confused. Things such as personalized clothing and the encouragement of personal belongings can be seen as having two major effects. First, they give the patient or resident a sense of identity, familiarity and security, and second, they help the staff to see that person as an individual with an unique history. The resulting change in staff behaviour is likely to be just as important as the rather small and relatively short-term gains in orientation.

One way of helping staff to see people as individuals and to improve their interactions is to ensure that detailed information is available on each resident or client. A detailed personal history form can be useful for this purpose.

Reminiscence has also been the focus of a good deal of attention and has, like reality orientation, generated much enthusiasm (Coleman, 1986). It is a common, though by no means universal, activity among older people, and can generate both positive and negative emotions. By drawing on the considerable past experiences of older people it can provide at least a valuable meaningful activity and, under careful guidance, be the means of psychological therapy.

INDIVIDUAL APPRAISAL

The relationship between cognition and emotion has likewise been shown to be of great value in enhancing well-being. There has been what can only be described as an explosion of work in psychological therapy, much of it soundly based on psychological knowledge and experimental evaluation (Woods and Britton, 1985). The techniques have the potential for application not only to frank disorder, notably anxiety and depression, but also to the promotion of positive adjustment to a wide range of life events. No doubt admission to long-term care could be included in this, but as yet this remains to be developed.

There is also the need to develop advocacy schemes similar to those being promoted in the care of those suffering from mental handicap. This would enable the interests of frail older people to figure more in the determination of care.

Personality and past history

Being rooted in the past, these may not seem to be amenable to change and therefore not directly relevant to the improvement of quality of life. However, they do have a very sigificant impact on how individuals adjust to different settings. Thus we should at very least give these weight in trying to provide the right sort of long-term care for individual older people.

Again, there can be special problems in the case of those suffering from dementia or other acquired brain damage. Such disorders can lead to considerable personality change and, as a result, a form of care which previously would have been rejected outright may now be the most suitable for current needs. We have to remain flexible in our approach not only so as to provide for the wide range of individual differences but also to allow for individuals to change over time.

THE ROLE OF MANAGEMENT

Good management is vital to the success of any complex enterprise. In the case of long-term care this includes monitoring that care and the implementation of change. There are very many ways of achieving this, but most involve some form of generating ideas and providing appropriate feedback to staff. The specific project may have almost any title – including Positive Monitoring (Porterfield, 1987), a Meritgram Scheme (Reingold et al., 1987), the introduction of Residents' Committees (Wells and Singer, 1988), or the use of a staff training programme (Open University, 1988).

Ultimately, promoting a good quality of life may be seen by some as best achieved by the introduction of performance-related funding. The studies of Kane and others (Kane et al., 1983a and b) have at least tackled some of the methodological issues which must be addressed if this were to be feasible. In particular they make the point that patient outcome depends on patient condition. Thus, any evaluation of care must take into account the initial level of function of those receiving care. Care must be evaluated as better or worse than expected for such clients if we are to avoid automatically rewarding those who provide care only for the least in need.

Whether this or some other approach proves to be possible and effective remains to be seen. For the present we must seek to consider all those things which may indicate quality of life and to ensure that these are central to our assessment of the outcome of the care which is provided.

CONCLUSIONS

By now it is probably clear to even the most optimistic reader that there is no easy answer to the question 'What is Quality of Life?' nor is there any single simple way of measuring this. We live and work in a real world where the benefit of compromise often outweighs that of pursuing the ideal. It is therefore reasonable to put philosophy temporarily to one side and to suggest which of the available approaches seem the most useful.

As there are several dimensions to quality of life, a short combination of measures seems best. Thus it is appropriate to choose:

1. A self-report measure either of mood (e.g. Beck *et al.*, 1961; Yesavage *et al.*, 1983), life satisfaction (Bigot, 1974) or happiness (Kozma and Stones, 1980)
2. A measure of behaviour or activity either from observation (Simpson *et al.*, 1981) or by the completion of an activity timetable showing the pattern of the residents' days each week.
3. A measure of the environment based on a checklist (Centre for Policy on Ageing, 1984) or a rating scale for social climate (Lemke and Moos, 1980)

Obviously it is also possible to use one of the comprehensive packages (Moos and Lemke, 1984a and b; Kane and Kane, 1981) but these are time-consuming and are likely to appeal only where there are personnnel available to spend quite a lot of time on their completion.

Whatever the situation it is clear that there is no excuse for not making at least some attempt to address the fundamental question 'How are we doing in providing a good quality of life for those under our care?'

REFERENCES

Abrams, M.A. (1973) Subjective social indications. *Social Trends.*, **4**, 35–56.

Adams, D.L. (1969) Analysis of a Life-satisfaction Index. *J. Gerontol.*, **24**, 470–474.

Andrews, F.M. (1974) Social indicators of perceived life quality. *Social Indicators Res.*, **1**, 279–299.

Andrews, F.M. and Withey, S.B. (1974) Developing measures of perceived life quality: results from several national surveys. *Social Indicators Res.*, **1**, 1–26.

Beck, A.T., Ward, C.H., Mendelson, M. *et al.* (1961) An inventory for measuring depression. *Arch. Gen. Psychiatry*, **4**, 561–567.

Bigot, A. (1974) The relevance of American life satisfaction indices for research on British subjects before and after retirement. *Age Ageing*, **3**, 113–121.

Botwinick, J., West, R. and Storant, M. (1978) Predicting death from behavioral test performance. *J. Gerontol.*, **33**, 755–762.

Braithwaite, V.A. and Gibson, D.M. (1987) Adjustment to retirement: what we know and what we need to know. *Ageing Society*, **7**, 1–18.,

Brennan, P.L., Moos, R. and Lemke, S. (1988) Preferences of older adults for physical and architectural features of group living facilities. *Gerontologist*, **28**, 84–90.

Brodman, K., Erdmann, A.J., Lorge, I. and Wolff, H.G. (1951) The Cornell Medical Index – Health Questionnaire. *JAMA.*, **145**, 152–157.

Centre for Policy on Ageing (1984) Home Life: a Code of Practice for Residential Care. Centre for Policy on Ageing, London.

Clark, A. and Fallowfield, L.J. (1986) Quality of life measurements in patients with malignant disease: a review. *J. Roy. Soc. Med.*, **79**, 165–169.

Coleman, P.G. (1986) *Ageing and Reminiscence Processes*, Wiley, Chichester.

Copeland, J.R.M., Kelleher, M.J., Kellett, J.M. and Gourlay, A.J. (1976) A semi-structured clinical interview in the elderly: the geriatric mental status schedule. 1. Development and reliability. *Psychol. Med..* **6**, 439–449.

DHSS (1976) A Life Style for the Elderly. HMSO, London.

DHSS (1980) Hospital Accommodation for Elderly People, Draft Building Note No. 37. HMSO, London.

Duke University Center for the Study of Ageing and Human Development (1978) Multidimensional Functional Assessment: the OARS Methodology, A Manual. The Center for Ageing, Durham, NC, USA.

Folstein, J., Folstein, S. and McHugh, P. (1975) Mini-mental state. *J. Psychiat. Res.*, **12**, 189–198.

Goldberg, D. (1978) *Manual of the General Health Questionnaire*, NFER-Nelson, Windsor, U.K.

Hall, J. (1976) Subjective measures of quality of life in Britain, 1971–1975: some developments and trends. *Social Trends*, **7**, 47–60.

Hamilton, M. (1960) A rating scale for depression. *J. Neurol. Neurosurg. Psychiat.*, **23**, 56–62.

Harris, H., Lipman, A. and Slater, R. (1977) Architectural design: the spatial location and interactions of old people. *Gerontology*, **23**, 390–400.

Havighurst, R.J. (1963) 'Successful Ageing', in *Process of Ageing: Social and Psychological Perceptors* (eds R.H. Williams, C. Tibbits and W. Donahue), Atherton Press, New York.

Holden, U.P. and Woods, R.T. (1988) *Reality Orientation: Psychological Approaches to the 'Confused' Elderly*, Churchill Livingstone, Edinburgh.

Jenkins, J., Felce, D., Lunt, B. and Powell, E. (1977) Increasing engagement in activity of residents in old peoples' homes by providing recreational materials. *Behav. Res. Therap.*, **15**, 429–434.

Kane, R.L. and Kane, R.A. (1981) *Assessing the Elderly: a Practical Guide to Measurement*, DC Heath, Lexington, MA, USA.

Kane, R.L., Bell, R., Riegler, S. *et al.* (1983a) Assessing the outcomes of nursing-home patients. *J. Gerontol.*, **38**, 385–393.

Kane, R.L., Bell, R., Riegler, S. *et al.* (1983b) Predicting the outcomes of nursing home patients. *Gerontologist*, **23**, 200–206.

Knapp, M. and Harrissis, K. (1981) Staff vacancies and turnover in British old peoples'homes. *Gerontologist*, **21**, 76–84.

Kozma, A. and Stones, M.J. (1980) The measurement of happiness: development of the Memorial University of Newfoundland scale of happiness. *J. Gerontol.*, **35**, 906–912.

Kutner, B., Fanshel, D., Togo, A.M. and Donovan, J.D. (1956) *Five Hundred Over Sixty*, Russell Sage Foundation, New York, USA.

Lawton, M.P., (1971) The functional assessment of elderly people. *J. Am. Geriatrics Soc.*, **19**, 465–481.

Lemke, S. and Moos, R. (19780) Assessing the institutional policies of sheltered care settings. *J. Gerontol.*, **35**, 96–107.

Lim, M.L. and Ebrahim, S.B.J. (1983) Depression after stroke: a hospital treatment survey. *Postgrad. Med. J.*, **59**, 489–491.

Lohmann, N. (1977) Correlations of life satisfaction, morale and adjustment measures. *J. Gerontol.*, **32**, 73–75.

Luker, K.A. (1969) Measuring life satisfaction in an elderly population. *J. Adv. Nurs.*, **4**, 503–511.

Meer, B. and Baker, J.A. (1966) The Stockton Geriatric Rating Scale. *J. Gerontol.*, **21**, 392–403.

Moos, R. (1980) Specialized living environments for older people: a conceptual framework. *J. Soc. Issues*, **36**, 75–94.

Moos, R. and Igra, A. (1980) Determinants of the social environments of sheltered care settings. *J. Health Soc. Behav.*, **21**, 88–98.

Moos, R. and Lemke, S. (1984a) *Multiphasic Environmental Assessment Procedure (MEAP): Manual*, Stanford University Medical Center, Palo Alto, CA, USA.

Moos, R. and Lemke, S. (1984b) *MEAP Supplementary Manual: Ideal and Expectation Forms*, Stanford University Medical Center, Palo Alto, CA, USA.

Murphy, E. (1982) Social origins of depression in old age. *Br. J. Psychiatry*, **141**, 135–142.

National Association of Helath Authorities (1985) A code of guidance for the inspection and registration of nursing homes. NAHA, London.

Neugarten, B.L., Havighurst, R.J. and Tobin, S.S. (1961) The Measurement of life satisfaction. *J. Gerontol.*, **16**, 134–143.

Nirenberg, T.D. (1983) Relocation of institutionalized elderly. *J. Consult. Clin. Psychol.*, **51**, 693–701.

Open University (1988) *Working with Mental Health Problems in Old Age*, Open University, Milton Keynes, UK.

Palmore, E. and Luikart, C. (1972) Health and social factors related to life satisfaction. *J. Health Soc. Behav.*, **3**, 68–80.

Pattie, A.H. and Gilleard, C.J. (1979) *The Clifton Assessment Procedures for the Elderly*, Hodder and Stoughton, London.

Peterson, R.G., Knapp, T.J., Rosen, J.D. and Pither, B.F. (1977) The effect of furniture arrangement. *Behav. Therapy*, **8**, 464–467.

Porterfield, J. (1987) *Positive Monitoring*, British Institute of Mental Handicap, Kidderminster. UK.

Powell-Procter, L. and Miller, E. (1982) Reality orientation: a critical appraisal. *Br. J. Psychiat.*, **140**, 457–463.

Raphael, W. and Mandeville,J. (1979) Old People in Hospital. King Edward's Hospital Fund, London.

Reingold, J., Grossman, H.D. and Burros, N. (1987) Merit Gram: a form of recognition in a long-term care setting. *Gerontologist*, **27**, 147–150.

Robinson, R.G and Price, T.R. (1982) Post-stroke depressive disorders: a follow-up study of 103 patients. *Stroke*, **13**, 635–641.

Rosow, I. and Breslau, N. (1966) A Guttman health scale for the aged. *J. Gerontol.*, **21**, 556–559.

Roth, M., Huppert, F.A. Tym, E. and Mountjoy, C.Q. (1988) *The Cambridge Examination for Mental Disorders in the Elderly*, Cambridge University Press, Cambridge.

Simpson, S., Woods, R.T. and Britton, P.G. (1981) Depression and engagement in a residential home for the elderly. *Behav. Res. Therap.*, **19**, 435–438.

Spreitzer, E. and Snyder, E. (1974) Correlates of life satisfaction among the aged. *J. Gerontol.*, **29**, 454–458.

Twining, T.C. (1988) *Helping Older People: a Psychological Approach*, Wiley, Chichester, UK.

Twining, T.C. and Allen, D.G. (1981) Disability factors among residents of old people's homes. *J. Epidemiol. Comm. Health*, **35**, 205–207.

Weihl, H. (1981) On the relationship between the size of residential institutions and the well-being of residents. *Gerontologist*, **21**, 247–250.

Wells, L.M. and Singer, C. (1988) Quality of life in institutions for the elderly: maximizing well-being. *Gerontologist*, **28**, 266–269.

Wing, J.K. and Brown, G.W. (1970) *Institutionalisation and Schizophrenia*, Cambridge University Press, Cambridge, UK.

Wolk, S. and Telleen, S. (1976) Psychological and social correlates of life satisfaction as a function of residential constraint. *J. Gerontology*, **31**, 89–98.

Wood, V., Wylie, M. and Sheafer, B. (1969) An analysis of a short self-report measure of life satisfaction: correlation with raters' judgements. *J. Gerontol.*, **24**, 465–469.

Woods, R.T. and Britton P.G. (1985) *Clinical Psychology with the Elderly*, Croom Helm, London.

Yesavage, J.A., Brink, T.L., Rose, T.L. *et al.* (1983) Development and validation of a geriatric depression screening scale: a preliminary report. *J. Psychiatr. Res.*, **17**, 37–49.

Ziller, R.C. (1974) Self other orientations and quality of life. *Soc. Indicators Res.*, **1**, 301–310.

Zung, W.W.K. (1965) A self rating depression scale. *Arch. Gen. Psychiatry*, **12**, 63–70.

Chapter 5

At home in hospital or nursing home?

Although there is an accelerating move away from hospital continuing care units towards 'home' or domestic-style accommodation in public and private nursing homes, patients are still not in their own homes. They are in care because they need the skills of the staff and their resources. In order to get that care they have to accept the status of 'patients'. Even those who appreciate the help they are given would rather be elsewhere. Some may not be convinced that they need care at all.

The patient admitted to an acute medical unit will temporarily give up certain rights in order to get better, but the patient in continuing care has no prospects of returning home and lacks clarity about long-term aims – doctors, nurses and the rest of the therapeutic team may be clear about the aims but often the patient is not. This makes it all the more important to look at the status of the patients and how long-term care reinforces their social dependency (Townsend, 1981). Where the end is uncertain, the means to that end have to seem sensible in themselves or the environment will be perceived as persecutory. Therefore, good practice in continuing care is increasingly putting emphasis on producing a home-like atmosphere in hospital and on the rights of patients (Norman, 1980). Certainly the situation has improved since Robb (1967) wrote so movingly. However, the Annual Report of the NHS Health Advisory Service (1987) shows that the hospital continuing-care sector still has a long way to go. The trouble is, as already stated, hospital is nothing like home. One aspect of living at home – perhaps the one that most justifies a person taking risks and staying at home against all the odds – is the ability to exercise some personal authority to match that of others, however powerful they seem. Home is what you own – psychologically if not literally. The importance of psychological ownership is evident, especially for those who are increasingly physically dependent and for whom the therapeutic task is to maintain their sense of identity and worth as people. What is important is that people who have to live in a nursing home or hospital for a long time should be able to make as many decisions for themselves as possible – and be consulted in decisions made

for them. These are the rights that are at risk when patients leave home
for hospital or nursing home.

WHAT DOES 'NURSING HOME' OR 'HOSPITAL' MEAN TO THE PATIENT?

We do not know? We can do our best to understand the patient's point
of view but we do not always get it right. Community Health Council
and Health Service Commissioner reports, Martin (1984), and Wickings
and Crown (1989) all provide eloquent evidence of failure to provide the
patient's needs and wants. If there is anything worse than ignoring the
patient's feelings it is taking them over, and assuming the right to
interpret their needs as the carers think fit.

The hospitalization of a patient may be seen in terms of making
relationships. This will occur constructively if patients and staff alike
are able to understand and appreciate each other as much as possible.
It helps if members of staff know in detail what sort of life the patient
led before admission. In elderly patient departments the consultants
may be in a privileged position since they may have made a domi-
ciliary visit and may even have been accompanied by a nurse or other
colleague. It is worth noting in case conferences how the quality of
debate can be affected if one or more of the participants knows the
patient at home, even for a brief visit. In contrast, the patient who has
been referred by another hospital department may be subtly deprived,
lacking the involvement of staff with the whole person. Staff therefore
need two types of information – medical, which relates to the person's
illness, and general, which relates to the patient's home lifestyle.
The nursing process obtains the latter information in a valuable formal
manner (Abrahams and Lamb, 1988) but some people can find it quite
intrusive.

It is important to recognize the radical shift that takes place in the
patient's life on admission to a nursing home or continuing-care unit.
The patient knows it but who else does?

> Day-to-day support for the chronically sick individual is provided
> mainly within the family network by untrained people without
> the knowledge or assistance of so-called caring agencies. In times
> of crisis, when their assistance is asked for, what is provided is
> mainly institutionally based and often inappropriate. (McCarthy and
> Millard, 1979)

> Moving into a facility diminishes control not only because the elderly
> person moves onto another's turf but also because the shock of the
> move assaults the memory and with it the capacity to function . . .
> the nursing home occupies the same place in the psyche of the

elderly today as the poorhouse and the orphanage had in the imagination of Victorian children. (May, 1982)

The way people come into a hospital or nursing home, and the decision to make that place their refuge, is such that the continuity of experience is often broken. The patient has really come, as it were out of the void. Staff may even feel it is necessary to keep a distance from what is outside to avoid a clash of values.

The services provided by the nursing home or continuing-care unit are better understood in the context of values in our society. The immediate family has been expected to, and often still does, take care of its elderly members either by itself or with help from neighbouring kin. Contrary values which emphasize the older person's achievement may be put aside and denied. The elderly are expected to keep pace and are judged as failing when they do not. While there has long been a trend to reinforce the advantages of family and community care, there are also demands, often made in very painful and stressful circumstances, for institutions to take over the problems of the family, by removing their infirm aged members who may view admission as equivalent to going into the workhouse. The hospital for the elderly patient is only one of a number of systems of care working in a confusing and ambivalent world of contrary values where the taking of responsibility for decisions may be as important as the content of the decisions themselves (Dartington *et al*, 1974).

It is relevant that this ambivalence of social values seems to have its internal counterpart with each individual patient. Continuing-care patients are those who neither get better nor die. Within each of them there is a valency or motivation to get better, to be active and independent, and a valency to give up, to be passive and to be dependent. The staff have to do all they can with these ambivalences and they are helped in this by having the personal history of the patient.

There are ways of recalling at least some of a patient's history. A nurse has described the advantages of getting away from form filling:

We found that many people were reluctant to respond to direct question and answer sessions, and if they did respond they usually gave very basic replies, which did not help us to build a true picture of their lifestyle. . . Afternoon tea-time proved to be the best occasion, when the informal atmosphere was encouraged by the nurse having a cup of tea with the patient. Magazines, photographs and personal belongings were excellent aids to prompting the patient to talk about himself. . . Photographs of family members led to discussion of home and family, and the presence of personal belongings gave an insight into the things which people like to have around to promote a home-like atmosphere. No notes were taken during the session, and we found it essential that all information was recorded in writing immediately afterwards. (Cairns, 1979)

If the staff could really have an image of their elderly patients as they remember themselves, many of the details of care which are outlined in checklists of good practice would have been done already. One such checklist is included in the appendix (Elliott, 1982); it discusses many significant areas of daily living and helps to interpret the hospital environment as it may look to patients. The theme of giving back to patients a sense of personal authority is explored in the rest of this chapter. This is a challenge for staff: 'How far do we dare let patients have the equivalent rights in hospital they have had at home?'.

RULES – SPOKEN AND UNSPOKEN

In any community there are rules. Who makes the rules, and what can be done to change those which frustrate development? There are rules that are in the interest of the patients, and others in the interest of staff. There are some rules that are not especially in the interest of patients or staff but are about the way things have been done.

Some patients have the reputation of being difficult. This may occur because of their unmet expectations, and because their behavioural response is an attempt to maintain personal control over the experience of being in hospital or nursing home. Frequently the nurses' response to regain control only exacerbates the situation (English and Morse, 1988).

Other patients are appreciated for the concern they show towards those who are caring for them. The most favoured patients are often acquiescent: 'I don't want to bother you dear.'.

It is not easy to avoid exploiting the good-natured patient, or curtailing the initiative of a difficult one. Yet the expectations of many patients are likely to be negative unless staff demonstrate the alternative. A nurse stopped to chat with a patient but she was not welcome: 'Go away. You are here to see I don't smoke.'. The assumption by patients that the staff are not there to help them to do things but to stop them is very unfair. However, being in an institution, be it a hospital or a nursing home, is a limitation on patients' freedom. They are being told that they are not capable of being independent and others know better. It is against this background that elderly patients are then asked to be positive about the therapeutic activities of the hospital.

Being in hospital is likely to be a frightening experience. Those who are working to make the place as benign as possible may accept that statement, but may not like the full force of its meaning. It is disturbing to be feared by those one is trying to help. It took a psychiatrist to turn the proposition around: 'Why are you angry at me?' he protested, 'I am not trying to help you'.

Those who now have to be in hospital may have lost some of their autonomy in the past because they were not given the facts on which to base their own judgement. Instead they were asked to do as they were told. A survey of unmet need would show however that increased dependence does not affect the individual's ability to know what he wants (Chapman, 1979).

The daily ward time-table has certain fixed points; for example, it is affected by staff duty rotas, and in particular the handover between night and day staff. However, if patients have to fit in with routines that seem efficient to staff, they may be seen to be unable to do things that they would be able to do in their own time.

What would happen if staff really felt that they had to fit in with patients? 'Will you see the doctor now?' If the doctor's round really looked like a home visit, then we might really say that the patient had retained psychological ownership of his world, however contracted and confined that had become. However, if the doctor talks of 'my beds', he is only acknowledging the reality of the politics of hospital life, and the patient is a displaced person, not at home in any sense at all.

The patients are not really going to be able to determine any aspect of their lives if the staff insist that they are there only as patients. Can patients 'own' their part of the hospital as well as the staff? This may require admitting that there is an implicit power struggle between patients and staff, and that this could be resolved in a way other than by the exploitation of one or the other. Hospital staff sometimes feel that they are having to undo the mistakes of other agencies. They may want to be sure that, in the implementing of rules that are consistent with a hospital culture, they are not repeating the mistakes of others.

WHO DOES WHAT? OPENING UP THE SOCIAL SPACE

Patients are not, and should not be, inmates of total institutions, where all aspects of their lives are determined by a very limited set of relationships. The greater the variety of the interactions that they are party to the less the danger that their lives are taken over. If their 'social space' is opened up then they will have more chance of living in an environment where they can retain some personal authority in their lives.

Social space allows individuals to develop relationships of some importance to the individual in the context of their life-style. Self-image is thus important in determining what social space has to be made available to the individual. It is not easily achieved, and safeguards protecting that space are easily eroded even after a short stay in hospital.

It is assumed, at least publicly, that the differing caring disciplines make a team which can produce impressive results. Although the disciplines are different, their functions can overlap. The doctor has his job to do and some of it may not be very different from what the social worker does. The nurse gives physical care but may offer some occupational therapy. It would be sad if these overlaps stimulated professional envy. However, the differences also allow those who work with the patient to take sides, focusing on different facets of the socio-medical aetiology of the patient's problems. Thus, the social-work role in hospital is sometimes seen as abrasive, questioning the establishment view in hot-headed advocacy of patient's rights, or as manipulative, speaking for that same establishment in getting patients to adjust to their circumstances. The advantages of, say, group work in helping patients to remain involved in their own lives has been an important contribution from social work in fact (Brearley, 1975). In the end it does not matter to the patient whether this is done by nurses, social workers, psychologists or whoever, as long as it is done well.

There is an inevitable waning of contacts with the outside world. Patients will have left behind a network of people who were significant to them. Some are more obvious and vigorous than others. Patients who have been members of an active church, for example, are less likely to be 'forgotten' when they go into hospital. However, some of those relationships are not going to survive the transition into hospital, so that hospital managers have a task in encouraging or recreating these networks with the outside world and overcoming the indifference of a community (Dartington, 1979).

What about the patients' families? Some are indifferent. Others love their own – for them it takes a mature attitude not to feel some sense of failure that the patient needs the care of the hospital or the residential home. It is a bewildering experience to seem to be a rejecting family. Where there is an old person who is part of the family, apparently integral to it, but making a mess in the house, preventing other members of the family from going away on holiday, causing unrest and rebelliousness in the children, it is easy to see how such a person could become a focus for problems, not all of their own making. Members of the family feel that they are denied the opportunity of coming to terms with their own problems, and hence see their problem only in terms of their relationship with the old person. Stresses can become unbearable over the years. Those who do not bother are not faced with the dilemma of those who have given every effort to maintain their old people as they think right, only to find that their care cannot prevent such deterioration that now means they can cope no longer. The caring itself has led to this most difficult rejection. What makes it seem even more difficult is that the decision feels like rejection on both sides, although made from the best motives, and apparently in the best interests of the old people.

Hospital departments may also reject patients. In all good faith an elderly patient and a psychiatric hospital may pass a disturbed and incontinent patient between their two institutions: all that they both agree is that the patient fits the criteria of the responsibility of the other. Similarly, the elderly patient hospital and the local authority may find themselves arguing about residential homes for those elderly for whom there is no obvious place, and who fit no ready-made criteria, so have to take up that most scarce of resources – a long-stay place in an institution (Dartington, 1980).

Long-stay staff often say that they are the 'end of the line'. It is part of their motivation that they can cope where families (and other agencies) have failed. It would be a different way of thinking for them to see themselves in collaboration with families to do their joint best for the elderly patient. This would not always work, but it would be a real move towards being 'like home' if patients were still able to exercise their personal authority towards their families, and family members understood this. The acceptance of families as an active influence in the lives of patients would also allow the staff to be themselves, and to care within the limits of their role.

Volunteers are potential agents for change: they can free patients and staff to be themselves. A paradoxical asset of volunteers is that they do not need any special skills. They are not a resource that should be used in a certain way or it will be wasted. In fact an opportunity has probably been missed if volunteers are made to fit into a ward regime as extra staff working under the nursing management. However, if they are doing what the patient wants, volunteers are doing well. In this sense they are like family, but with the important difference that they do not share a family history with the patient. Consequently, they should not suffer the idiosyncratic feelings of guilt and rejection that sometimes inhibit family involvement in the care of their old people. Sometimes volunteers are enough like family that they can do some of the personal care of patients. Indeed, where some long-stay wards are understaffed volunteers may be made welcome as surrogate staff, though they did not volunteer to sort out laundry for example.

In both their material and spiritual life, patients may have their own preoccupations. It is difficult to hear what they really want if what they are suggesting directly or indirectly seems strange or disturbing to others. When people refer to religion and patients, very often they are talking about death and dying, and the chaplain may find that he is assumed to be the expert on death. What patients really want is going to be different in every case. Some want to sort out their affairs, some fear pain more than death. For some religious faith is strengthened or weakened as they approach the end of their lives. Some take a matter-of-fact attitude that is shocking to those who are trying to protect their sensibilities. The example of the hospice movement in allowing people to accept their own death must have implications for all kinds of care. Certainly the patient who is suddenly not there, and not talked about, offers a very depressing, even cruel, vision of what others can expect when they die.

How patients manage their money is also a test, not only of their ability to think for themselves, but of the ability of others to let them think, especially when what they want to do seems irrelevant, wasteful, unrealistic or embarrassingly generous to others. So patients often do not manage their money at all. They may have lost the ability to do so, and their pensions add up to a fund for a non-existent future. The counselling or social work that would reverse this process is time-consuming, difficult, and is seldom undertaken.

Ordinary relationships between people sustain their idea of themselves as normal. The segregation of the sexes is sometimes seen to be in the patients' own interests, on the grounds that they do not want to be bothered, or out of respect for their privacy. These seeming advantages, however, just serve to confirm to the patient their dependent position. The mixing of the sexes is not only natural, but can prevent decline in standards of ordinary human behaviour.

The question of privacy is not solved by segregation. Privacy means that the individual can be private, not just that the ward is closed to visitors, or is single-sexed. The physical environment can make privacy almost impossible. Visitors should never have the experience of passing doorless or curtainless toilet cubicles. Patients should never be toileted in full view of the staff. Those living in modern continuous-care units should come to expect en suite toilets to each bedroom area.

It should not be too much to expect that modern continuing-care units have a kitchen which patients can use or have staff to follow their instructions. The freedom to make one's own cup of tea, or to offer a cup of tea to a visitor or a friend – one of the last freedoms held on to by a dependent old person at home – is likely to be lost instantly in the transition to being a patient. There should also be some choice in the food, and there should be some flexibility in the arrangements for eating and taking refreshments.

Direct-care staff are not the only ones who have to understand what life is like for elderly patients in hospital. The staff may have to educate those in charge of 'hotel services', about how elderly patients can be actively involved in determining their lifestyles. The management task would be to decide what outcome is wanted and then to provide the necessary conditions to bring it about (Miller, 1978). One could imagine a gardener sitting down with a patients' committee to discuss spring planting. This could be viewed as an impossible interference in the gardener's work, or a valuable contribution to job satisfaction.

Those responsible for hospital units for elderly patients may say that they are already doing some of these things, or that others are far-fetched. They will be able to think of some patients for whom such ideas would be inappropriate, or others, who despite their disability or mental confusion, would benefit if some of these far-fetched ideas could be put into practice. It should be possible to act on some of the ideas, and not rely entirely on the new NHS nursing homes to adopt some of these 'advanced' policies.

QUALITY OF LIFE IN A CONTINUING-CARE WARD

The ideas expressed in this chapter assume a wish to maintain and improve the quality of life for people who have to *live* in hospital and are not making a temporary stay as patients. 'Quality of life' is a more complex and elusive aim than 'standards of care'. Staff may want to integrate the two, so that they may feel they are maintaining the quality of life of patients by emphasizing standards of care, such as cleanliness, bed-making and so on. It would be helpful to devise objective measures of quality of life, but the essential factor has to be subjective – how patients feel about the environment in which they live. The criteria used in making that judgement on their behalf – how much privacy they have, or personal possessions, or choice of activity – are also subjective. Quality of care will depend on the degree of fit between patient's expectations and needs, and what they actually receive (Challis and Bartlett, 1987).

The disengagement theory of ageing (Cumming and Henry, 1961) has some advantages if it stops well-meaning activists putting elderly patients through an assault course of social and physical activities in the course of an ordinary day; some old people, like anyone else, sometimes want to be left alone. On the other hand the activity theory (Maddox, 1963) also has some advantages if it stops us thinking that only people in a day room doing nothing but staring into space are necessarily content.

Why not ask the old people themselves? This is certainly worth doing, although there are difficulties about such an obvious tactic. Form-filling and questionnaires run the risk of being counter-productive, adding to such feelings of persecution that patients already have and encouraging them to give the answer they think is required. Even informal inquiries may get a bland response that obscures more than it reveals.

It is always possible that staff would prefer not to hear some of the depressing thoughts of their patients. They are trying to do their best in circumstances far short of ideal, and instinctively they want their efforts to be appreciated. If patients were to be openly critical they would be thought of as ungrateful. There are many patients who understand this and would not like to make a fuss, however bitterly they may report their feelings to others, or to family or friends.

A useful survey (Raphael and Mandeville, 1979) took account of both patients and staff. Some conflict of interests between them is to be expected. Patients, for example, prefer small rooms, and staff have a liking for larger ones. Doctors dislike cot sides more than either patients or nurses. Patients have very different needs for social contact with each other. Staff are more critical, it seems, of the physical environment than patients, who put down inadequacies in their life to shortage of staff.

If it is not possible to depend on patients to state clearly what is in their best interests then the staff should develop a clear idea on their behalf of what they are trying to achieve. Talking about quality of life only keeps the discussion in very general terms because it is not easy to be specific about what we mean. Staff need to agree amongst themselves a norm by which their practice might be assessed.

MAKING CHANGES

At the present time many health and social policies are aimed at privatizing continuing care. It is argued that these will improve standards of care for those in long-stay accommodation, reduce the financial burden on the NHS allowing the elderly patient services to concentrate their expertise on acute and rehabilitation patients (Lewis and Wattis, 1988). It is implied that privatizing means de-institutionalization and better care/efficiency (Knapp, 1988) especially since the public sector applies standards to the private sector which it would not often care to apply to itself. It can therefore be argued that care is better in the private sector. That this is a simplistic view is clear from American experiences where there have been scandals in private nursing homes, half of whom provided their care in life-threatening situations in at least one aspect (Davies, 1986). Many of these problems arose because the responsibility for financing the parameters of care and proving quality, while preventing and punishing fraud and abuse, were fragmented between agencies at all levels. British experience with private nursing homes is also not without its problems (Challis and Bartlett, 1987). However, change can take place in the public sector – although it is perceived as persecutory if imposed from above. It is less threatening if carried out by the staff themselves out of their knowledge of what is possible. They may have to research the workload and re-order their priorities in order to create more social space for patients staying in hospital. This is the bottom-up approach to change.

The implementation of new practices, especially to the extent that improving patient care required changes in professional roles and attitudes, commonly provokes considerable resistance among staff. This is because of the disruption of established ways of working and social relationships entailed, the guilt that may derive from the unfavourable reflection of past activities which innovation often implies, and the challenge which change constitutes to existing systems of defence against anxiety embodied in traditional practices. These difficulties are particularly likely to arise in efforts to improve the care of elderly patients. It follows that groups of staff engaged in innovation often require considerable support from management if they are to overcome these resistances to change, and successfully work through the emotional issues involved, particularly if this is to be achieved without the innovating group being psychologically 'split off' from other groups of staff in their hospital (Towell and Dartington, 1978). It also follows that it is not helping patients to be independent to let them give up their say in matters concerning them. When a patient says 'Whatever you think, dear', whether it is about what to wear, what to eat, or what to do, he or she is trying to be helpful. Primarily the staff are there to help the patient, not to think for them. This is a difficult concept to put into practice.

MOTIVATING STAFF TO CHANGE

Working practices to allow patients independence can be achieved by group discussions with a facilitator to lead the debate while containing feelings which may be aroused. Issues which may need to be discussed include: the importance of negative feelings towards family or community and justifying one's own way of working in the hospital; the satisfaction of keeping people alive while avoiding the question 'What are they living for?'; the dependence that staff have on patients gives meaning to their work; the wish to counter the depression and futility of the world outside, as one sees it, by displaying optimism and hope in the hospital setting. This may seem unnecessarily psychological to those trained in physical medicine, but some questioning of this kind would be supportive to those who want to look at existing practices and wonder how they might have done differently. Anyone who has worked in the health service will know that change can take place. What is needed is to ensure that change is for the better.

REFERENCES

Abrahams, R. and Lamb, S. (1988) Developing reliable assessment in case-managed geriatric long-term care programs. *Quarterly Review Bulletin* **14**, 179–86.

Brearley, C.P. (1975) *Social Work, Ageing and Society*, Routledge and Kegan Paul, London.

Cairns, J. (1979) Treating long-term patients as individuals. *Nursing Times*, **75**, 1058–9.

Challis, L. and Bartlett, H. (1987) *Old and Ill*, Age Concern, Mitcham, London.

Chapman,P. (1979) *Unmet Needs and the Delivery of Care. A Study of the Utilisation of Social Services by Old People*, Bedford Square Press, London.

Cummings, E. and Henry, W.(1961) *Growing Old: the Process of Disengagement*, Basic
    Books, New York.
Dartington, T. (1979) Fragmentation and integration in health care: the referral process
    and social brokerage. *Sociol. Health and Illness*, **1**, 12–39.
Dartington, T.(1980) *Family Care of Old People*, Souvenir Press, London.
Dartington, T., Jones, P. and Miller, E.J. (1974) Geriatric Hospital Care. Tavistock
    Institute of Human Relations (unpublished).
Davies, B. (1986) American lessons for British policy and research on long-term care
    of the elderly. *Quart. J. Soc. Affairs*, **2**, 321–55.
Elliott, J.R. (1982) *Living in Hospital*, 2nd edn, King Edward's Hospital Fund, London.
English, J. and Morse, J.M. (1988) The 'difficult' elderly patient, adjustment or malad-
    justment. *Intern. J. Nursing Studies*, **25**, 23–39.
Health Advisory Service.(1987) Annual Report. From NHS Health Advisory Service,
    Sutherland House, 29–37 Brighton Road, Sutton, Surrey, England.
Knapp, M. (1988) Searching for efficiency in long-term care: de-institutionalisation
    and privatisation. *Br. J. Soc. Work*, **18**, 149–71.
Lewis, R. and Wattis, J. (1988) Continuing care of old people: a medical viewpoint.
    Ageing Society, **8**, 189–209.
Maddox, G.L.A. (1963) A longitudinal study of selected elderly subjects. Activity
    and morale. *Social Forces*, **42**, 195–204.
Martin, J.P. (1984) *Trouble in Hospital*, Blackwell, Oxford.
May, W.F. (1982) Who cares for the elderly? *Hastings Centre*, **12**, 31–7.
McCarthy, M. and Millard, P. (eds) (1979) *Management of Chronic Illness*, King
    Edward's Hospital Fund, London.
Miller, E.J. (1978) Autonomy, dependency and organisational change, in *Innovation
    in Patient Care: an Action Research Study of Change in a Psychiatric Hospital* (eds
    D. Towell and C.J. Harries), Croom Helm, London.
Norman, A.J. (1980) *Rights and Risks*, National Corporation for the Care of Old People,
    London.
Raphael, W. and Mandeville,J.(1979) *Old People in Hospital*, King Edward's Hospital
    Fund, London.
Robb, B. (1967) *Sans Everything*, Nelson, London.
Towell, D. and Dartington, T. (1978) Encouraging innovations in hospital care. *J.
    Adv. Nursing*, **1**, 5–23.
Townsend, P. (1981) The structured dependency of the elderly. *Ageing Society*, **1**, 5–25.
Wickings, I. and Crown, J. (1989) Proof of the pudding. *Health Serv. J.*, **99**, 1070–1.

APPENDIX

Coming into hospital. Check list from *Living in Hospital* (Elliot, 1982) reproduced by
    kind permission of the publisher. King Edward's Hospital Fund for London.

1. How are new residents made to feel welcome?
2. Is there reasonable privacy for admission procedures?
3. Is the new resident introduced to other residents?

Daily timetable

4. May residents go to bed at a time of their choice?
5. May residents rise when they like?
6. Subject to treatment considerations, may residents wash and dress when they
    choose?

7. May residents, who are able, make drinks when they like?
8. May residents go and lie down when they fancy a nap?
9. Does each resident have his own outer clothes?
10. Does each resident have his own underclothes?
11. Do residents choose their own clothes freely, from a good range?
12. Does each resident have his own wardrobe?
13. May residents, if able, launder their own clothes?
14. Is there an adequate laundry and dry cleaning service for resident's clothes?

Hairdressing

15. Are residents encouraged to go to an outside hairdresser?
16. Does the visiting hairdresser attend to difficult or antisocial residents?

Personal spending money

17. What steps are taken to make sure that all residents benefit to the full from the allowances to which they are entitled?

Food and dining arrangements

18. Is the menu for residents variable and unpredictable?
19. Do residents have a genuine opportunity to choose from a menu?
20. May residents indicate how much food they want?
21. Are residents permitted to provide food to suit their own taste?
22. Is there a dining room, or recognized dining area, in the ward?
23. Are the table settings homelike?
24. May residents help themselves?
25. Do staff ever sit down with residents for a meal?
26. Are residents ever permitted to organize for themselves a festive meal to mark some special occasion?

Noise

27. Are residents with transistor radios asked to use an earpiece?
28. Is the volume of the ward radio or television kept down to a level acceptable to the residents?
29. Are staff mindful, when they are talking in the ward, that they are in a place which is, in effect, the residents' only home?

Washing, bathing and toileting

30. May residents decide for themselves when and whether to wash?
31. Are relatives encouraged to help with washing and toileting?
32. Are residents afforded due privacy for bodily functions, even when the ward is closed to visitors?

A place of one's own

If a resident has a single room:

33. Are there any limitations on when he is allowed to use it?
34. May he bring in any furniture or furnishings of his own?
35. Is a reasonable domestic untidiness and clutter permissible?
If a resident is in an open ward:
36. Is the ward arranged in such a way that each resident has a small piece of territory which is his to control, as though it were a single room?
37. Do staff respect the human need of all residents for a place of their own?

Worthwhile

38. Are residents, who are able, given the opportunity to undertake work of any kind?
If so:
39. Does the work help the resident community?
40. Are residents encouraged to offer their old skills, or to learn new ones?
41. Is there a fair system of payment for work done?

Recreation: holidays and outings

42. Is there somebody responsible for a full programme of widely varied recreational activities?
43. Is encouragement given to those who wish to pursue minority interests?
44. Are residents enabled and encouraged to take part in planning the recreational programme?
45. Does the programme include special items for those confined to bed?
46. Is use made of volunteers in developing the recreational programme?

Further education

47. Has the hospital exploited fully the basic right of *all* its residents to the whole range of further education services?
48. Do tutors from the local polytechnic/college of art/adult education department come to the hospital?
49. Have residents easy access to the public library service?
50. Is it possible for a resident to obtain regularly the newspapers or journals of his choice?
Is there a real encouragement to residents to retain or develop an interest in:
51. Art?
52. Music?
53. Literature?
54. Hobbies?
55. Current affairs?
56. Are younger adult residents encouraged to pursue formal studies, and are they given adequate facilities and privacy for this?

Gardens, flowers and animals

57. Have residents easy access to, and is appropriate seating provided for, a garden, lawn, terrace, or similar area?
58. Are well-behaved pets allowed to visit residents?
59. Are residents encouraged to grow their own plants, or to tend the ward plants?

60. Do residents have any opportunity to care for birds or pet animals?
61. Do residents ever have the chance to look at wild life, to walk in woodlands and meadows, to sit by the river?
62. Are residents who wish and are able, encouraged to go out to the local church?
63. If residents cannot go out, is there an attempt to bring church members to them?
64. What arrangements are made to cater for different denominations and religions?

Choosing your neighbour

65. Is care taken to try to ensure that, wherever choice is possible, each resident has ward neighbours who are congenial to him?
66. If husband and wife are both in hospital, is it possible for them to share accommodation if they wish?

Mixing the age groups

67. Are older residents, when they wish it, given the opportunity of the company of young people?
68. Does someone see that those without family or friends receive occasional visitors?
69. Are younger residents allowed plenty of social interchange with visitors of their own age group, even though their boisterousness may disturb the calm of the ward?
70. Is there a real opportunity for the residents of one ward to mingle with residents of different age groups, or different medical conditions, or of the opposite sex, from other parts of the hospital?
71. Do inpatients and day patients mix freely?
72. Does the hospital afford the opportunity for men and women to meet together in their daily lives – for example, at meals, in the day room or workshop?
73. Are there any areas of the hospital where integrated living accommodation is available?
74. Has the hospital authority given clear guidance to hospital staff about the degree to which sexual relationships between long-stay residents are permissible?
75. Is there an opportunity for men and women residents to meet in privacy, and without subterfuge?

Persistence of imagined rules

76. Are the staff or residents working to any hospital rules which no longer need apply?
77. Are residents conditioned or inhibited by rules which do not officially exist at all?
78. In what ways are the rules of the hospital aimed at developing each resident to his full potential?

Links with former life

79. Are residents, including the disabled or bed-bound, easily able to keep in touch with home by telephone?
80. What planned efforts are made to help residents keep in contact with the world they used to live in?
81. How frequently are arrangements made for trips home?

Relationships with other residents

82. Are residents encouraged to help other residents, in however small a way?
83. Are residents encouraged to help in small domestic chores, such as dusting, washing-up, or making tea?
84. Are residents, particularly the mentally ill or mentally handicapped, given the chance to do voluntary jobs in the outside community?
85. Is there a residents' committee?
86. Are residents encouraged to organize social events amongst themselves?

Relationships with staff and family; counselling

87. In what ways are attempts made to reduce social distance between professional staff and residents?
88. Are family relationships developed by staff as a possible therapeutic strength?
89. Are members of the family encouraged to take a hand in caring for their own resident member?

Problems which require medical and nursing intervention

90. When specialist medical or nursing procedures become necessary, are these explained in advance to the resident, in understandable terms?
91. When the resident becomes more frail, or incontinent, is he helped to discuss with understanding staff his anxiety, insecurity, and feeling of demoralization?
92. Even when a resident is quite helpless, do staff still respect his dignity and his personality and avoid treating him as a baby?

Staff morale

93. Does the health authority, through its members, officers and ways of working, consistently demonstrate a concern with maintaining the morale of staff in their difficult task?
94. Are study days, inter-hospital visits and other forms of relevant in-service training arranged regularly?
95. Is there genuine machinery through which staff of all grades and professions can express their collective views?
96. In what ways does the health authority listen to the views of staff and respond to them?
97. Are junior staff encouraged to discuss their problems frankly with seniors?

Influence of the management system

98. How far does the management system make provision for participation in decision making by staff at all levels?
99. What methods are used to help staff work together in a truly multidisciplinary way?
100. What steps are taken to ensure that managers put the interests of residents first when making decisions?

Chapter 6

Nursing care

INTRODUCTION

A picture painted by Hubert von Herkomer, RA, in 1878 shows a group of old ladies in what appears to be the large hall of an institution. It is entitled 'Eventide' (Figure 6.1) and illustrates succinctly the attitudes of society to elderly people at that time. Although there are charming, though toothless, smiles on some of the faces, the general impression is one of hope abandoned and apathetic acceptance of what the bleak, comfortless room offers.

There has, in recent years, been much progress in caring for elderly people requiring long-term care. Many innovative and interesting experiments have taken place such as the experimental units at Portsmouth, Fleetwood and Sheffield (HMSO White Paper Cmnd 8173, 1981). One of the units evaluated in this document is Jubilee House, Portsmouth (Chapter 19). NHS nursing homes with private room and personal space have been developed which greatly increase the possibility of improved care and more dignified living conditions for elderly people. However, with increasing financial constraints and the growing elderly population, it is more important than ever that the care is appropriate, of a high standard and is value for money. The elderly are the biggest single care group and they are the main users of all services (Garrett, 1983). It is therefore important that their needs are taken into account when planning all services. Skilled nursing and recognition of elderly people's needs will enable as many elderly people as possible to return to their homes for as long as possible. Developing complications delay transfer home; the longer old people are dependent the more difficult is the transition home as well as the danger of social support networks at home collapsing. These factors were highlighted by Sir Roy Griffiths in 'Community Care: Agenda for Action'.

MANAGEMENT OF CHANGE

Managers and staff working within continuing care units will frequently

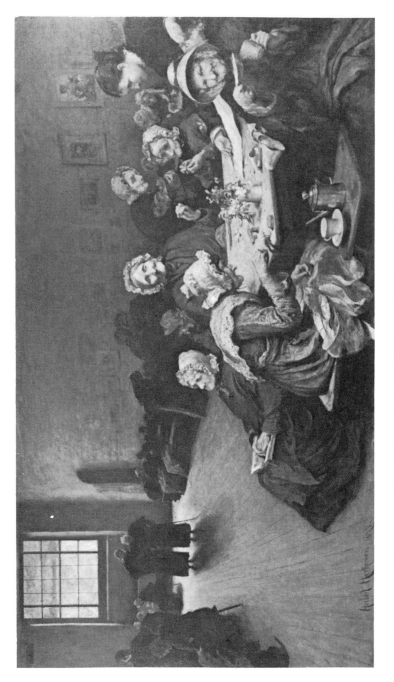

Figure 6.1 'Eventide', a painting by Hubert von Herkomer showing the care of the elderly in the late 19th century.

come across practices and attitudes that they wish to change. Changing attitudes is a very difficult process but it helps to know the reasons why staff resist change in order to prepare strategies to overcome this resistance and change behaviour. Managers have a responsibility to create a working environment that is conducive to change and questioning practices. Staff working in continuing-care units need a work culture that encourages, questions, initiatives and a reflective evaluation of work and practice. This needs supportive and helpful managers who are committed to the elderly. There need to be good channels of communication that give staff opportunities to meet and share experiences. Change is becoming increasingly a way of life in the National Health Service. When handled badly there are always adverse effects on the service. Organizational change causes major upheavals to individuals: this may cause stress which, if not handled well, will cause disillusionment and alienation. This in turn will generate conflict to which most of the energy will be given. Patients no longer become the primary focus for staff, and standards will invariably suffer. It must be recognized by managers that change is traumatic as the individual is always striving towards a balanced state. Nobody likes imbalance, and this produces stress and tension (cognitive dissonance). People will handle change better if they feel in control and are participating fully rather than being driven by change over which they have little control.

Any attempts to change attitudes or practice will provoke anxiety. It is helpful to be able to recognize the factors that may be barriers to change. Stating the desire to change implies criticism of present practice. There may well be fear of the unknown and a lack of confidence, knowledge and skills to carry out the change. Initially, change causes workloads to increase and mistakes often happen. There may also be too much emphasis on the benefits and not enough recognition of the problems and difficulties. Managers need to support their staff and plan the change well.

Managers must secure staff commitment for change in order to be successful. Rogers (1972) states that for nurses to be effective as change agents 'the target group must be aware of the innovation; and it must be persuaded of its value; it adopts the innovation; and it continues to use the innovation after its initial adoption'.

THE ENVIRONMENT FOR CONTINUING CARE

Elderly people who require continuing care were most often placed in long-stay wards that were no longer considered modern enough for acute services. Thankfully, this practice is gradually being overtaken by developments, although for some of us not nearly quickly enough. Some consideration and thought to the environment will not only give the elderly more dignity but will halt the negative image of long-term care that nurses often have. It is an area where nurses can be very fulfilled

and achieve a real understanding of what individualized care can mean
(Appendices 1 and 2).

It is important that the environment is acceptable to patients and relatives; their opinions need to be sought. If a ward is to be used it is helpful
for colour to be used to convey function and identify the different areas
so that they can be easily recognized. Elderly people should be able to
see out of the window, whether they are in bed or a chair. Many who
have faulty vision will require brighter reading lamps than others.

Elderly people often feel cold; their temperature should be monitored
with thermometers, and heating must be available on a cold summer's
day. Radiators and hot-water taps should be protected; every bath and
shower needs a locally adjustable mixing valve to provide a blended water
temperature not exceeding 43°C.

The ward or nursing home requires items that stimulate interest and
provide a homely look, such as large clocks, fish tanks, etc. Pets too can
give a lot of pleasure if properly cared for.

ADEQUATE BED-SPACE

All patients need their own personal space. The minimum critical dimension in each bed area within the multi-bed area is 2500 mm x 2900 mm
for each patient. They need space for their own commodes and aids,
and should always have immediate and constant access to their belongings. This is only the minimum space and should never fall below
this requirement. Extra beds with no lights or other services or their
own curtain tracking should never be erected. Not only is this very un-
satisfactory from the patient's point of view but it can also become a
hazard if this bed blocks fire escapes and exit routes.

TOILETS AND PRIVACY

It is essential that dignity is respected at all times. Patients' toilets require
space, and doors should be kept closed during use. Patients in bed must
always be screened completely when using a bedpan, made comfortable
and not left for a long time. They should always be offered a bowl to
wash their hands and made comfortable afterwards. Some patients in
a ward may find using a commode more convenient, but they must be
able to use it with the curtains drawn around. It is a very poor unit indeed
that allows patients to be exposed during toileting or bathing. This
indicates a lack of respect for the individual, and any vigilant nurse will
be careful that good practice and standards are maintained at all times.

Ideally each patient should have his or her own toilet with aids to match
the individual's disability. If shared, the minimum number of toilets should
be one for each three patients. No patients should have to walk more

than 12 m, and a commode should be available at the bedside for night-time use. Consideration over toilet arrangements will do much to lessen incontinence and constipation which gives added discomfort and distress.

BEDS, FURNITURE AND EQUIPMENT

High low beds will be required for all elderly patients. Mattresses will need to be replaced every four years, and all individual wheelchair foam cushions every 1–2 years, depending on make. All aids for mobility, such as frames, wheelchairs and commodes for the night, will need to be kept around the patient's own personal space. Patients should be allowed freedom of movement and be able to return to bed whenever they wish.

There should be a wide variety of chairs of a domestic appearance. All patients are not the same size, so there will need to be a variety of chairs to fit height. Styles should also show a range, such as: some high-backed and winged, some with padded arms and filled-in sides. There may well be instances where patients may require a chair to their own specification. There are no circumstances however where elderly people need to be placed in tilted restraining chairs.

Noise can be a big problem for elderly people. Ideally, patients should have control over their own television and wireless which should never be left on continuously for the benefit of the staff. There needs to be a quiet room or corner provided for those who wish to be quiet or to talk quietly to relatives. Much can be done to eliminate unnecessary noise by maintenance of doors and trolleys. The attitude of staff is important; they need to be sensitive and to be able to observe the times when patients require peace and quiet.

Wards or nursing homes will require their own hoist to lift heavy patients, but all the nurses will require training in the use of the hoist in order to maximize its effectiveness.

PERSONAL SERVICES FOR THE ELDERLY PATIENT

There needs to be, within every unit, a planned programme of relevant social activities for all wards and nursing homes. Every patient needs the opportunity to pursue interests, such as painting, music and craftwork. Adult education teachers may well be required to supervise and encourage this work. Live entertainment, outings and special-occasion parties are all important as these and other events will be required to overcome boredom and to act as a substitute for activities that may no longer be possible. Newspapers and periodicals need to be delivered daily, including mother-tongue publications for those patients from ethnic minorities who request them. Patients will need to have control of their own money in order to pay for any additional items and services they require.

Full personalized clothing, including underclothes, are necessary for every unit, which should have a small laundry attached in order that clothes are well cared for and returned to the owners promptly and in good condition. Patients or relatives can be asked to bring a selection of clothes in order that patients may have a choice. A visiting hairdresser and a barber are necessary additions. Patients residing in nursing homes may be able to visit local facilities if wheelchair access is possible.

THE ORGANIZATION OF NURSING CARE

Following the acceptance by the Government of the Griffiths Report on Community Care (Community Care: Agenda for Action) the responsibility for purchasing continuing care will become the responsibility of the local authority. Continuing care may be purchased for elderly people in a wide variety of settings, depending on what is locally available in the health authority, voluntary sector and the private sector. A high degree of medical intervention is not required for long-stay units, and with the expansion and changing of provision for this group there is every opportunity for nurse-led units to flourish.

The difficulty in producing a more domestic and home-like environment in a hospital block has led to the development of smaller units away from the major hospital complex. This has often resulted in the sister in charge becoming the manager and holding the budget for the entire facility, not just the nursing expenditure. As the sister's role changes this also leads to the examination of the way nursing care is delivered. The need for the elderly patient to have more autonomy, and with more non-directive forms of nursing care, the introduction of primary nursing into the unit comes to the fore. Primary nursing was first introduced in America by Marie Manthy. There are five basic concepts to the primary nursing system (Castledine, 1985):

1. The assessment of the patient by the primary nurse who carries out the care when on duty.
2. The associate nurses carry out the care planned by the primary nurse when she is not on duty. The primary nurse has a 24-hour responsibility for the patient through the written directions on the care plan.
3. Patient involvement, wherever possible, is important for providing and achieving goals.
4. There should be an improvement in communication between the nurse and other members of the health care team.
5. Because of the greater involvement there should be better discharge planning, patient teaching and family involvement.

There is more involved in the implementation of primary nursing than simply moving from team to primary nursing. The concept of a therapeutic nursing care involving a partnership and dialogue with the patient would appear to be an ideal organization for elderly patients requiring continuing care. This new partnership of care would lead to more patient choice and be manifested in practices such as the sister and nurses on the unit not wearing uniforms.

One important aspect of primary nursing is what Manthy called 'visibility'. The one essential requisite is that the patient should know who the nurse is. Helpful methods to establish this are boards giving photographs and names of nurses, information leaflets and a photograph of the primary nurse and patient together (Wright and Wills, 1988).

Registered nurses will need to be supported by health-care assistants. This enables skilled nurses, who are a scarce resource, more time to be involved in nursing care. These health care assistants will, in the future, undertake recognized basic training modules and will receive further training within their unit of work, but the registered nurse remains, at all times, accountable for the delivery of nursing care to the patients (UKCC, 1989).

The care plan

Assessment of the elderly patient requires a nursing history. It is very important that nurses explain the reason for the interview so that the patient is aware that the information will be required for the formation of the care plan. The elderly are not used to being interviewed and some may become very anxious, but once a good rapport has been established, information can be gained informally during general nursing interventions and conversations over a period of time.

The planning of care should be a joint exercise between the nurse, patient and, if appropriate, his family. Involving the patient signifies respect for his right as an individual to have a say in his own health care. Problems identified need to be placed in priority order and goals identified. These goals must be realistic with regard to the patient's individual capabilities. Ongoing evaluation of care is necessary.

A monthly disciplinary review is a useful practice whereby different professionals can review the patient together in order to solve problems and to aid the patient to maximize his potential for enjoyment of life.

Skill mix

The impending demographic changes in population make it imperative that we consider how nurses are deployed. It is wasteful to employ highly skilled people for work in which their skills are unused. The deployment of staff must be cost-effective and matched with service quality. Manpower levels for long-stay units need to be planned and related to number of patients, dependency of the patients, standard of service to be achieved, annual leave, sickness and absenteeism, time for education and training, time spent in meetings, time spent on quality assurance activities, level of support staff available, and delegated general management responsibilities. The number of nurses will depend on how the unit is to be organized and whether the unit is considered a facility with its own budget. A senior nurse carrying general management responsibilities and 24-hour continuous responsibility can become the manager. This manager would need to be supported by an F-grade sister who leads the clinical team. If the ward is being organized around primary nursing there would need to be one primary nurse with the necessary experience and skills for eight patients (Pearson, 1988).

ILLNESS IN THE ELDERLY

Elderly patients frequently show signs of more than one disorder with atypical presentation that requires careful investigation of the underlying symptoms. The three major reasons for admission to a long-stay unit are: intellectual failure, instability, and immobility and incontinence. Many elderly patients have a mixture of all three which makes their support at home difficult and increases their dependency on others.

There are many causes of confusion, some of which are hard to explain. The onset of an acute confused state may be abrupt and it may be very difficult for relatives to understand what is happening. Confusion may also distress other patients and staff who are not used to dealing with it. Any physical or emotional stress can trigger off the problem. Some common causes are: inadequate cerebral oxygenation, congestive cardiac failure, cardiac dysrhythmias, fluid and electrolyte imbalance due to diarrhoea and vomiting and faecal impaction, trauma such as head injury or fractured neck of femur, any infection, or a change of environment. Careful investigation of the cause, and nursing interventions aimed at minimizing the confusion, such as one nurse to care for the patient during the span as well as careful explanation of any procedures, will do much to reduce the effect of the confusion.

Dementia, in which there is progressive impairment, is often a problem and will affect not only the personality but the individual's ability to care for himself or herself.

INCONTINENCE

Urinary incontinence should not be considered the inevitable consequence of aging. Catheterization should be the last resort rather than the first. Incontinence needs investigation and diagnostic facilities. Temporary incontinence may occur in response to a urinary tract infection, acute illness, immobilization, confusion, sedation, impacted faeces and a new and stressful environment. Correct diagnosis and management may well make all the difference to the elderly person. When considering catheterization the risk versus the benefit should be carefully evaluated. Elderly people often have a low fluid intake as they often become less thirsty with age. If they are suffering from urinary problems they may wish to restrict fluids further so aggravating the problem. An increased fluid intake should therefore be encouraged. A note needs to be kept of intake and urinary output and the times when patients are incontinent in order to plan action. Access to toilets, a commode at the bedside at night, consideration of the height of the toilet and presence of safety rails as well as privacy, all need to be assessed.

Support to patients who have difficulty in maintaining continence needs to be given by a continence advisor who will discuss with the patient and the patient's nurse the most appropriate management policy and the aids that are required and acceptable to the patient. A record needs to be kept on the patient's record of progress and satisfaction with care, support and aids offered.

MOBILITY AND IMMOBILITY

Elderly patients often suffer from defective balance and are unable to right themselves. This leads to falls, and fear of falls – which in turn often causes immobility. Many elderly patients admitted to a long-stay unit are immobile. However, with the provision of a safe environment and an appropriate mobility aid, such as a Zimmer frame, walking stick

Table 6.1 The pressure sore Risks Assessment-Scoring System

General condition	Mental state	Activity	Mobility	Incontinence
4. Good	4. Alert	4. Ambulant	4. Full	4. Not incontinent
3. Fair	3. Apathetic	3. Walks with help	3. Slightly limited	3. Occasionally incontinent
2. Poor	2. Confused	2. Chairbound	2. Very limited	2. Usually/urine
1. Very bad	1. Stuperous	1. Bedfast	1. Immobile	1. Doubly incontinent

A score of 14 or below means that the patient is at risk and requires an individual prevention programme. Patients who suffer from neurological diseases, such as Parkinson's disease and multiple sclerosis, are particularly vulnerable, as also are patients who have sustained a fractured neck of femur. Assessing the patient on admission is necessary, but the patient should be reassessed if any new condition should arise. For instance, a urinary tract infection, chest infection or impacted faeces will increase the risk, and the pressure sore prevention programme will need to be reappraised. A wide range of support systems must be available within every unit for the elderly, and some of the most suitable aids are as follows: Large cell ripple mattress; Pegasus Airwave bed; Spenco mattress/Polycare mattress; water beds; sheepskins; small bed cradles; chair cushions. (From Norton *et al.*, 1962, with permission.)

or tripod, some may have the confidence to try and ambulate, thus reaching a level of achievement, however small.

PREVENTION OF PRESSURE SORES

Elderly patients are very much at risk in the development of pressure sores. They cause pain and can seriously impair health and well-being. Nearly all pressure sores can be prevented. Most occur during an acute illness, but some patients will always be at risk, and the nurse needs to be aware of these patients and other events that make the patient's risk increase. All patients need to be assessed on admission. There are several assessment scoring systems available, the best known being that of Norton *et al*. (1962) (Table 6.1).

CARE OF THE DYING PATIENT

Death must simply become the discreet but dignified exit of a peaceful person from a helpful society, without pain or suffering, and ultimately without fear. (Aries, 1977)

The challenge of nursing the elderly in any continuing care unit is to maximize the quality of life that there is. Inevitably, though, patients will die, and it is the recognition that a patient is dying and the sensitive and appropriate care given that will allow death to follow the aims quoted from Philippe Aries, above.

Elderly patients should have access to the many specialist services, including pain relief, that are now in operation in many districts. Health districts should have their own manual relating to administrative procedures and symptom control. This manual should be compiled with help from the community so that wishes and customs of the ethnic minority groups are recorded and adhered to. Patients may feel the need to sort out their affairs and ask advice about making a will. Any local Citizens' Advice Bureau can give information and help. Relieving distressing symptoms as they occur will require skilled nursing. There should be a nurse working on the ward who has completed the care-of-the-dying course who can act as a source of support and advice.

One of the main problems with dying patients is that of anorexia where the main aim will be to enable the patient to feel he is taking enough nourishment. Small portions of suitably prepared food should be served whenever the patient can eat, not necessarily at mealtimes. Liquidizing foods and offering Complan and build-ups may also help. The dietitian's advice should be sought in these situations.

Good oral hygiene is very important as a sore mouth is miserable. Daily inspection of the mouth with a torch should be carried out. Oral candidiosis frequently affects these patients and requires prompt attention. A dry mouth can be eased by chewing gum, pineapple chunks or lemon drops. It is best to give small frequent drinks or small pieces of ice to suck.

Lack of normal diet, immobility and pain-relieving drugs frequently induce constipation. Whenever opiates are prescribed a regular aperient, such as Dorbanex, will be required.

Nausea and vomiting are also common distressing symptoms but it is better to find out the cause first before prescribing the most appropriate anti-emetic.

The management of a cough depends upon the general state of the patient. Productive coughs require humidification, bronchodilators and physiotherapy. A non-productive cough will require an anti-tussive, such as codeine linctus, methadone or morphine.

Breathlessness can produce anxiety, fear and tension; all possible causes should be considered. Small doses of Diazepam may help to reduce anxiety. If the patient is accustomed to oxygen this can be continued but it may alarm some patients if suddenly introduced and may make them very claustrophobic.

It is very important to believe patients whenever they say they are in pain, and react accordingly. Pain can be increased by anxiety and fatigue. There may also be an accompanying depression and a feeling of isolation. Elderly patients' pain is often relieved well with small doses of Diamorphine repeated frequently rather than less-frequent larger doses. Regular injections can be replaced by a syringe driver which will administer a steady dose over twenty-four hours. A good night's sleep is important in order to cope with the next day, but above all the dying patient requires comfort and support from family and staff. No patient should automatically be placed in a side room but their wishes need to be considered. Some will enjoy the peace of their own room, others may prefer a more open spot.

Nurses need to make time to sit and listen; information may have to be given more than once. Relatives need to feel involved in order to cope with the grieving process later on. Nurses need to remember that hearing and the sense of touch often remain until the patient dies. It is a comfort if someone stays with them holding their hand. They will know that they have not been left alone. Caring for relatives must not be forgotten after the patient has died. Their own circumstances will be known by a caring nurse and they may need the services of a bereavement counsellor.

THE NEED FOR AND ENJOYMENT OF FOOD

One of the major interests of elderly patients can be the food they are offered or choose. Food is very important, not only to the maintenance of health but also to add interest to the patient's day. The food needs to be nourishing, and meet the recommended daily amounts for nutrients. A high-fibre diet with a good fluid intake – one to one-and-a-half litres per

day – will help prevent constipation and dehydration. Special consideration needs to be given to nutrients which can be deficient in the elderly,
such as vitamin C. Fresh fruit and fruit juice should be available every
day. Vegetables should not be overcooked. These measures should also
ensure a good folic acid and potassium intake. Vitamin D may need to
be given as a supplement if patients are unable to get out in the sunlight.
B vitamins are essential for mental health. In some cases other medication prescribed will increase the need for these to be supplemented.

There should always be a choice of food; not all elderly people require
a soft, bland diet. Consideration must be given to elderly patients from
the different ethnic groups within the community. Vegetarian diets may
be required. Types of food certain groups wish to avoid must be known
and replacement meals should be acceptable and be adequate in nutritional value.

The presentation of food is very important, and it should look appetizing. Food must be served at the correct temperature; for example, hot
food must be served hot. Patients should be encouraged to send food back
that has not been served at the correct temperature. Clean tablecloths and
napkins should be available at every meal. Patients in bed should have a
tray. A full range of condiments should be available as sense of taste is
often enhanced with sauces and relishes. Specially adapted cutlery, aids
and drinking utensils should always be available for all patients who
require them.

Elderly people require time to eat and enjoy meals. Meals should
be served in an unhurried manner and there should be no pressure
placed on patients to take meals at any one particular place. The
evening meal should not be served before 6 pm as this will leave an
unacceptably long gap before the next meal. Special teas, birthday
cakes and treats that can be shared by all act as welcome social occasions. Alcohol should be available as well as beer, Guinness and
sherry for those with poor appetites, and will be much appreciated
by elderly people who have regularly had a drop to drink throughout
their lives. Brandy and hot milk is often much safer and more effective
than sleeping tablets.

PATIENTS' MONEY

A clear policy must be established in every unit which outlines the responsibility of staff for the management of patients' finance. The appointed
officer can assist the patient in managing their pension and benefits and
make banking arrangements for them. Medical assessment is required
if there is any doubt about the patient's mental ability to make decisions
about money. Patients should have constant access to regular amounts
of money which they keep with them and use as they wish.

QUALITY OF CARE WITHIN A CONTINUING-CARE UNIT

The aim of caring for the elderly within continuing-care units must be to deliver services to elderly patients viewing them as people in need of holistic individual care with the end objective of optimizing welfare and maximizing well-being. Each unit needs to identify a method for regular audits linking this to the planning and financial cycles. There should be action plans with responsible individuals named to see the improvements through. Progress can be checked every six months before the annual assessment commences again (Lang, 1976).

A quality assurance programme can be conceptually viewed as a cycle of activity with five principal states (Figure 6.2):

1. Agreement of values through philosophies
2. Identification of standards and criteria
3. Measurement of standards
4. Making interpretations
5. Choosing and taking courses of action

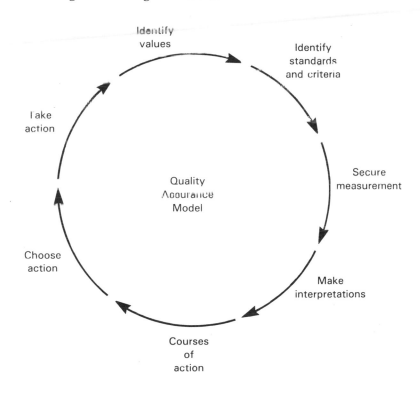

Figure 6.2 Lang's Quality Assurance Model.

STANDARD SETTING

A very important part of the quality assurance programme is the setting of standards. There are three levels of standard setting:

1. *At the national level.* These are universal and generic standards and can be said to promote a philosophy of care. They are general statements of beliefs, values, ideologies and professional codes of conduct.
2. *At the district level.* These are statements of good practice to which patient care is aiming. They provide guiding principles and can be target setting, so setting the scene and getting everyone going in the right direction.
3. *At local level.* Where the care takes place. These are dynamic standards. They need to be owned and formed by the practitioners of care at the clinical level. It is important that they are measured and are achievable. A standard must therefore be observable, achievable, measurable and desirable. A standard needs to be agreed by practitioners to be the necessary standard to achieve the goals for the patient.

Standards at clinical level

These are best defined by the Donabedian method of structure, process and outcome components.

1. *Structure.* These are the organizational standards, whatever is required to provide the standard of care specified – for example, staff, equipment, tools, materials, systems and information. Within the structure we should be looking, therefore, at some of the following points:

   Do the staff have the knowledge, skills and attitudes?
   Have we the staff with the appropriate skills available?
   Is the environment suitable?
   Does the organizational system make the standard possible?
   Is all the relevant information provided?

   The structure standards should be the responsibility of the practitioners and managers. They are important as there is little chance of the standard being achieved without achieving the structure standards first.
2. *Process Standards.* These refer to the delivery of care, the method, the assessment, the procedure, the tools and techniques used, the resources that are used, and the evaluation of the level of competence of staff carrying out the standard.
3. *Outcome.* The result of the care and what is expected and desirable. This should be described in a specific and measurable form.

Examples of the practical application of standards at a clinical level are the prevention of pressure sores and promotion of continence, details of which follow.

STANDARD STATEMENT FOR THE PREVENTION OF PRESSURE
SORES (City and Hackney Health Authority, 1987/8)

Every patient within the health authority identified as being likely to
develop pressure sores will have an individual prevention plan.

Structure criteria

1. The nurse will be able to assess the patients using the Norton Score.
   This assessment will be carried out on admission and at least weekly
   by completion of a patient-at-risk form (Appendix 3).
2. The nurse will recognize precipitating factors which will increase
   the risk.
3. The nurse will have knowledge of all support systems and those
   most suitable for individual patients.
4. General managers and nurse managers will forward plan and budget
   for equipment needs.
5. The nurse will have 24-hour access to all essential equipment.
6. The nurse managers will provide workshop facilities for cleaning
   and maintenance of equipment.
7. The nurse managers will organize the mattress replacement programme and record yearly.
8. All staff caring for patients will have had in-service education relating
   to safe lifting techniques and use these techniques.
9. The health authorities practice on pressure area care will be present
   on every ward and health authority premises and will be known
   and understood by all staff.
10. The nurse caring for the patient will know when and where specific
    help for patients' problems can be obtained, e.g., dietitian,
    physiotherapist, pharmacist, continence adviser.
11. Computing facilities will be available for measuring outcome.
12. The nurse will be responsible for updating her own knowledge on
    recent research.

Process criteria

Nutrition

1. The nurse will, at the beginning of each shift, inform the patient of
   the fluid intake goal for the shift.
2. The nurse will encourage intake up to x ml per day (amount specified
   daily for the individual patient).
3. The nurse will offer assistance with drinking when needed.
4. For the patient who is unable to take oral fluids the nurse will
   administer fluids via the route as prescribed.

5. The nurse will, on admission, if the patient's condition allows, obtain dietary information from the patient and ensure diet needs are met on a daily basis.
6. The nurse will obtain professional advice and instructions from the dietitian and physician when dietary needs are not met.
7. The nurse will observe for signs of dehydration within two hours of each shift. Signs of normal fluid balance are:
    (a) the skin and mucous membrane have good turgor and are not dry;
    (b) there is no postural oedema on patients eyelids, legs and sacrum;
    (c) there are no signs of raised jugular venous pressure, i.e., the neck veins are flat when the patient is resting and the neck turned to one side;
    (d) the patient's urine is not scanty and concentrated;
    (e) the patient's pulse rate and rhythm are normal, or, if abnormal, can be attributed to other factors.

Elimination

8. The nurse will, on admission, if the patient's condition allows, obtain history of bowel habits. Bowel movements will be recorded daily.
9. The nurse will record all intake and output hourly for those patients who require strict monitoring of fluid balance.
10. For those patients who are incontinent, the nurse will offer the bedpan or commode two- to four-hourly.

Care of the skin

11. Within the first two hours of the shift, the nurse will observe the skin for changes in the normal colour, e.g., erythema or blanching.
12. The nurse will provide perineal care for the patient after each voiding if the patient cannot do this for himself.
13. In the event of a patient being incontinent of urine and/or faeces, the nurse must wash the area after every episode and dry thoroughly. Barrier substances such as oil, silicone or zinc base may be useful, but each patient must have their own tube.
    The nurse will also refer to the continence advisor and to the continence policy.

Mental state

14. The nurse will assess the patient's mental status on admission.
15. The nurse will devise programmes, on admission, which will assist the patient to become familiar with his/her surroundings.

Activity – mobility

16. The nurse will change the patient's position, usually two-hourly or more often if necessary. However, the patient nursed on a Pegasus Airwave Bed or Clinitron bed will require only occasional changes of position for comfort.
17. The nurse will discuss at all times with the patient and other members of the team the use of appropriate support systems to be included in the care of the patient.
18. The nurse will inform the patient before changing position.
19. The nurse will ensure that staff are aware of correct turning techniques before turning the patient.
20. The nurse will ensure correct lifting techniques are used.
21. The nurse will obtain advice and assistance from other professionals in devising ambulatory programmes.

Drugs

22. The nurse will be aware of drug side-effects, and any must be reported immediately to the senior nurse and physician.
23. In the event of a patient developing a pressure sore, or the pressure sore deteriorating, the nurse will grade the sore immediately and thereafter weekly.

Outcome criteria

1. The patient's fluid and electrolyte balance will remain within normal limits at all times.
2. The patient will not experience constipation or incontinence of urine.
3. The patient's skin will remain intact at all times.
4. The patient will not experience muscle atrophy, joint deformities, pathological fractures and contractures.
5. There will be no deterioration of the patient's mental state as assessed on admission.
6. The patient will not be fearful or anxious.
7. The patient will be able to verbalize his or her needs depending on his/her mental state.

Outcome standards – patient satisfaction

1. The nurse provided adequate information before carrying out each procedure.
2. The nurse asked for patient's opinion, where appropriate, before using available support systems.

3. The nurse explained to the patient why certain procedures had to be carried out.
4. The nurse answered any questions asked by members of the patient's family or friends.

Measured outcome

The success of the prevention plans and the incidence of pressure sores will be measured weekly:
1. Patients identified as being at risk and the condition of the patient.
2. Nursing interventions.
3. Patient-support systems.
4. Incidence of pressure sores with severity grades recorded.

STANDARD STATEMENT FOR THE PROMOTION OF CONTINENCE AND MANAGEMENT OF INCONTINENCE
(City and Hackney Health Authority, 1987/8)

Structure criteria

1. The nurse will have knowledge of measures for maintenance of continence and knowledge of prevention of incontinence.
2. Incontinence will not be accepted as an inevitable problem.
3. Full assessment and investigation of incontinence will be carried out to determine the underlying cause.
4. The Continence Advisor will be available to give advice on the maintenance of continence to those at risk and give support to patients who are incontinent and to their carers, e.g. nurses, relatives, friends.
5. Aids and appliances are readily available for the patient.
6. Aids and appliances are regularly reviewed for suitability, comfort and effectiveness.

Process criteria

1. The nurse will give patient care with maintenance and/or prevention in mind.
2. The nurse will explain to the patient the causes of incontinence.
3. Investigations should include: full history from patient, or relatives or carer if appropriate, documented in the Nursing Kardex.

Urinary incontinence

4. A continence chart should be completed indicating frequency and volumes, if possible for at least five days.
5. Physical examination of (i) genitalia, observing for any rashes or

exoriation. In women, observe for signs of vaginitis or obvious prolapse (ii) rectum to exclude constipation.

6. Urinalysis, should be performed: if protein and/or blood present, mid-stream specimen of urine should be sent for microscopy culture and for sensitivity. If glycosuria is present, BM Stix performed.

Faecal incontinence

7. A record is kept of when the faecal incontinence occurs.
8. Rectal examination is performed to exclude faecal impaction, weakness in the anal sphincter or any abormality.

Urinary and faecal incontinence

9. Blood tests may be requested by medical staff to exclude any related abnormalities, e.g., diabetes mellitus, raised urea and electrolytes from outflow, obstructure, etc.
10 If none of the above reveals a diagnosis, medical staff may request urodynamic investigation for urinary incontinence, sigmoidoscopy or radiopaque X-ray for faecal incontinence.
11. If appropriate, referrals may be made to specialists, e.g., urologist, gynaecologist, geriatrician, continence advisor, occupational therapist, physiotherapist, etc.
12. The continence advisor is contacted for advice, education and support.
13. Where treatment is unsuccessful, effective individual management is commenced. The nurse will ensure that a suitable aid/appliance is obtained for the patient.
14. Staff ensure, where possible, that patient's opinions and feelings regarding aids and appliances are made known to the person supervizing the delivery of care.

Outcome standards – patient satisfaction

1. The nurse will be able to instruct patients in the promotion of continence and prevention of incontinence. For example, where indicated, the patient may be instructed how to perform pelvic floor exercise.
2. The patient and staff understand that incontinence is a sign/symptom of an underlying disorder.
3. A record of progress is kept and evaluated at each change of shift. Results of physical examinations and analyses are documented in the Nursing Kardex. Abnormalities are reported to the medical staff.
4. Faecal incontinence is documented in the Nursing Kardex unless a specific bowel chart is available in the unit.

5. Diagnoses are made following investigations, and appropriate specialists are contacted to offer advice.
6. Support is received from continence advisor for advice regarding continence and incontinence.
7. Aids and appliances are evaluated for performance and comfort. The staff obtain them for the patient without difficulty.
8. The person supervizing the delivery of care, e.g., the district nurse, ward sister or HNS, liaises with the continence advisor regarding aids and appliances. The continence advisor reviews the contract items and others with the Regional Health Authority's Specialist Group.

REFERENCES

Aries, P. (1983) *The Hour of Our Death*, Penguin, London.

Castledine, G. (1985) Defending the all rounder. *Nursing Times*, **81**(38) 22.

City and Hackney Health Authority (1987) Achievable standards of care for the elderly patient cared for in the acute assessment wards, continuing-care wards, nursing homes and day hospitals within the City and Hackney Health Authority. Project Paper 72, King Edward's Hospital Fund for London, re-printed CHHA 1989.

City and Hackney Health Authority (1987/1988) Unpublished examples of standard setting.

City and Hackney Health Authority (1988) Pressure area care for the City and Hackney Health Authority.

Garrett, G. (1983) Chapter 15, forward planning – something must be done about it. *Health Needs of the Elderly: the Essentials of Nursing*, Macmillan, London, pp. 107–9.

HMSO White Paper Cmnd 8173 (1981) Retirement, a time of opportunity, in *Growing Older*, HMSO, London.

Lang, N. (1976) *Issues in Quality Assurance in Nursing, ANA Issues in Evaluative Research*, American Nursing Association, New York.

Manthy, M. (1980) *The Practice of Primary Nursing*, Blackwells, Oxford.

Norton, D., McLaren, R. and Exton-Smith, A.N. (1962) An Investigation of Geriatric Nursing Problems in Hospital. The National Corporation for the Care of Old People (now the Centre for the Policy on Ageing), London, re-issued 1975, Churchill Livingstone, London.

Pearson, A. (1988) *Primary Nursing: Nursing in the Burford and Oxford Nursing Development Units*, Croom Helm, London.

Rogers, E.M. (1972) *Change agent, Clients and Change*. In Creating Social Change. (eds G. Zaltman, P. Kotler and I. Kaufman.) Holt, Rinehart and Winsten, New York, pp. 194–213.

UKCC (1989) *Exercising Accountability*, UKCC, London.

Wright, S. and Wills, G. (1988) Getting to know you. *Nursing Standard*, 26 November.

FURTHER READING

Royal College of Nursing and British Geriatrics Society, 1975 (revised 1987) *Improving Care of Elderly People in Hospital*, RCN, London.

APPENDIX 1

Guidelines for the provision of residential continuing care
(To be used in conjunction with DHSS Building Notes)

Environmental and physical

(a) Living space:
variety of chairs, tables, spare chairs for visitors, curtains, carpets, colour pictures, clocks, calendars, shelves for ornaments, library books, magazines and newspapers: indoor gardening, flowers, fish-tank, bird-cage.
Non-smoking area, quiet area.
Quick and easy access to WCs and wash-hand basins.
Hand rails around walls.

(b) Dining area:
variety of tables – size and shape, space for wheelchairs at tables, suitable dining chairs, table mats, cloths, menu cards, flowers, condiments, teapots, water jugs for each table, space for eating alone if desired, chairs for those helping with feeding if necessary, hand rails around walls.

(c) Activity space (combination of (a) and (b) if necessary):
Self-care facilities – safety kettle and heater ring, access to cutlery and crockery etc., lockable bar facilities, storage area with cupboards for games, equipment television, radio and tape machines, photographic and screen equipment, telephone on trolley, large tables for art and handicraft and games.

(d) Bed area:
individualized space by the provision of room dividers or curtains, adjustable height beds, mobility space, wardrobe lockers with accessible mirror and personal drawers, carpets, non-slip mats, rotating discs to aid transfer from bed if appropriate, bed head variable light controlled locally, socket for individualized radio and television headphones, call-bell, cantilevered bed tables with drawer.

(e) Bathrooms:
choice of free-standing, wall-fixed, sitting or adjustable baths; shower bath in spacious, warm, well-draining area, shower chair, combination of hand shower with bath, space for movement of hoists, handrails; bath seats, bath aids, shelves for toilet articles, hooks for clothes, warm towel rails, razor points, mirrors, hand-basins at height for wheelchairs, easy-turn taps, cupboards for local stores and bath cleaning materials, hair-washing sink, laundry containers, call bell.

(f) Lavatories:
space for wheelchairs and walking frames, centrally placed pedestal with hand rails which fold back against wall, recessed toilet roll holders for both leaf and rolls on both sides, small hand-washing sink, liquid soap, disposable towels and bucket, door handle and bolt which can be opened from outside in emergency, engaged sign, call bell.

(g) Dirty disposal room:
bed-pan disposal unit or washer, bed-pans and urinals, urine-testing equipment, slop-hopper, bucket sink, wash-hand basin, dirty laundry containers and space for bags.

(h) Treatment room:
clinical equipment in cupboards, sterile supplies and disposal facilities, medicine trolley and locked lotion cupboard, special apparatus – oxygen and suction, wash-hand basin, etc.

(i)   Personalized clothing area – away from residential area if possible but sufficiently near to provide daily individualized service, washing and drying machines for small items, ironing equipment, labelling and repair facilities; all this equipment should be suitable and well-placed for use by the residents themselves.

(j)   Staff areas:
        cloak and changing room with toilet facilities; office with information boards, rest room with drink-making machinery if it is not possible for staff to reach central provisions; teaching area with books.

(k)   Storage space for equipment, aids, wheelchairs, hoists, disposable goods, games, etc.

APPENDIX 2

Questions to be asked about the quality of life for patients in continuing care

Yes/No   Action

1.   Do staff take time to listen and try to understand what life in the group is really like?
2.   Have residents a mini-home area which is their own place with their own things?
3.   Can they be alone and private in this or some other place?
4.   Can they give refreshments to their relatives or friends at their own wish – by inviting them to tea which they have provided, etc.?
5.   Have they private control and do they handle their own money?
6.   Do they have the opportunity to choose and buy their own clothes – from shops, visiting dealers or from mail orders?
7.   Can they see relatives, friends, priests, solicitors and others in private and at any time?
8.   Are there facilities for achieving their best in creative and physical activities:-
        music, art, sports, games, gardening, writing,
        debating, hobbies, craftwork, pottery,
        weaving, spinning, etc.?
9.   Is there a committee formed by the residents to discuss and define their wishes regarding the organization and activities of the group? Are they encouraged to appoint their own honorary officers, keep notes and follow up the suggestions put forward?
10.   Is there a catering committee on which residents are represented and do they have a choice of menu?
11.   Do residents take part in domestic and cooking activities as far as they are able, being given full responsibility for certain duties, e.g. dusting their own areas, shelling peas, etc.?
12.   Are residents informed and consulted about changes in decoration or furnishings, about official visitors, changes in staff or any other plans for the unit?
13.   Are there areas for non-smokers, non-television addicts or Brahms' lovers?

14. Are outings arranged to places of interest, shops?
15. Are invitations issued by the residents to other groups and organizations to come to their home?
16. Are the residents involved in efforts to help other people, e.g. Oxfam, British Legion?
17. Are holidays and exchange visits arranged by and for residents?
18. Is full attention paid to enabling residents to make full use of all their senses:-
    sight, hearing, speech, smelling, touching, feeling, decision-making
19. Is the protection of personal dignity and privacy given the highest priority in the provision of such physical help as is needed?
20. Are residents and their friends aware of the method of making a formal complaint?

APPENDIX 3

REGISTER OF PATIENTS WITH, OR AT RISK FROM, PRESSURE SORES

HOSPITAL................ WARD............. NO. OF PTS.   WEEK   SIGNED..........
                                          ON WARD...... ENDING.........

PATIENT DATA

SEX M/F HOSPITAL NO. .... SURNAME .... FORENAME................. D.O.B. ....

DATE OF ADMISSION .... MAIN DIAGNOSIS .... SPECIALTY ....
DATE OF DISCHARGE ....

NORTON SCORE (PLEASE CIRCLE)

GENERAL CONDITION	MENTAL STATE	ACTIVITY	MOBILITY	INCONTINENCE
4 GOOD	4 ALERT	4 AMBULANT	4 FULL	4 NOT
3 FAIR	3 APATHETIC	3 WALKS WITH HELP	3 SLIGHTLY LIMITED	3 OCCASIONAL
2 POOR	2 CONFUSED	2 CHAIRBOUND	2 VERY LIMITED	2 USUALLY/URINE
1 VERY BAD	1 STUPEROUS	1 BEDFAST	1 IMMOBILE	1 DOUBLY

TOTAL NORTON SCORE =

SORE DATA

A. Did patient have
   sore(s) on
   admission?   Y/N

   Site(s)   Grade(s)

SITES	GRADES
1 SACRUM	1 DISCOLOURATION
2 BUTTOCKS	BLISTER
3 ISCHIA	PERSISTENT REDNESS
4 HIPS	2 SUPERFICIALN SKIN LOSS
5 HEELS	3 LOSS OF TISSUE TO
6 MALLEOLI	DERMIS+/– SURROUNDING
7 KNEES	DISCOLOURATION
8 SPINE	4 CAVITY INTO SUBCUTANEOUS
9 SHOULDERS	TISSUE OR DEEPER
10 OCCIPUT	
11 ELBOW	
12 OTHER	
(STATE)	

B. Did patient develop
   sore(s) after
   admission?   Y/N

   Site(s)   Grade(s)

TOTAL NUMBER OF SORES =

SUPPORT SYSTEMS   AIDS   (PLEASE CIRCLE)

SUPPORT SYSTEMS	AIDS	
1 CLINITRON BED	1 VAPERM MATTRESS	10 HEEL FLEECE
2 EGERTON TURNING BED	2 POLYFLOAT MATTRESS (TALLEY)	11 BED CRADLE
3 LOW AIR LOSS BED	3 PEGASUS ALTERNATING AIRWAVE	12 PILLOWS
4 BEAUFORT WINCHESTER	4 LARGE CELL RIPPLE MATTRESS	13 ELBOW PROTECTOR
5 OTHER WATER BED	5 BUBBLE PAD RB	14 HEEL PROTECTOR
6 OTHER (STATE)	6 SPENCO MATTRESS	15 MONKEY POLE
	7 POLYCARE MATTRESS	16 HOIST
	8 BEAUFORT BEAN MATTRESS	17 OTHER (STATE)
	9 SACRAL FLEECE	

Did you have difficulty in obtaining these?   Y/N
If yes, please state which...................................

OTHER DATA (PLEASE CIRCLE)

NUTRITION	DRUGS	CONSTIPATION	HYGIENE/SKIN CARE
1 IVI	1 TRANQUILLISERS	4 NO	1 GOOD SELF CARE
2 N/G FEEDS	2 HYPNOTICS	3 TREATED	2 ASSISTED WASH
3 ORAL FLUIDS (Self Admin)	3 SEDATIVES	2 CONSTIPATED	3 BLANKET BATH
4 ORAL FLUIDS (Nurse Admin)	4 ANALGESICS	1 IMPACTED	4 WOUND/SKIN CARE
5 TOTAL PARENTERAL NUTRITION	5 STEROIDS		5 TOPICAL CREAMS/
6 SOFT DIET (Liquidised)	6 HYPOGLYCAEMICS		LOTIONS/POWDERS
7 NORMAL DIET (Trolley)	7 VITAMINS		6 OTHERS (STATE)
8 SPECIAL DIET	8 OTHER		
9 SPECIAL DIETARY SUPPLEMENTS	9 ANTIBIOTICS		

Chapter 7

Nutritional care of the long-stay patient

Nutritional deficiencies can occur all too often with residents in long-stay care, and it is necessary to be alert to this possibility. Experience in a long-stay hospital in South London highlights problems where, in 1980, low concentrations of plasma ascorbic acid were found. A vitamin-C-enriched drink was arranged for all the patients, yet three years later a case of clinical scurvy occurred, and in a further three years one third of all the patients were found to be deficient in vitamin C (Fenton, 1989). This and other investigations into the nutrient intakes of elderly patients in hospital show how many factors can be involved (Jones *et al.*, 1988). Hence, time spent identifying and monitoring the links in the chain from the kitchen to the actual meal consumed should help to avoid potential nutritional problems for the patient.

There have been several well documented dietary surveys of the elderly, both at home and in residential care (DHSS, 1972, 1979; Exton-Smith *et al.*, 1972; Davies, 1981). Collectively, the results (of averaged figures for the groups of people studied) show that they tend to meet the recommended amounts of nutrients required by groups of individuals. However, their intakes of energy (kilocalories) are consistently low. It is important to remember that, although the tendency is for the groups studied to meet their nutritional requirements, some individuals within these groups do not reach these goals and can be on the verge of a nutritional deficiency. A further factor is that the lower energy intake means that the nutritional density of the food consumed must be high to meet the needs of these people.

Individuals coming into long-stay care may have been having a poor diet previously as a result of a multitude of problems which have led to their need for care. They can, therefore, already be 'at risk'.

The current recommended daily intake of nutrients for the elderly are given in Table 7.1 (DHSS, 1979).

Studies which measure how much food is eaten, and the consequent nutrient intake, do not take into account whether the food was actually absorbed by the body. Nutrients are often less well absorbed as age increases, and in addition certain drugs can interfere with their

Table 7.1 Recommended daily intake of nutrients for the elderly

	Men		Women	
	65–74	*75 and over*	*65–74*	*75 and over*
Energy (kcal)	2400	2150	1900	1680
(MJ)	10.0	9.0	8.0	7.0
Protein (g)	60	54	47	42
Thiamin (mg)	1.0	0.9	0.8	0.7
Riboflavin (mg)	1.6	1.6	1.3	1.3
Nicotinic acid equivalent (mg)	18	18	15	15
Ascorbic acid (mg)	30	30	30	30
Vitamin A retinol equivalent (µg)	750	750	750	750
Calcium (mg)	500	500	500	500
Iron (mg)	10	10	10	10

Vitamin D. There is a footnote stating: 'Adults with inadequate exposure to sunlight, for example those who are housebound, may need a supplement of 10 µg daily.'.

absorption. There are, however, some residents in long-stay care who are very thin despite eating well and obtaining their daily requirements of nutrients. The reason for this is not, as yet, understood. Many factors need to be considered, therefore, when planning meals for residents in long-stay care:

1. An awareness of the nutritional state of the resident prior to admission.
2. The nutritional requirements of the individual.
3. The nutrients which need particular attention.
4. Physical problems which affect eating and swallowing.
5. Factors which affect appetite.
6. Food preference and long-term food habits.
7. Religion.
8. Drugs which interfere with absorption of nutrients.
9. Mealtimes and the social environment.
10. The menu-planning process.
11. Observation of the amount of food consumed.
12. Requirements for special diets.

MEALS

Mealtimes must not be regarded as a quick half-hour slot three times a day which interrupts ward routine.

The meal period should be considered as a social, pleasurable occasion by both staff and residents. Meals are one of the familiar routines of a lifetime, linked to memories of the past, and their regular occurrence is a familiar landmark which breaks up the day. Only too often drug rounds, staff mealtimes, shift changes, pressure from kitchen staff for the return of equipment, makes this a rushed time and those people who need to take time over their meals, together with those who need help with feeding, can suffer.

MEALTIMES

The timing of meals should allow some flexibility if at all feasible, particularly over the timing of breakfast. Breakfast is a meal which is usually popular and well eaten. It should be late enough so that those residents who wish to be dressed, have time to do so. If flexibility is not possible, the spacing between mealtimes needs careful planning. It is not acceptable to have the last food of the day at 5 pm. Suggested times are:

Breakfast	8.00 am to 9.00 am (flexible where possible)
Mid-morning drink/snack	10.00 am to 10.30 am
Lunch	12 noon to 1.00 pm
Mid-afternoon drink	3.00 pm to 3.30 pm
Cooked tea	5.30 pm to 6.30 pm
Evening drink/snack	8.00 pm to 9.00 pm

CHOOSING THE MEAL

A planned menu should be available in advance, and wherever possible residents should be encouraged to take part in choosing their meals. It is an excellent plan to have a system of collecting residents' ideas for dishes they would like included; this may be arranged through a catering committee, where suggestions and discussions on meal service can take place, or in a smaller unit it should become part of the routine procedure. There are many favourite recipes which the elderly enjoy, and dishes such as tripe and onions and sweetbreads are popular.

The menu choice may be written on individual menu cards, and here relatives and friends visiting can help in making the meal choice. If the resident has problems in reading the menu it is very important that it is still discussed with them. For those unable to make a choice, records must be kept of individual food preferences obtained from the individual or their relatives. It should be possible to order a varied size portion and this should be negotiated with the catering department so that staff are familiar with the portion sizes offered.

If a bulk meal service is used the choice will still be made in advance but the meal, and hence portion size, will be served by nursing staff.

However the meal is served, the important fact is that the residents are almost totally reliant on the nurse/helper for what, how and when they eat.

For the meal to be an enjoyable event, food must be served at the appropriate temperature as well as being varied, tasty, nutritious, attractive to the eye and of the right consistency.

It is good to encourage visitors to be involved at mealtimes. This can make the meal more of an occasion, and extra help is thus available to ensure that food is eaten and liquids taken. Even participating in a cup of tea or coffee after the meal can make the meal more pleasurable.

WHERE SHOULD RESIDENTS EAT?

The ideal is for people to have their meals away from the bedside which is associated with sleeping, washing, toiletries, medications and other routines of the 24-hour day. Preferably there should be a separate dining area for those who can get up and sit at tables for their meals. The tables should be small so that there is a social atmosphere. Less mobile residents may be in a day room with their individual tables. In this way the only people who sit by their beds for meals are those who wish to.

Coloured, attractive tablecloths should be obtained, with bright coloured napkins. It is possible to have some of the tablecovers plasticized so that they can be used inconspicuously where spills may occur. With good sized napkins it should not be necessary to use bibs, which can be degrading for the elderly. Flowers on the tables make a great difference.

Eating aids can make a great difference to how much of a meal is consumed. Hand tremors can be a real cause of insufficient food being eaten. Non-slip place mats, or suction pads can help to hold the plate in place. The handles of cutlery can be difficult to grip for those with arthritic hands, and slip-on rubber handles or grips help here. Plate rims or guards stop food sliding off the plate and some of the china companies make attractive deep plates with a lip. Beakers or cups with a slanted base or two-handled cups can help, and a flexistraw can make those who cannot hold a cup more independent when they wish for a drink. Such aids are often a better solution than a feeding cup with a spout.

An occupational therapist can assess patients with particular problems and should have a range of aids which can be tried. Alternatively, The Disabled Living Foundation can provide these aids.

PREPARATION FOR THE MEAL

Always check whether a visit to the toilet is needed before the meal. A disrupted meal can otherwise result and the desire to continue eating later is diminished.

See that the residents are comfortably seated, whether at the table, in a lower chair, or in bed, and that their special eating aids are ready. If help is needed with feeding be sure to keep the meal hot until the nurse or helper is ready to help.

MEAL SERVICE

In the dining area it is advantageous to serve the main protein (meat, fish, egg, cheese dish) directly onto individual plates and to have serving dishes of the vegetables and potatoes with a jug of gravy separately. In this way there is an element of choice and decision (with guidance) for the resident. Cruets should be available, and so should a jug of water or a fruit drink.

For those unable to make a choice, serve the meal directly onto the plate with care over the portion size. A large meal can be quite overwhelming and have an unfavourable effect on the appetite. It is much preferable to have a system where a second helping is available.

For elderly people it is helpful to see that any pre-wrapped items of food (butter and/or cheese portions) are unwrapped, otherwise there is a danger that they will not be eaten.

If the meal service is a centralized tray system, the complete meal will come on a tray from the catering department. These meals, however, still need attention before they are given to the patient. It may not be immediately obvious which food is to be eaten first, so some re-arrangement of the tray may be necessary. Ideally, the dessert should not be served until the main course has been eaten. Familiar accompaniments are important, such as vinegar with fish and chips, mint sauce with lamb, and horseradish sauce with beef. If the eyesight is poor, try to ensure that the resident can recognize the food – and where it is on the plate. Relating this to the face of a clock is one way of doing this.

HOW MUCH FOOD IS EATEN?

It is an essential part of the meal service procedure to observe how much food has been eaten by the individual. It is very unusual to find all plates completely cleared, and hence a judgement needs to be made as to whether a meal replacement or a supplementary drink is necessary.

MENU PLANNING

The menu should be planned in advance to cover a period of at least three weeks to ensure that it is not monotonous. A choice should be available to cover the need for different textures or religious preferences – as well as likes and dislikes. Plain food with familiar names should be used. Traditional dishes such as the Sunday roast are important. A lighter choice should be available for those residents not wishing for a main meal, such as omelettes, salad or toasted sandwiches. There should be flexibility in the menu so that events such as special birthdays, local cricket matches, Royal occasions, Halloween and similar events can be enjoyed.

When planning menus many points need to be taken into account. These include: seasonal availability of foodstuffs, the diversity of cooking equipment (bearing in mind the different requirements for any one meal) and staff capabilities. In all, the menu should be looked at for the colour and attractiveness of dish combinations; we all know of meals of steamed white fish with mashed potato and cauliflower, followed by rice pudding, yet with thought it is easy to insert some colour.

The caterer, nurses and helpers should all work together to ensure that the residents are getting the essential nutrients from their food.

CATERING SYSTEMS

In the light of technology, changes are occurring in the kind of catering systems used in long-stay units. Three main systems, or a combination of these, may be found:

1. Conventional cooking: food is prepared and cooked in the normal manner.
2. Cook freeze: cooked dishes may be purchased ready frozen *or* cooked and frozen on the premises using special freezing equipment. The food is held in freezers and re-heated, preferably in special ovens until the correct temperature is reached.
3. Cook chill: food is cooked, then chilled in a purpose-built unit under careful quality control. It is held at 0–3°C (for a maximum of five days). The food must be kept chilled at this temperature until re-heated quickly in ovens or special food trolleys with careful timing. These meals must be consumed without delay after heating and there should be clear instructions provided by the caterers.

The cook chill and cook freeze methods enable more flexible use of staff, and by using good cooking practices and quality control, can provide food of a good nutritional standard provided procedures are closely adhered to and monitored regularly (DOH, 1989).

VEGETARIANS

There are many reasons for people requesting vegetarian meals, and it is important to find out exactly what foods are eaten. It may be for religious or moral grounds, but the term can also be used when people find some foods not to their liking or difficult to eat.

Vegans are strict vegetarians. They do not eat animal products, and their meals will need to be based on vegetables, pulses and cereals. It is wise to ask your local dietitian to advise on the nutritional adequacy of these meals.

Lacto-vegetarians do not eat meat, poultry, fish or eggs, but they will take milk, cheese, yogurts and other milk products. Some lacto-vegetarians will also eat eggs.

A vegetarian diet can be healthy, but it is necessary to include a wide variety and good mixture of cereals, pulses and vegetables for the main meals. Milk should be increased to one pint daily. For further details refer to the references at the end of this chapter.

RELIGION AND FOOD PREFERENCES

Strict Hindus and Sikhs will not eat foods which have involved the taking of life. They are therefore usually vegetarian. Milk and yogurt can be consumed.

Muslims will not eat pork, bacon or ham. All meat must be ritually slaughtered (known as Halal). Kosher meat is acceptable to many Muslims. Ramadan is a major festival, and during the month of Ramadan all Muslims must fast from dawn to sunset. The date varies each year according to the Muslim calendar. Special exemption from fasting during this period is allowed for chronically ill people, who could be adversely affected.

Judaism. Orthodox Jews are not permitted to eat pork (or any products of the pig). They may eat beef, lamb, chicken or turkey if the meat has been ritually slaughtered and prepared. It is then known as 'Kosher'. Cheese, eggs, fish (apart from shellfish) are acceptable. Meat and milk must not be served at the same meal, or used together in cooking, i.e. a milk-based pudding may not follow a meat dish. Kosher meals can be obtained frozen. These will have been ritually prepared. Care must be taken to keep saucepans, plates, serving utensils separate so that the food is not contaminated in any way with non-Kosher ingredients. For further information see references at the end of this chapter.

HEALTHY EATING

Food and Health policies are being introduced widely because healthy eating can help to prevent not only heart problems but other conditions such as constipation, other bowel conditions and obesity. The nutritional guidelines behind these policies are based on reducing the amount of fat, sugar and salt consumed and increasing the amount of fibre-rich foods.

WHICH OF THESE ARE RELEVANT FOR THE LONG-STAY ELDERLY RESIDENT?

It is helpful to increase the amount of fibre taken to improve bowel function and to help prevent constipation and conditions such as diverticulitis.

The other changes being encouraged are not relevant for this population. Fats should be reduced only if excess weight is a problem. They are an essential source of energy, and as we have seen, it is difficult to obtain enough energy from the amount of food eaten in this age group. Fats are also a source of fat-soluble vitamins. Skimmed milk is not normally recommended for use in drinks or in cooking for long-stay elderly people. Care must be taken to see that food policies using skimmed milk do not automatically include long-stay units for the elderly.

SUGAR

Sugar should also be reduced only if there is a diabetic patient or a resident with a weight problem. Too much sugar in a concentrated form, i.e., a lot of sugar in cups of tea, can dull the appetitie.

SALT

Salt should be reduced only in individual cases if there is a medical reason. Palatability is extremely important, and indeed, some elderly people can be harmed by reducing their salt intake too much.

NUTRIENTS WHICH NEED PARTICULAR ATTENTION

Vitamin C

Foods containing vitamin C should be consumed daily. The main sources are fruit and vegetables. It is well-known that a shortage of vitamin C over a period of time leads to scurvy and this does still occur – even in hospital. Signs of mild vitamin C deficiency are an increased tendency to bruise, poor wound healing and general apathy. The vitamin is very easily destroyed: it is soluble in water and destroyed by heat. There will be negligible amounts of the vitamin left in vegetables which have been prepared well in advance, held in water, overcooked and then delayed in transit before being consumed. Bicarbonate of soda, which is sometimes added to keep the vegetables a good green colour, destroys the vitamin and should not be used.

The best sources of vitamin C are: oranges, grapefruit, mandarins (and their juices); blackcurrant juice/drink; raw tomatoes and lightly cooked green vegetables; potatoes, depending on how they are cooked (jacket potatoes and chips are not cooked in water and hence retain more of the vitamin). If an instant potato powder is used it is essential to use a brand with vitamin C added.

The quality of the fruit or vegetable used is vital in relation to the amount of vitamin C it contains. Badly bruised, wilted, stale vegetables have low levels of the vitamin as it is destroyed on bruising and storing.

Frozen vegetables are generally a good source but dried vegetables (unless fortified with the vitamin) will contribute negligible amounts.

Citrus fruit juice or fresh fruit should be consumed at least once a day. Vegetables, fresh or frozen, should be eaten at least twice a day. This should provide the minimum of 30 mg a day.

Note: A glass of 'natural' fruit juice, or a blackcurrant drink, should be given daily to all long-stay residents in view of the uncertainty as to how much of the vitamin has been destroyed during cooking, and prior to serving.

Vitamin D

Too little vitamin D causes disturbances of bone and calcium metabolism and may lead to osteomalacia (Exton-Smith, 1988). The main way of obtaining enough of the vitamin from natural sources is from the action of sunlight on the skin (to convert precursors into the active form cholecalciferol).

It is not easy to obtain the necessary amount of the vitamin purely from food with this age group, because it is found only in a limited range of foods. The elderly who are in residential care (and those who are housebound) are thus likely to have low blood levels of the vitamin. Every opportunity should be taken to encourage residents to be outside, to use balconies or to sit by open windows. Even a mixture of partial sun and shade is beneficial.

The main dietary sources of vitamin D are: oily fish, such as sardines, pilchards, kippers, tuna and salmon; eggs; table margarines: these are fortified with vitamin D, but not all bulk catering margarines are; liver, including paté, liver sausage, faggots; some yogurts, evaporated milks and malted milk drinks have vitamin D added, as do some breakfast cereals. Therefore, sandwiches made with table margarine and spread with fillings of sardines, pilchards, liver sausage or paté, are useful ways to provide vitamin D.

There is some interest currently being shown in the possibility of fortifying milk puddings, custards and other desserts with vitamin D; this would be very helpful for the house-bound person and those in long-stay care with less access to sunlight.

An intake of 10μg daily is needed, and evidence suggests that only about one-quarter of this can be obtained from natural foods for this group of people.

Supplements of vitamin D for long-term immobile residents should be seriously considered (DHSS, 1979).

Iron

There are many reasons why the elderly may become anaemic. A survey of hospital patients (DHSS, 1970) showed that 27% of male and 32% of female patients were anaemic. Anaemia can be due to haemorrhoids, diverticulitis, hiatal hernia, peptic ulcers, malabsorption, a depressed appetite, or reliance on a limited selection of convenience foods. A good dietary source of iron is necessary. Sources of iron include the following: red meats such as beef, lamb, corned beef, black pudding; liver, kidney – or derivatives such as paté, liver sausage; dark green vegetables, peas, beans, lentils; dried fruit such as apricots and prunes; wholemeal bread and flour; eggs; fortified wholegrain breakfast cereals.

Not all iron is well absorbed by the body, and taking a form of vitamin C (such as orange juice) at the same meal will help this.

Folate

A deficiency of folate can often show as soreness of the mouth with a burning sensation of the tongue. Continued low blood levels lead to megaloblastic anaemia, changes in the nervous system and neuropathy. Mental changes may be observed before the anaemia appears, such as confusion, depression and apathy. The cause of these low levels may be due to a low dietary intake, malabsorption or impaired effectiveness of the vitamin. Folate in food is very easily destroyed by exposure to sunlight, heat and cooking. A low vitamin C intake can affect how available the folate is to the body. Sources of folate include the following: liver, including paté and liver sausage; kidney and other offal; green leafy vegetables (remember overcooking and keeping hot destroys folate); peas and beans; oranges and bananas; yeast extracts, Bovril, Marmite; bread.

Fibre

Constipation can be a problem for people who are less mobile and for those who include very little roughage in their meals. On the whole, the elderly tend to avoid foods with a good fibre content because of long-term habits or because they prefer soft, textured foods. It is preferable to try to adjust the diet to include more fibre than to resort to laxatives which can interfere with absorption of some nutrients.

The fibre content of the diet can be increased by: using 100% wholemeal bread or a white high-fibre bread for those who do not like wholemeal bread; serving wholemeal cereals such as Branflakes, Weetabix, Shredded Wheat, Readybrek or muesli; offering high-fibre biscuits, such as digestive or bran type; cooking with a mixture of half wholemeal and half white flour for pastry, pies, scones and fruit crumbles; encouraging the eating of more vegetables, and boiling or baking potatoes in their skins; adding pulses such as peas, beans and lentils to stews and casseroles; using wholegrain spaghetti and brown rice; including more fruit, both fresh fruit and in desserts. Dried fruits such as prunes and apricots are rich in fibre.

As a last resort, pure bran can be added to porridge or other foods such as soups. Care needs to be taken when introducing bran as it can cause flatulence unless introduced slowly. Start with two teaspoons of bran a day and increase up to two tablespoons. It is essential to see that sufficient fluids are taken as the bran absorbs a significant amount of liquid. Pure bran can interfere with the absorption of nutrients such as calcium, iron and magnesium; for this reason it should not be used for long periods.

The daily requirement of fibre is 25 to 30g – depending on the previous intake. Such an intake of fibre can be achieved by consuming one portion of a high-fibre breakfast cereal; three slices of wholemeal bread; one medium-sized potato, cooked in its skin; one portion of peas (two tablespoons), or of baked beans or corn; one portion of fruit; two digestive biscuits or one wholemeal scone – or a dessert made with a mixture of wholemeal flour.

Fluid

Fluids are essential, and it is important to ensure that sufficient is taken. It is too easy to become dehydrated, with the ensuing problems. The elderly can be reluctant to take fluids if they have incontinence problems, particularly when this is at night. In this case, adjust the times when fluids are given to the earlier part of the day. Insufficient fluids may be taken because fluids are not easily accessible, or because the drinking cup or glass cannot be held firmly.

Too few fluids will encourage constipation and can lead to renal problems. At least eight cups of liquid should be taken daily. These can include tea, coffee, water and fruit juice.

FACTORS WHICH AFFECT THE CONSUMPTION OF FOOD

Resistance to changes in eating habits

The reasons for resisting change may be due to long-held beliefs about food, to old wives' tales about foods which are 'acid' and foods which are 'binding', and people who have remained on strict diets long after the condition has been resolved.

Lack of taste

With aging, there is a progressive loss of the number of taste buds per papilla on the tongue. The ones lost initially are those of the anterior tongue which detect sweet and salty tastes, whilst those which detect bitter and sour tastes increase. This alters sensitivity to tastes, and strongly flavoured, highly seasoned food is a must.

Poor oral hygiene can mask taste perception, whilst decreased appreciation of aroma also makes food seem less appetizing.

Respiratory problems

Emphysema and bronchitis and other respiratory problems can affect eating, and supplements may be needed.

Dentition

All too often dentures may be missing or inadequate. Whilst this must be attended to, it is too easily assumed that denture-less people need only minced and mashed food. The gums, however, have usually hardened, and most textures of food can be masticated. The important point is to see that meat is tender, and that large pieces are cut up; even dessert apples can be eaten if sliced. It is wrong to assume that only sloppy food can be eaten.

Swallowing problems

Swallowing problems may be due to: facial weakness, which can result in poor lipseal and difficulty in retaining food, liquids or saliva in the mouth; difficulty with jaw movement and swallowing; loss of swallowing reflex; inability of the tongue to propel food and liquids to the back of the tongue, or to clear food from the cheeks or from the teeth and gums; loss of protective reflex.

With swallowing problems there is a high risk of aspirating thin liquids and, therefore, textures of food must be watched. Chilled thick drinks are often managed more easily than hot, thin drinks. Liquids can be thickened easily by using products such as Carobel (Cow and Gate Ltd). Moist food with a firm *consistent* texture should be given.

Some differing textures are hard to consume – for example: cornflakes and milk; soup with pieces in it, e.g. minestrone; dried fruit in cakes; dry biscuits (dunking in tea helps).

When a soft or pureed meal is needed, care should be taken. It is too easy to thin down the meal to a dilute consistency and hence provide few nutrients and little energy. A food processor is useful for adjusting textures without having to add a diluting liquid. Pureed/soft meals must be presented attractively. The meat, vegetables and potato should be served separately – not mixed together as a soup. Simple ideas such as a nest of pureed potato with the pureed meat in the centre is more attractive than all merging into each other.

Small amounts should be given frequently as the recipient will usually tire easily.

Positioning is important for people with swallowing problems: they should be upright with the head tilting slightly forwards. Ideally they should be assessed by a speech therapist so that help is given in improving the swallowing reflex.

Depression, apathy and confusion

All of these conditions lead to lack of interest in food and to a depressed appetite. Alcohol, such as a glass of sherry before meals, can act as a stimulant.

Dementia

People with dementia may not remember when or whether they have eaten. They are also unable to express any feelings of hunger that they may have. A regular routine is important. Care is needed in seating these residents at mealtimes so that they do not cause too much disturbance to others. They need prompting to eat when their attention wanders, and if they are restless and unable to sit for any length of time it may be necessary to give them food which they can take away – such as sandwiches and finger-type snacks. In this case, nourishing supplementary drinks are essential to ensure that sufficient nutrients are consumed.

When patients lack the ability to feed themselves, constant help and observation of problems are essential. Being fed is not pleasant, as the recipient is not in control of the amount or speed of food given. If care is not taken, food will cool quickly. An upright posture is again essential when assistance with feeding is needed.

INTERACTION OF DRUGS AND NUTRIENTS

Effect on appetite

Drugs which will decrease appetite include the biguanides (Metformin, Phenformin); Indomethacin; digitalis; glucogon; and cyclophosphamide.

Drugs which increase appetite include the sulphonylureas (Tolbutamide, Chlorpropamide, Glibenclamide); phenothiazine (Largactil); the benzodiazepines (Valium, Librium); anabolic agents (Durabolin); insulin; and alcohol.

Nutritional interaction

Drugs should be checked with care as they may interact with nutrients. Some examples are given – the drug being followed, in brackets, by the nutrient(s) affected: thiazide diuretics (sodium, potassium); anticonvulsants (folic acid, vitamin D); antacids (phosphate); purgatives (potassium, vitamin K); aspirin (iron); and tetracyclines or corticosteroids (protein metabolism).

Dietary modifications

It is helpful to have those residents who are on modified diets for medical reasons, sitting at the same table in the dining area. In this way it is easier to keep a watch on those who use sugar or need an artificial sweetener, or need skimmed milk and other variations.

Weight problems

Simple adjustments can be made to meals for those residents with a weight problem. Even a slow loss of weight, or halting an increase in weight, can be beneficial. If a strict diet is necessary for medical reasons, a dietitian should be involved in adapting this for the individual.

The following foods should be avoided – each of the foods being followed, in brackets, by foods which can be provided as alternatives: sugar in any drinks (artificial sweeteners, low-calorie soft drinks); jam, marmalade (savoury spread, Marmite, Bovril); snacks between meals (fresh fruit); fried foods and pastry (grilled, steamed or baked dishes); excess butter or margarine (low-fat spread, fortified with vitamin D); rich or starch puddings, sweets and chocolates (fresh fruit, or fruit tinned in natural juice, diet yogurt, egg custard, milk pudding with artificial sweetener).

Diabetic diet

Most elderly diabetic patients can be treated with a 'no-added-sugar' diet. Those who are on oral hypoglycaemic agents or insulin injections may need their diet to be individually tailored by a dietitian.

Patients who are treated by diet alone and are overweight would follow the same advice as given above for people who are overweight.

A 'no-added-sugar' diet for those who are not overweight avoids sugar or glucose in drinks; jam, marmalade, honey, syrup, sweetened puddings, cakes and sweet biscuits; it encourages a high-fibre diet by including wholemeal bread and cereals.

Remember that regular meals are important for patients with diabetes. For those who are on oral hypoglycaemic agents or insulin, meal replacements should be made with a drink or other suitable food. The dietitian will give you a suitable list.

Low-fat diets

Low-fat diets may be needed for medical reasons. The following foods should be avoided – each of the foods being followed, in brackets, by foods which can be provided as alternatives: all fried foods (grilled, baked, steamed dishes); fatty meat, including paté, sausages, corned beef (lean meats, chicken, turkey); pastry and pies; oily fish (white fish: cod, haddock, plaice); eggs; cheese (cottage cheese, low-fat curd cheese); ordinary butter and margarine (low-fat spread, fortified with vitamin D); ordinary milk (skimmed milk); ice cream (sorbet, jellies); malted milk drinks (tea, coffee, fruit juice); cream soups (consomme, vegetable soups); chocolates (boiled sweets, peppermints).

Note. A low-fat diet is lower in energy than an ordinary diet, and this must be compensated for by increasing the amount of bread, potatoes, cereals and sweet foods provided. If a low-fat diet is continued for more than three months, fat-soluble vitamin supplements will be required.

High-protein diets

High-protein diets may be needed for a variety of reasons. The patient may be poorly nourished, or may have increased need due to infections, poor wound healing or pressure sores. Protein comes mainly from milk, cheese, eggs, fish and all kinds of meat. Vegetarians will rely on cereal sources such as bread, cereals and pulses (peas, beans and lentils).

The main problem can be one of a poor appetite, and it is essential that the energy intake is adequate in order to get the advantage of the higher protein intake.

Extra milk-based savoury sauces can be given with meat or fish dishes, and on vegetables. In addition, desserts should be made with a milk basis, or with custard or evaporated milk – or an egg added. Meals and drinks can have additional protein added by mixing two tablespoons of skimmed milk powder to each pint of milk and then using this milk mixture as ordinary milk.

Supplements

Supplementary drinks should be used for replacing meals not eaten, or for extra nourishment between meals. These can be either home-made, by adding milk powder to milk and using for flavoured drinks, or with flavoured ice cream for milk shakes, adding to cream soups or milk shake syrups, and so forth. Alternatively, powdered supplements can be obtained in sachets to add to milk; these include Complan (Crookes Products Ltd), Build Up (Carnation Health Care) or similar. Some companies make sip supplements which come in individual containers in a variety of flavours. The range available is constantly being added to.

It is important that supplements are not given just before meals, as this will reduce the amount eaten at the meal.

REFERENCES

Davies, L. (1981) *Three Score Years . . . and Then?* Heinemann Medical Books, London.
DHSS (1970) First report by the panel on nutrition of the elderly. Report on Public Health and Medical Subjects No. 123. HMSO, London.
DHSS (1972) A nutritional survey of the elderly. Report on Public Health and Medical Subjects No. 3. HMSO, London.
DHSS (1979) Nutrition and health in old age. Report on Health and Social Subjects No. 16. HMSO, London.
DHSS (1979) Recommended daily amounts of food energy and nutrients for groups of people in the UK. Report on Health and Social Subjects No. 15. HMSO, London.
DOH (1989) Chilled and Frozen. Guidelines on Cook-Chill and Cook-Freeze Catering Systems. HMSO, London.
Exton-Smith, A.N., Stanton, B.R. and Windsor, A.C.M. (1972) Nutrition of housebound old people. King Edward's Hospital Fund for London, London.
Exton-Smith, A.N. (1988) Nutrition in the elderly, in *Nutrition in the Clinical Management of Disease* (eds J.W.T. Dickerson and H.A. Lee), pp. 133–37, Edward Arnold, London.
Fenton (1989) Some food for thought. *Health Service J*, **99**, 666–7.
Jones, Eleri, Hughes, R.E. and Davies H.E.F. (1988) Intake of Vitamin C and other nutrients by elderly patients receiving a hospital diet. *J. Hum. Nutrit. Dietet*, **1**, 347–53.

FURTHER READING AND REFERENCE BOOKS

Asian Patients in Hospital and at Home. A. Henley. King Edwards Hospital Fund for London, London.

Davies L. and Holdsworth, M.D. (1979) A technique for assessing nutritional at risk factors in residential homes for the elderly. *Journal of Human Nutrition,* **33** 165–9.
The Home Assessment kits discussed in this article are available from The Gerontology Nutrition Unit, Royal Free Hospital, London NW3.
Catering for Minority Groups. Catering and Dietetic Branch, DHSS. HMSO, London.
Chilled and Frozen. Guidelines on Cook-Chill and Cook-Freeze Catering Systems. HMSO, London.
Eating a Way into the '90s. A handbook for those concerned with providing meals for the elderly. Nutrition Advisory Group for the Elderly (NAGE). British Dietetic Association, Birmingham.
Health Service Catering – Nutrition and Modified Diets. Catering Dietetic Branch, DHSS, HMSO, London.
Three Score Years . . . and Then? Louise Davies. Heinemann Medical Books, London.

Chapter 8

Ward furniture and equipment

Whilst concentrating upon the medical and nursing care of any patient it is easy to forget that much can usually be done to improve that patient's life by changing his environment. Successful living is surely dependent upon a state of equilibrium between the patient and his environment. After disease or injury this equilibrium is disturbed, and all therapy should be directed towards its re-establishment. Improvement in the patient's condition sometimes proves very difficult because of the severity of the disease. In these circumstances modification of the environment may provide the key to improvement in the quality of life. A major part of our environment is the furniture around us, and this is particularly true for the patient admitted to long-term care in a hospital, nursing home, local authority home or rest home. In addition, special equipment will be needed to overcome particular difficulties for the patient and for the staff caring for him. It is with these aspects that this chapter is concerned.

BEDS

There are two conflicting considerations to be borne in mind in the choice of a bed for a patient in long-stay accommodation. If the patient is able to get in and out of bed, then the bed must be of such a height from the ground that the patient can sit on the edge of the bed with his feet on the ground. The shorter the patient, the lower the bed will need to be. However, the nurses or care assistants will find such a low bed difficult to make, and nursing a patient in a low bed gives rise to back strain. A much higher bed is therefore favoured by the staff. In hospital this problem is overcome by having beds of adjustable height, and the same solution could be adopted in a nursing home.(Figure 8.1). People come in different shapes and sizes, and this applies to the staff as well as the patients. In any long-stay accommodation it may be wise therefore to provide a selection of different beds. Some should be adjustable, whilst others may be the height of a bed at home for those patients who are being rehabilitated. The mechanisms for altering the height of the bed

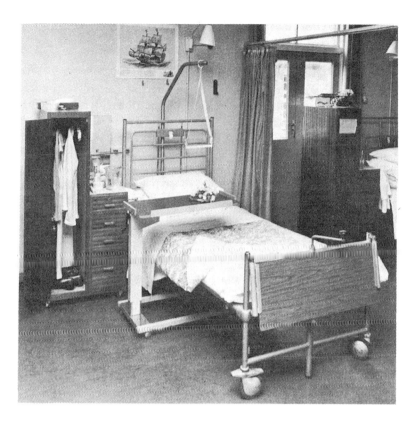

Figure 8.1 Adjustable height bed with continental quilt.

vary from one manufacturer to another. On older beds there is a detachable handle which elevates or lowers the bed by means of a screw. More recently an hydraulic system has been used and this is operated by a foot pedal. This tends to be somewhat jerky in raising the bed, but it is smoother when the bed is being lowered.

It is essential that the wheels or castors are capable of being locked, so that the bed does not move either when the nurses are attending to the patient or when the patient is sitting on the edge of the bed.

All hospital beds are fitted with an adjustable backrest to give support when the patient is sitting up. These built-in backrests are preferable to separate supports which are placed on the bed and which are often used in a patient's home. The integral backrest must be easily adjustable by a nurse, preferably using one hand, and it must not retract suddenly when leant back upon by a heavy patient. Other beds have an electric motor which can raise the head end of the bed or lower the foot end. This has the advantage that it may be controlled by the patient, giving him a measure of independence. The controls can be managed even by a patient with crippling deformities of the hands. The lowering of the foot end of the bed is of great value to those who prefer to sleep sitting up because of respiratory or cardiac disease.

The choice of bedding is important. The mattress should be firm, particularly at the edge in order to give the patient good support. On all modern beds the base of the bed is a solid sheet of metal. Upon this is the mattress, which previously was an interior-sprung one, fitted closely so that it could not slip. More usually now the mattress is made of foam plastic, often in several layers as in the 'Vaperm Mattress'. Another design is the 'Talley Mattress', which is made of foam in two distinct layers; the upper layer is deeply cut, forming a pattern through its three-inch depth, while the lower layer, which is bonded to the upper, is entire. The sides are made of separate strips of more solid foam, stuck to the sides of the two layers, providing firm edges. The whole is contained in a nylon fitted cover. This type of mattress is very comfortable and is greatly favoured by nurses for the frail thin patient.

When the prevention or treatment of pressure sores is required, an alternating pressure mattress may be used on top of the ordinary mattress. This consists of two sets of air-filled tubes running alternately. By means of an electric pump under the bed one set of tubes is inflated whilst the other is deflated. The process is then reversed. With the alternation from one set of tubes to the other the area of the patient that is supported is changed regularly. The best diameter for the tubes is not agreed, but those of wider bore are favoured now.

A variation of this is the Air Wave System used for the 'Pegasus Mattress', which has two layers of air-filled cells. There are three sets of horizontal wide-bore tubes in each layer, each set being deflated in rotation.

For some patients who have pressure sores, or who are at great risk, such as paraplegics, a water-bed may be used. (Figure 8.2). It consists of an impermeable membrane single-cell sack filled with water, at a thermostatically controlled temperature of 37°C and circulated by a pump under the bed. There are two main types – the shallow water bed and the deep bed. The shallow bed has a thicker outer membrane which is filled fairly taut by the water. When the patient lies on this mattress it shapes itself to his contours, in a similar way to a foam mattress, with the patient lying on the surface. In contrast, the deep water-bed has a very large thin outer membrane which is only partially filled with

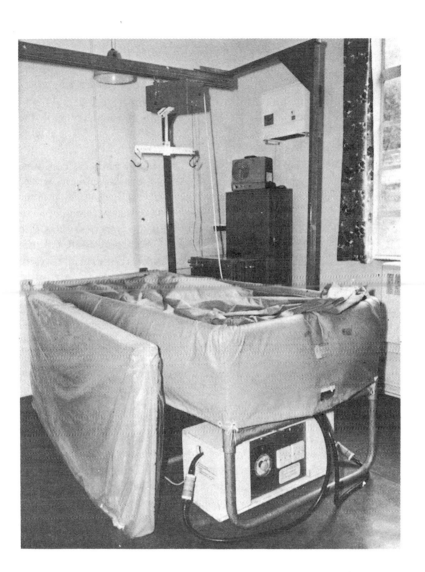

Figure 8.2 A Beaufort-Winchester water-bed with hoist and gantry.

water, so that the membrane on the upper surface is loose. The patient lying upon this mattress sinks into it as though floating on his back in the sea with only his head and toes above the surface. In both cases the objective is to spread the weight of the patient over the whole of his back area – shoulders, back, buttocks, thighs and calves – thereby reducing the pressure to a few ounces per square inch. Both beds are useful, but it is found that the warm water and the plastic membrane provoke sweating and the smell of human secretions can be quite fierce and offensive. For this reason, and because many elderly patients are worried by the floating sensation, water beds are less often used than formerly.

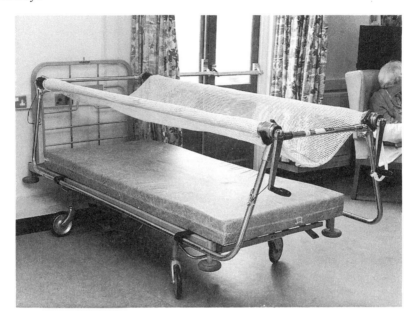

Figure 8.3 A net bed.

Net beds (Figure 8.3) are now popular for nursing the patient who is liable to develop pressure sores. The patient lies on a mesh net which adopts the shape of the patient's lower surface. The net, which is of considerable width, is wound on two long rollers, one on each side of the bed, supported upon a superstructure attached to the ordinary bed. The rollers are controlled by two handles at the foot of the bed. By rotating the handles in opposite directions the patient may be elevated or lowered. Once in the raised position, the patient may be turned from one position to another by one nurse turning the two handles in the same direction. This is a great advantage where the nurses are busy or in short supply, such as at night. There are disadvantages to the net bed however. The patient is suspended a long way above the ground and may feel insecure. If the net is fairly loose between the rollers the patient's shoulders are pushed together and this restricts respiratory movements. If, on the other hand, the net is too taut the patient loses the supporting effect and spreading of his weight, and his sense of vulnerability is increased without any sides to the 'hammock', being so high from the ground. The pressure of the mesh upon the patient's under surface produces a pattern on the skin which is transient. For nursing procedures the patient is lowered onto the bed below.

As a general rule, pillows need to be firm, except perhaps for the top pillow. Elderly patients need many pillows, especially if they have any cardiac or respiratory disease. For support in bed an inverted V-shaped pillow has been made. The point of the V is placed behind the patient's head, and the two wings of the pillow then support the patient on either side. This is of help to those with a marked dorsal kyphosis. The V-shaped pillow may be useful for a hemiplegic patient. One wing of the pillow is placed liked an ordinary pillow behind the patient's head and neck. The other half lies down the hemiplegic side supporting the paralysed arm and hand. A patient who is well-supported by pillows can do far more in bed unaided than the patient who has slipped down or to one side surrounded by soft pillows.

The traditional bedding of sheets, blankets and an eiderdown can be very restricting for the patient, especially if well tucked in by an enthusiastic nurse. Most beds are still made in this manner involving much work for the attendants. Continental quilts are now much more popular and have been used with the precaution of a waterproof cover. They have proved surprisingly popular with older patients and with the staff, who welcome the easier, quicker bed-making. A top sheet is used under the quilt. The patient is kept warm without undue pressure from the bedclothes and is able to move in bed more easily. This may prove a factor in the prevention of pressure sores. Polyester sheets allow the patient to move more easily but may provoke sweating which can, in turn, encourage breakdown in elderly thin skin. Similarly, plastic sheeting placed under the lower sheet may hasten pressure sores in those patients who are incontinent of urine and/or faeces. The bedclothes should be made of material that is fire-retarding. This is especially true when the patient smokes. Indeed, all the materials around, such as curtains, chair coverings and even the patient's clothing should be fire-resistant. The majority of hospital beds have a shelf at the lower end to support the bedclothes when they are turned down whilst the bed is being made. This shelf either folds down when not in use or can be retracted into the base of the bed.

When sheets and blankets are used, and it is necessary to keep the weight of the bedclothes off the patient's leg, either because of a hemiplegia or because of arthritis, a bed cradle may be used. Bed cradles are not popular with a number of patients because their feet feel cold in the space beneath the cradle. Care must be exercised in the choice of bed cradle to ensure that there are no sharp edges and that there is an adequate distance between the two arms. This must be large enough for the depth of the mattress and the length of the patient's feet. This is significant when the patient is a tall ex-policeman!

To protect the vulnerable areas of the sacrum, hips, buttocks and heels from pressure, artificial sheepskins, which are washable, may be used. Pads of plastic foam are useful in the same way. One of these, the Lennard pad, is designed to be wrapped around the patient's ankle to keep both malleoli and the heel off the bed at all times. A tubigrip sock may be placed over the patient's heel to prevent friction sores. Pads of foam cut to the appropriate size can be used between the patient's knees, particularly in those with severe rheumatoid arthritis. Pads may be cut and scooped out to fit particular parts of the patient's anatomy such as the elbow. A useful cushion for use with the very deformed patient consists of a large number of fine polystyrene beads and air in a plastic cover with a valve. The cushion with the valve open is shaped to the body so that the patient is comfortable. When the air is extracted from the cushion with a vacuum pump, the cushion forms a perfect cast of the part of the patient needing support.

The use of cot-sides is controversial. If an ill patient is restless, or if a patient is paralysed down one side, it is felt by some that cot-sides should be used. For most patients however the presence of cot-sides is very disturbing. Newton's third law of physics should be borne in mind – to every action there is an equal and opposite reaction. If a patient is placed in a cage it will only provoke increased exertions for escape. There can no longer be any mental hospitals that employ padded rooms for the restraint of manic patients; they recognize that such restriction is counterproductive. In the same way cot-sides should not be used unless there is no other way of keeping the patient from falling out of bed. In the past thirty eight years that I have practiced elderly patient medicine, two patients under my care have fractured their skulls falling out of bed over cot-sides, and more have fractured their arms, collar-bones or legs. The effect of finding themselves confined behind bars has an adverse effect on patients and is very distressing to relatives and friends.

For patients with a hemiplegia, arthritis of the hips or knees or an amputation, an overhead pole, attached to the frame of the bed, with a handle on a chain or strap will be helpful. (Figure 8.1). By using his good arm (or arms) he can lift himself into the sitting position, or he can lift his buttocks off the bed to relieve pressure or to help his attendants. This often enables the patient to be assisted by one nurse rather than two. In a similar way 'a rope ladder', with wooden rungs, attached to the foot end of the bed, will make it possible for some patients to pull themselves from the lying to the sitting position unaided.

For patients who have to be nursed flat in bed it is possible to fix mirrors in suitable places to enable them to see what is happening around them or the view from the window.

BEDSIDE LOCKERS

One of the worst features of long-term care in an institution is the loss of nearly all of the patient's personal treasures. For any patient therefore a good bedside locker is a vital place in which to keep the few personal belongings that remain. Whether the locker is also required to accommodate his clothes depends upon the arrangements in the ward or home. If it does, then it will need a higher section for hanging up his outer clothes. It is probably better if these and the patient's undergarments are stored in a separate wardrobe. Access to the locker needs to be easy for the patient to manage both from a chair and from bed. The locker should not have fastenings on the doors that are difficult for elderly hands to open. Most patients find it is easier to store their things in a drawer rather than behind a flap that gives access to a deep compartment, which is dark and whose recesses are beyond the patient's reach. If the locker has castors, they should not allow it to move too easily if the patient leans upon it for support. Many falls are precipitated by pieces of furniture moving away under the patient's weight. Nurses and care assistants should remember to ask the patient's permission before delving into his personal locker.

If it is possible it is best not to have a bedside locker at all, but to use the patient's own chest of drawers from his home.

CHAIRS

The choice of a chair for the individual patient assumes great importance when it is borne in mind that the greatest part of the patient's waking hours will be spent in it. The variation in height and size of patients from the tall to the very small and from the obese to the very thin demands a considerable variation in the height and size of the chairs needed. Unfortunately, very many chairs in everyday use are badly designed and bear little relationshp to the actual shape of the human body. The back of the chair needs a bulge in its lower half in order to support the normal lumbar lordosis. In the same way it needs a shallow depression in its upper half for the normal thoracic kyphosis. A chair that needs a pillow for the back is badly designed. The height of the back of the chair may be short or tall. The chair with the tall back, which supports the patient's head is usually favoured by the long-term patient for sitting in for prolonged periods. The shorter back may be better if the patients are sitting around a table having a meal or playing card games. The seat must be comfortable, but not so soft that it sags under the patient's weight. We have all had the experience of sitting in a so-called 'easy chair' or on a sofa with the seat so low that we are sitting about one foot above the floor with our knees higher than our buttocks. Such chairs tend to have short low-set arms. Even for an athlete such chairs present a problem when the time comes to get up! Such chairs must be avoided in the care of the elderly.

The arms of the chair need to be of the correct height from the seat to support the patients arms when sitting, and they should also protrude forward of the front of the chair so that the patient can place his hands on the front of the arms to push himself up into the standing position. If the arms are not high enough, the patient, especially an arthritis sufferer, will be quite unable to rise from the chair. He will push himself up only to find that his legs are still flexed, although his arms are straight. From this posture it may be impossible to complete the manoeuvre into the standing position. For the immobile patient the chair arms will be required as support, particularly if he has a hemiplegia. Some arms are padded, others have wooden tops, and some have the sides filled in. Open sides to the chair are often better for the more active patient.

The height of the seat from the ground will depend upon the height of the patient and whether or not the patient is mobile. A patient who is able to rise from the chair will need the seat 17 to 20 inches (42 to 50 cm) from the ground. These views on the design of chairs are supported by the findings of workers in biometrics and ergonomics.

The mobility of the chair will depend upon the need to transport the patient from one place to another. Many chairs should not have castors, in particular those for mobile patients. Others will have castors at the front and rubber tips to the rear legs. These rear legs may be raised with a lever, bringing a set of castors down so that the chair may be moved. Such a chair must be rigid, and must not move when the castors are raised.

There are chairs which can be adjusted in height. The legs are telescopic, are changed in length by moving the inner tube out of or into the outer tube to produce the correct height, and are then fixed with a peg. Although stable when there is plenty of overlap between the inner and outer tubes, these chairs tend to be unstable when in the higher positions. By having the front legs longer than the rear legs it is possible to obtain a chair whose seat slopes backwards.

Controversy surrounds the use of chairs that tip back and may be locked at various angles of tilt. The chairs are favoured by some nurses for those patients who tend to slip forwards in an ordinary chair. This sliding in the chair is assisted by the smooth waterproof plastic upholstery with which they are usually covered. The actual tilting of the chair often frightens the patient, particularly if it is jerky. There is no doubt that prolonged backward tilting in a chair provokes a tendecy for the patient to lean backwards when standing. Such tilting chairs should be avoided for those patients who are being taught to stand or to walk again. As many patients as possible should be in this category, even amongst those in long-term nursing accommodation.

To assist patients, in particular those with severe arthritis, to rise from a chair, an ejector seat may be useful. This may be built into the chair, or it may be a separate seat placed on the seat of an ordinary chair. This ejector seat is hinged at the front and is pushed up by springs, the strength of which may be varied according to the weight of the patient and the amount of assistance he needs to get up. When he sits on it the seat locks in the down position. When he wishes to rise, the lock is released by a lever at the side enabling the springs to push him into the erect posture. An automatic lifting chair is worked by a powerful electric motor with a control built into one arm of the chair. Such a chair can also lower the patient from the standing to the sitting position. Some electric lifting chairs also have a reclining back and an elevating foot rest separately controlled.

For those at risk of developing pressure sores, or those with sores, a number of special cushions are available. These may be filled with foam or have alternating pressure in tubes similar to the alternating pressure mattress already described. Water-filled cushions are used, but many nurses prefer a dry flotation cushion filled with air contained in seventy-two separate cells (Figure 8.4). Sheepskins are simple but effective. For those who slide forwards in their chair a wedge of foam deeper at the front may discourage this and protect the pressure areas.

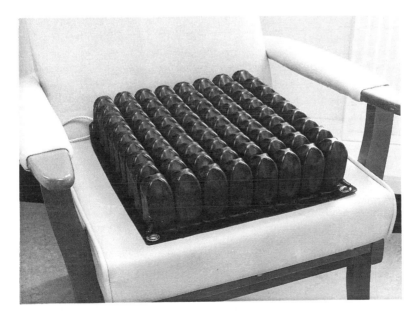

Figure 8.4 A Ro-ho dry flotation cushion.

When sitting for prolonged periods in a chair with their feet on the floor patients develop dependent oedema. This may be helped by a footstool which may have one of two functions. A low footstool raises the feet so that the backs of the patient's thighs do not press on the front of the chair restricting the venous return from the legs. Alternatively, the stool may be of a height equal to that of the seat of the chair thus keeping the legs straight and parallel with the ground. It is essential that any stool must be stable and must not wobble. Dependent oedema may also be treated by an air-filled cuff that envelopes the foot, the calf and most of the thigh. The air pressure in the cuff is reduced and elevated alternately to provide a pumping action encouraging the removal of the oedema.

TABLES

Whilst sitting in a chair the patient will need a table for meals and other activities. Some favour a table attached to the chair, so that it is completely stable; others feel that this is too restricting and recommend a cantilever table, the counterbalancing foot of which goes under the chair. On a tipping chair any table which may be attached should itself be able to be adjusted to a level position. Such a fixed table is favoured by some as a method of keeping the patient in his chair, particularly if he is mentally confused and likely to fall if attempting to rise and walk unaided. In practice such a restriction tends to provoke an adverse reaction in such a patient, increasing his restlessness (remember Newton's third law). Any table attached to the chair must be capable of being removed easily or swung to one side so that the patient may be helped from his chair to use the lavatory or commode. Some patients who are apathetic like to lean forward onto a pillow on a table across the front of the chair, and in this case the fixed table would seem the wiser choice.

Apart from tables for use when in a chair, tables will be needed for use when in bed. Such tables, usually cantilever (Figure 8.1), should have horizontal side sections and a tilting centre section to support a book. There are a series of clamps, poles and adaptors allowing items such as mirrors, book holders and trays to be attached to beds or bedside tables (Orange aids). Other tables are needed for communal meals and for occupational therapy. Such tables should be extremely stable, with a leg at each corner so that they do not shift if a patient uses one for support when walking, or if one is clutched at to prevent the patient who has lost his balance from falling down. Nearly all tables have sharp edges and corners that present a hazard to the patient who momentarily loses balance whilst walking. Theoretically, a rounding of the edges and corners might reduce the damage done by a blow from such a fall. Small flimsy tables must be avoided altogether. Sitting four patients around a square table promotes conversation and makes playing card games or other activities easy. If patients sit around the walls of a room, side by side, conversation with a neighbour is not easy when they cannot look at each other directly. This is made doubly difficult if the patient has arthritis of the cervical spine, as so many elderly patients have. Conversation involves the eyes and not just the tongue.

WHEELCHAIRS

Many arthritic patients, and some who have had one or both legs amputated, are able to regain a measure of independence once they have mastered the control of a wheelchair. Self-propelled wheelchairs have a set of small rotatable wheels and a pair of large wheels with an outer rim upon which the patient pushes with his hands. The large wheels should be at the back if the patient is able to transfer on and off the chair. Some other patients find propulsion easier if these large wheels are at the front because of the difficulty in putting their arms and hands back to grasp the top of the outer rim. For the patient with arthritis, in particular rheumatoid arthritis, the outer rims may be fitted with pegs like a capstan. These pegs at regular intervals make it much easier for the patient to propel the chair despite the lack of any firm grip in his hands. For the hemiplegic patient wheelchairs may be obtained with either right-handed control or left-handed control of both wheels. Normally there is a separate brake with a lever on each side on the chair. For the hemiplegic patient a brake acting on both wheels may be operated by a lever on the appropriate side. If the patient will be sitting in a self-propelled wheelchair for most of the day, it should have a foam cushion and an appropriately raised backrest to provide adequate support. The footrests are fitted with hinges at the side so that they can be flapped upwards when the patient is getting in or out of the chair. The footrests can also be rotated sideways but are usually fixed in the forward position by small locks. These locks can be operated by a small lever by the nurse or assistant.

For patients who are unable to control a wheelchair for themselves, a chair pushed by an assistant can give welcome mobility outside in the garden or town. Such wheelchairs usually have four small-diameter wheels, and tend to be quite difficult to manoeuvre because of the difficulty in steering.

There are several designs of mechanical chairs relying upon an electric battery, which needs to be charged regularly. The chair is controlled by a lever which is pressed down to start and is moved from side to side for steering. It is moved back for reversing. These chairs are ideal for many severely disabled people including those with severe arthritis of the hands, wrists and arms.

As with a motorcar, wheelchairs require regular servicing. A drop or two of oil on moving parts makes work for the patient minimal. The brakes in particular need regular adjusting to ensure that the wheels really are locked when the brake is on. The tyres are usually pneumatic and need regular pumping up – a soft or flat tyre increases the work of propulsion considerably. The footrests often cause trouble by dropping off at inopportune moments after the chair has been in use for some years. Many wheelchairs are capable of being folded flat so that they take up less space when stored or placed in the boot of a car.

HOISTS

The heavy or severely disabled patient presents a problem to the nursing

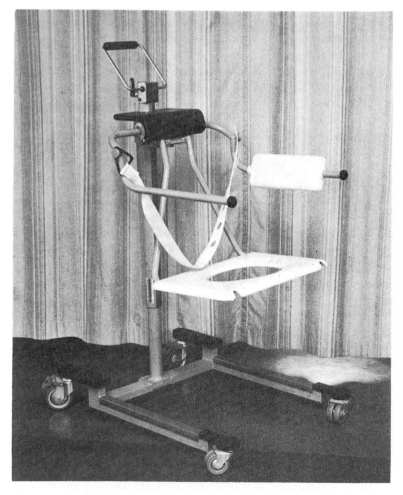

Figure 8.5 An Ambulift hoist with slings and chair attachment.

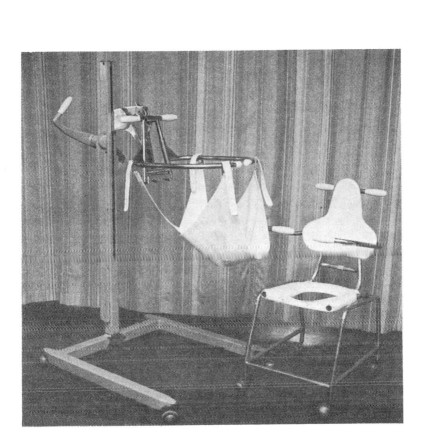

Figure 8.6 An Argo hoist showing how the patient sits sideways.

staff or assistants when he needs lifting from the bed, from a chair or into the bath. In a modern factory heavy weights are not lifted by hand but are transported by mechanical means. Nurses should not be expected to risk damaging their backs with such heavy manual work in what is already a tiring job. Nurses and assistants need to become familiar with the use of hoists. These may be fixed or mobile. It is very valuable in any long-stay ward to have an electric hoist suspended from the ceiling over the centre of one or more beds. This hoist moves on a rail bolted to the ceiling joists. It is used with slings which vary in design but which mostly have a wide band across the patient's back and under the arms. A second wide band passes under the thighs, leaving the lower back and buttocks between the two slings so that the patient is hoisted in the sitting position. A similar fixed hoist is valuable over a water-bed or over a bath. An electric hoist can also be mounted on a tripod frame which can be used over the patient's bed and which helps to move the patient from his bed to a commode or chair alongside. This is a very valuable piece of equipment in the patient's own home.

There are several types of mobile hoist (Figures 8.5 and 8.6), all with long cantilever legs, which are wide enough apart to fit one on each side of a bath, but equally not too wide apart to prevent going through doorways. The lifting of the patient is achieved either by an hydraulic pump or by a geared chain drive controlled by rotating a lever. These hoists are manually operated. The patient will be supported in slings similar to those for the fixed electric hoist, or he may sit on a plastic seat with movable supporting arms on either side. Nurses find that hoists, with familiarity, are a very great help with many patients. It must be recognized that patients at first find the slings uncomfortable, and being moved suspended in the hoist can be frightening. Nurses need to be reassuring to the patient when using a hoist on a patient, especially for the first time.

TRANSFERS

It is not always appropriate or possible to employ a hoist when a patient is lifted in the bed or from the bed to a chair or commode. Although two nurses are well able to lift a patient without any special device, there is a blue plastic sling with hand holds at each end which is very useful (Figures 8.7 and 8.8). If slipped under the patient's thighs it makes lifting easier for the nurses and often more comfortable for the patient.

Transferring a patient from his bed to a chair or commode can be difficult. If the patient is quite unable to help himself the blue plastic sling may be used. Other patients are able to help to some extent, but are not able to stand. For these a shuffleboard, which is a smooth piece of timber, sloping from the bed to the chair is used. Supported by the nurse, the patient sits on the edge of the bed at the upper end of the board and manoeuvres himself down the board onto the chair. It can be used, but seems less successful for the return journey. For those patients, who are able to stand by the bed with help but cannot walk, a turntable on the floor may be employed. Once the patient is standing on the turntable he can be rotated round from the bed

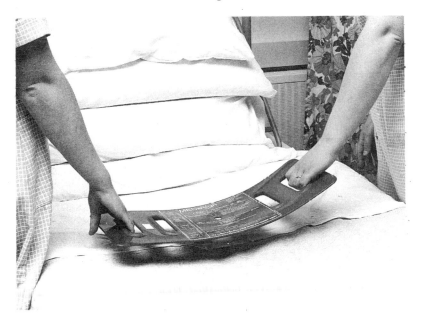

Figure 8.7 A Medesign patient handling sling.

until his back is opposite the chair, into which he can then be seated.

When a patient, who cannot walk, needs to be moved up and down stairs each day a stair-lift may be used. This is custom-built for the staircase and has a seat moving slowly on a rail at the side of the stairs. It is electrically operated, and so is quite smooth, but many patients find it frightening at first and need reassurance.

WALKING AIDS

The number of patients in long-stay accommodation, who are able to walk, may be small, but many more will be able to stand and take a step or two with help in order to loosen stiff muscles and joints. To use a walking stick needs a strong grip and wrist, both of which do not exist in most of these patients. A tripod or tetrapod stick is much more stable and is more widely used. It is interesting that the modern metal tetrapod stick is a development of the wooden four-legged stick originally designed by the late Dr Marjorie Warren and made by the hospital carpenter for the rehabilitation of hemiplegic patients more than fifty years ago. For those patients able to grip with both hands a lightweight walking frame is the best walking aid as it is really stable. It is useful too, by way of support, when the patient stands up from a chair albeit with help.

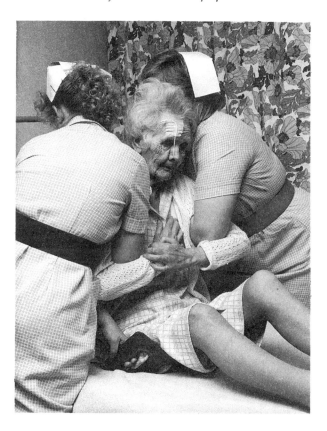

Figure 8.8   A patient being lifted on handling sling.

Occasionally a patient finds a walking frame with wheels on the front legs is easier to manage than the ordinary frame that must be lifted up and moved forward every couple of steps. If the patient has a poor grip in his hands, the walking frame may be fitted with gutter supports for his forearms and vertical handles for his hands to hold.

It is not wise to issue an adjustable stick to a patient for permanent use since any such device is less stable than a solid one. The higher the stick is adjusted the less stable it becomes. This stricture also applies to an adjustable walking frame and to adjustable crutches. The proper use of an adjustable stick is to measure the height of stick that the patient requires. A wooden stick can then be cut to this height and marked with the patient's name. For the elderly, crutches are best avoided altogether, whether the crutches are used in the axillae or with gutters for the patient's forearms. If used in the axillae, palsies may be caused by pressure on the nerves. The patient who loses his balance, when using crutches, is unable to save himself from falling since he is effectively splinted on either side. The resulting fall will be severe, either onto his face or backwards.

For an amputee, a necessary standing or walking aid is an artificial limb. It is true that many long-stay above-knee amputees reject their prosthesis because the back of the socket cuts into the back of the stump when they are spending most of the day sitting in a chair. For some, the wearing of their artificial limb, often a pylon, makes them feel more complete and enables them to stand between chair and bed and walk a few steps. For the double amputee the wearing of one or both prostheses makes it much easier to sit in a chair without the danger of toppling forward. For the long-stay patient, as his stump shrinks, the socket needs lining with soft leather or padding in order to prevent it causing pain by pressure, particularly on the front of the pelvis, or chafing by movement between the stump and the socket.

BATHS AND SHOWERS

After an old person has been managing, or rather failing to manage, alone, one of the greatest joys of being admitted to hospital or to a home is that of being clean again. He may not have been able to have a proper bath for years because of his disabilities. Getting into and out of an ordinary bath is difficult, and with slippery bath surfaces, a wet body and a smooth floor, the chances of falling are great. Similarly, from the nurse's viewpoint, baths and bathrooms are problem areas unless careful consideration is given to the difficulties that arise in handling a wet naked disabled patient. When the patient is being rehabilitated the design of the bath must suit him or her, but when he or she requires long-term care it is the convenience of the nurses or care assistants that should be paramount.

The ordinary domestic bath has its bottom near the floor and has high sides. It is usually installed with one side against a wall. In a hospital or home the bath should be shallower, with its bottom well above the floor. It should be free-standing, with its head only against a wall and with free access to both sides and the end, with plenty of space for manoeuvring around it. It should not be boxed in at the sides, allowing the nurse's feet to go under the edges of the bath and the feet of the mobile hoist to pass on either side of it. Fixed metal handles at the sides of the bath are best avoided as they are additional hazards to the patient's perineum whilst getting into and out of the bath. Non-slip strips may be stuck onto the bottom of the bath to prevent the patient from sliding down from the sitting position in the soapy water. If the patient finds it difficult to lie flat in the bath, and because of arthritis finds the sitting posture easier, then a wooden seat that fits down in the bath may be used. The taps should be simple and unobtrusive but can be fitted with special handles to make them easier to use with arthritic hands. A shower attachment with a hose fixing onto the taps is useful for hair washing.

There are several special baths designed to assist the entry of a disabled person. One of these, the Medic bath, has a water-tight door and is made so that when in the bath the patient is in the sitting position. The door is closed and the bath filled with water at the correct temperature. After bathing the water must be emptied out before the door can be opened and the patient removed from the bath to be dried. Even in a heated bathroom it is not easy to keep the patient warm whilst the bath is filling and emptying.

Another design is the Parker bath, which is able to tip backwards and forwards. With the bath in the upright position the deep foot end is filled with water. The patient sits in the upper part of the bath, swings his legs round into the lower end and the door is shut. The bath is slowly tipped into the horizontal position so that the water flows around the whole patient. When washing is completed the bath is tipped back into the upright position again, the door is opened and the patient lifted out of the bath for drying before the water is drained out. The tipping process takes only a few seconds and, providing the nurse is standing by the patient, it does not seem to cause any alarm. The only criticism is that the mechanism for tipping back is rather jerky.

There are also designs for a cantilevered bath which can be raised and lowered. With the bath in the lowest position it is filled with water and the patient helped into the bath. By an automatic hydraulic mechanism the bath is raised to a convenient height for the nurse to wash the patient. The bath is lowered again so that the patient can be lifted out for drying. It is easier to manage the patient if the hoist has a chair in which he is transported and which can be lowered into the bath with him. For the patient who cannot sit up a stretcher attachment on the hoist allows the patient to be moved and bathed with the minimum of disturbance.

Showers are more familiar to younger people than to the elderly patients of today. As the years pass they will be more popular. For the disabled a shower taken in the sitting position in a warm bathroom may be the easiest way of washing all over. A chair made of wood, such as teak, is better than a cold metal or plastic one, and is less slippery. The shower spray is best held in the nurse's hand rather than fixed overhead. It may be that a shower is the easiest way to clean a patient after faecal incontinence. A bidet is also available for this task.

Washbasins for patients in long-stay accommodation should be of simple design, mounted at a height suitable for use from a wheelchair, and the taps should be easily turned on and off with arthritic hands. Washbasins need to be near to the lavatories, preferably in a lobby between the lavatory and the corridor.

Electric points for shavers need to be mounted within reach of a sitting patient with a mirror at a suitable height.

LAVATORIES

It is said, not without justification, that old people are obsessed with their bowels and micturition. This is easy to understand when the bowels are sluggish and there is urgency of micturition due to lessening of the power of control. The majority of old patients would be continent if they could, and are distressed when they lose control. In any long-stay accommodation there should be plenty of lavatories, preferably one for every four patients. At certain times of day, such as first thing in the morning and after main meals, they will all be needed. One of the commonest causes of incontinence is delay in getting to a lavatory. The design of lavatories must emphasize the needs of disabled patients. Lavatories should not be 'the smallest room', for much space is needed for a wheelchair to enter and manoeuvre round. There must be space for attendants to help transfer the patient and attend to him. The door should open outwards and may be better divided into two narrower doors. Privacy is essential for the comfort and dignity of the patient, so the doors should reach from floor to ceiling and should not have a window in them.

The height of the lavatory basin with the seat down should be the same as that of the wheelchair and of the correct height for a Sanichair to pass over it. This is of particular importance when a male patient is on the Sanichair lest the genitalia are pinched between the two seats. A higher lavatory basin will be needed for patients with severe osteoarthrosis of their hips and knees who cannot sit in a fully flexed position. For these there are shaped plastic seats of various heights that fit onto the lavatory basin itself and are washable.

Supporting bars near the lavatory basin are important. Many of the designs for these are very poor and can be dangerous, precipitating a fall if the patient rises unaided. Any supporting bar must be stable, firm and without wobble. Thus, mobile bars are to be avoided, such as those that hinge up onto the wall beside the seat and cistern with a hinged leg that comes down when it is brought forward into position. The leg of such 'supports' has no attachment to the floor and is consequently unstable. A tubular metal frame screwed into the back wall and into the floor is better, but care must be taken to ensure that the two bars are wide enough apart for the Sanichair to pass between. A better arrangement is a pair of bars, designed by Dr John Agate (Ipswich, Suffolk, England), which slope upwards and forwards from beside the lavatory basin to the roof (Figure 8.9). These are made firmer by a horizontal bar back to the wall behind the basin. Not only are these bars rigid but they

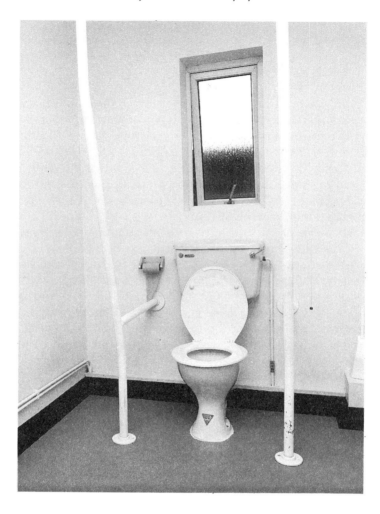

Figure 8.9 A lavatory with Agate bars.

also enable the patient to move from the sitting to the standing position by pulling on one or both poles, however tall he may be. There must be sufficient space alongside the lavatory basin outside any bars for the nurse to attend to the patient after defaecation. There should be lavatories not only in the ward area, and opening off the day rooms, but it is wise to have one near, or in, each bathroom.

Sanichairs and commodes are most useful. The Sanichair is used to move the patient rapidly from the ward or day-room to the lavatory. It must have firm arms at the sides to support the patient, and efficient brakes on its wheels. There is usually a rack under the lavatory type seat for a bedpan, which should be in place for all patients with precipitancy. There should be a footrest for the patient's feet, and this may be retractable. Similar considerations apply to a commode with regard to the need for rigid arms, and the commode should be immobile or fitted with good brakes.

FLOOR COVERINGS

It goes without saying that the floors in any area for elderly patients must be non-slip. An aspect that is often forgotten is that the floor should not look slippery to the patients as this will undermine their confidence when trying to stand or walk. Most floor coverings seem to be made of vinyl which may well be non-slip but appears shiny. If the patient has the usual plastic-soled shoes and the vinyl is dusty, the dust adheres to these shoes which then have little grip on the floor. For particularly hazardous areas like bathrooms and lavatories vinyl may be obtained with grains of carborundum embedded into its surface to enhance grip.

There is debate about the best surface for the floor of the sitting room or day-room, where the obvious objective of trying to make it as homely and comfortable as possible with a carpet, must be weighed against the need to have a surface that can cope with spilt drinks, urine and faeces on occasions. There are nylon carpets that can washed but they may become stained and offensive looking unless cleaned throughly and regularly. Alternatively, carpet squares may be laid, and these may be moved about and replaced as any deteriorate. Rugs are popular because they make a more homely atmosphere but they are liable to slip especially if a patient treads at one end. This is particularly true if they are on a vinyl surface: The smaller the rug the more likely it is to slide away; these latter are often called, with justification, slip mats!

LIGHTING

Increasing age generally produces a diminution in visual acuity. It is necessary to have a good level of illumination not only in the ward and sitting room but also in the corridors and sanitary annexes. This light is best diffused or indirect, for too bright a direct light causes a glare, which can worry patients, particularly those with a cataract. When a patient wishes to read or do handiwork an adjustable table-lamp which throws a pool of bright light onto the work, not at the patient, is preferable. This light in conjunction with a hand-held magnifying glass will often assist those with poor sight more than a new pair of glasses.

Bright sunlight through the window either in the bedroom or sitting room can dazzle elderly patients. Venetian blinds provide a way of obtaining good illumination without direct light.

MISCELLANEOUS EQUIPMENT

When one considers how much each patient has abandoned on entering a long-stay institution, every effort should be made to make the environment as comfortable and personal as possible. Is there any valid reason why pieces of furniture such as a chest of drawers or a favourite chair should not come with him from his now abandoned home? Private rest homes and nursing homes often do this, but National Health Service long-stay wards and Local Authority Welfare Homes seem reluctant to follow suit. The patient's personal pictures and photographs should be hung on the walls. Uniformity of beds, lockers, chairs and tables should be avoided, for the patients would value having their own familiar furniture reminding them of the past.

Many patients have personal radio or television sets so that they can choose their own entertainment. Tastes in music and other programmes differ but it is certain that the continuous 'pop music' played in most long-stay accommodation is to very few patients' tastes, being for a younger generation altogether. A point worth consideration is the design of the controls on personal radios, for many sets on the market have small control knobs on slides that are difficult for a weak or deformed hand to manage. Pre-set stations with simple buttons to press on and off are better. For television, remote infra-red ray controls are now a very great help. For the deaf patient it is only fair, on him and on other patients, if the sound from his set is passed into light-weight earphones, rather than disturbing everybody.

It is, alas, true that there are many pieces of ward furniture and equipment that are produced although they are quite unsuitable for a variety of reasons. In view of the expense involved it is wise to have a discussion involving all the members of the health care team before any new items are purchased. Similarly, such a multi-disciplinary approach is needed for the design of new accommodation for the elderly, whether this is a hospital ward, a nursing home, a rest home or special housing in the community.

The fact that the ward is to the long-stay patient *his* home must never be forgotten.

Chapter 9

Communication with patients in residence

What is communication? We hear the word bandied around so much these days. This is the age of the satellite, of electronic telecommunication which can transmit messages across continents and the universe. We are able to say a few sentences to an anonymous ear and know that it will be received in writing by someone sitting in an office on the other side of the world. We are able to programme computers to give us the results of complicated equations and questions. All these important functions have one thing in common – they begin with a human being.

Communication skills develop from birth. Very few of us are able to remember how we learned the ability to express ourselves in response to other people. Linguists and psycholinguists have described in detail the development of human communication, but for most of us, however, there has never been the need to analyse the changes in voice inflection that can totally alter the meaning of a word or the sequencing of words that can change a statement into a question. It is only where there is a breakdown in the flow of understanding and expression that the alarm is raised and frustration begins both for the receiver and transmitter.

Communication skills are taken for granted in most normal healthy individuals but the underlying processes can be extremely involved and complicated. A look at a simple model of these skills shows some of the complex procedures necessary to complete the chain (Figure 9.1). This

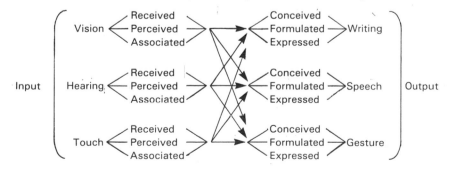

Figure 9.1 Communication. (Adapted from Porch, 1971, with permission).

diagram does not illustrate olfactory or kinaesthetic senses but it may be true that all things we hear, see, touch, smell or feel in movement can be expressed in one or more of several ways.

A speech therapist is trained to look at all aspects of communication and to assess the abilities as well as the breakdowns. Although many patients in long-term care are several years post onset, there is evidence to demonstrate that further intervention is beneficial. Helm-Estabrooks and Ramsberger (1986) demonstrated the positive effects of further therapy for patients with dysphasia of five to seven years duration. For many patients with speech and language difficulties following an acquired neurological incident, it is the residual skills which have to be practised and made proficient if there has been irreparable damage to the more commonly used methods of communiction. This may involve teaching someone to use an electronic communicator or a sign language such as the British Sign Language or Amer-Ind.

COMMUNICATION PROBLEMS FOLLOWING NEUROLOGICAL DAMAGE

Dysphasia

This refers to all aspects of language including comprehension of spoken language, verbal expression, reading, writing, spelling, numerical relations and telling the time. Ideas, plans, thoughts, beliefs and wishes are usually expressed in spoken or written words which should be responded to by apposite speech, writing or gesture. The dysphasic patient will often have a mixture of problems affecting understanding and expression and each dysphasic person will be different. Difficulty may be predominant in one aspect of language and not another. For instance, there may be no difficulty in understanding what is heard and yet there may be a problem following written material or a specific difficulty in naming objects and people.

As each dysphasic person is different, it is important to have an awareness of the patient's difficulties because it will make communication easier and decrease everyone's frustration. Although dysphasia is commonly found in patients with a right-sided hemiplegia, it can occur in patients with a left-sided hemiplegia and also in some patients with no paresis at all. Dysphasia may result following cerebro-vascular accident, head injury, tumour, and in patients who have had neurosurgery.

In the elderly population dementia can also occur, and a major problem for all those involved in the care of some elderly stroke patients is the differential diagnosis of dysphasia and dementia. It is not an easy diagnosis to make but it is important to clarify the patient's position to ensure correct long-term management and intervention by all staff. One of the first essentials is a clear and detailed history of the patient's communication abilities and behaviour before being assessed by the caring team. It may be that the dysphasia has a sudden onset if it is symptomatic of a catastrophic cerebro-vascular accident. However, if a patient has had a series of transient ischaemic attacks, the communication breakdown may be gradual and insidious in its effect on general ability. Patients who are ultimately diagnosed as demented will often have a history over several months of deterioration in communication skills as well as general behaviour. Functions such as memory and concentration may be affected in a demented patient but the same may be true of someone who is dysphasic and who no longer has the language skills to control his environment. A detailed speech and language assessment can be useful in differentiating between dementia and dysphasia. The irregular breakdown of skills in a demented patient, e.g., correct structure of sentences but distorted content, may begin to give some clues for diagnosis. Although far from being conclusive, the degree of frustration and anxiety, which are so often present for the dysphasic, may be a useful indicator. Observing response to therapy will also provide valuable information where the patient attempts to respond to help and achieves success in alternative methods of communication.

Dysarthria

In literal terms, dysarthria means distorted articulation and could therefore result from non-neurological causes such as cleft palate or faulty dentition, but it is more commonly associated with defective articulation owing to neuromuscular disorders. As articulation is the result of a complex process of control and co-ordination of movement of the organs of articulation, any disorders affecting the muscles may reduce the intelligibility of speech. There may be omissions, substitutions and distortions of speech sounds. Rhythm, intonation, stress and speed of utterance can be affected, and as the primary use of the muscles of speech is eating, chewing and swallowing may also be impaired. Drooling may be present, and the voice may be distorted if laryngeal muscles are involved. Dysarthria following a cerebro-vascular accident is found more commonly in patients with left-sided hemiplegia but may occur with right hemiplegia or in some patients with no paresis.

Neurological classification of dysarthria is related to the neuro-muscular system involved. Therefore dysarthrias may have distinct features depending on the site of the lesion. An upper motor neurone lesion may produce a spastic dysarthria, e.g., following certain types of cerebro-vascular accidents or development of motor neurone disease. A lower motor neurone dysarthria may follow a Bell's palsy, and speech will be slurred due to unilateral facial weakness. The dysarthria found in extrapyramidal disorders such as Parkinson's disease results in a weak, monotonous voice with rapid repetitions of syllables and words. Cerebellar dysarthria, such as can occur in multiple sclerosis, is slurred speech with staccato rate and scanning of the utterances. Articulation in dysarthria may range from being weak and indistinct with a soft voice to a specific staccato rate with explosive voice quality.

Dyspraxia

Dyspraxia of speech is a disorder of articulation where the patient may have difficulty in voluntary control of the organs of articulation in the absence of muscle impairment. Chewing and swallowing may be quite normal but the patient will have great difficulty achieving the specific postures for speech.

INTERVENTION

The speech therapist's role with the elderly has greatly expanded in recent years. Therapists have an obvious role in the assessment and treatment of specific disorders resulting from neurological impairment. However, our knowledge of communication has led to involvement in promoting and improving communication for elderly individuals in the hospital environment. Many therapists are involved in Reality Orientation groups for the elderly confused. More general communication groups are also run, involving both the speech impaired, and other elderly patients who would benefit from social contact and encouragement to communicate.

Lubinski (1981) stated that 'communication and its disorders are inextricably related to the environment in which they occur'. Therefore, when considering intervention more general factors affecting elderly patients' ability to communicate will be discussed together with specific aspects of therapy.

Physical factors

Eyesight and hearing often deteriorate in the elderly, and this may cause increased social isolation even in those patients who do not have specific communication problems. It is important, therefore, that spectacles and hearing aids are checked regularly for cleanliness and suitability. Hearing aid moulds are prone to becoming blocked with wax, and batteries need to be changed regularly. Ill-fitting dentures have a marked effect on clarity of speech and can cause a normal-speaking individual to become unclear. Patients should be encouraged to wear their dentures as this will not only boost morale but will assist during eating.

Swallowing problems are common in patients with neurological disorders such as cerebrovascular accident and Parkinson's disease. Each patient requires a detailed assessment to establish at which stage of swallowing the problem is occurring. Management will require input from a number of professionals including medical staff, radiology, dietitians, physiotherapists and nursing staff. Following assessment, treatment may take the form of specific rehabilitative techniques carried out by the speech therapist, e.g., thermal stimulation to aid a delayed swallow reflex (Logemann, 1983). However, other factors such as positioning and altering the consistency of the diet, may have an equally crucial role. Patients with dysphasia will require close attention to ensure that they maintain adequate oral hygiene. Weakened muscles and reduced sensation can cause food to be lodged in the mouth, and the development of ulcers will not only cause discomfort but may lead to a reluctance to eat.

Decreased mobility is a further physical factor increasing isolation. Immobile patients who rely on others in order to change position are limited in the choice of people with whom they can communicate. Care should be taken when positioning patients so that their wishes and needs are considered It is extremely frustrating for the elderly to be aware of other people in the room but be unable to see or hear them because they are too far from their neighbour.

Environmental factors

Lubinski (1981) defines the environment in which many elderly find themselves as: 'a communication-impaired environment'. She describes this as 'a setting in which there are few opportunities available for successful meaningful communication'. The effect of such an environment will be equally depriving for the normal-speaking individual as it is for the communication-impaired.

Anyone who has spent any time in hospital will be familiar with the feelings of insularity. A hospital is a world by itself, governed by routine and procedure. Much of this uniformity is vital to the patient's care and well-being and protects people from outside stresses so that all their energies are concentrated upon recovery. However, for those patients who require long-term care, prolonged exposure to the day-to-day environment of a hospital ward can be disorientating. The result is often withdrawal into silence and inactivity. How often do so-called 'normal' people ask themselves 'What day is it today?', 'What is the date today?', 'What time is it now?'. Reality Orientation aims to provide an environment where patients are constantly provided with such stimuli to assist their orientation. The technique is primarily used with the elderly confused. However, the principles should also be applied by everyone caring for patients who are at risk of losing touch with their environment. Daily routine in a ward can often reinforce orientation for patients when meals are brought at a regular time, or they always have a bath on Wednesdays, etc. However, many patients appreciate the extra stimulation of being told these basic facts, and it can encourage them to use their own initiative to read the newspaper for example, or check the day and date. Barnett-Douglass (1986) demonstrated the success of using the principles of Reality Orientation in a group setting, to improve both the orientation and communication of the elderly in residential homes. Lubinski (1981) states that 'if the environment is static and unchanging, there will be few reasons to talk'. Therefore taking a patient to a window so he can look out at the world or taking him/her to the hospital shop may promote a reason for discussion.

Becoming a long-stay patient does not necessarily mean an end to thoughts and ideas, and for many old people it is immensely reassuring and stimulating to be asked for an opinion on some matter. Even those with communication difficulties are able to share in these sorts of discussions. Patients with residual abilities in any form should be encouraged to maintain and use their skills. In an environment where day-to-day needs are anticipated, patients with speech handicaps may have little opportunity or reason to communicate. Failing to anticipate can lead to the individual experiencing success at communicating, e.g., he or she may be able to gesture how many sugars they want in their tea, or point to where an item is on their locker. Providing situations in which patients are able to convey a message successfully can do much for their self-esteem and will promote further attempts.

Mealtimes are a natural social setting and can provide an excellent opportunity to stimulate discussion. They can revive memories for many different recipes and methods of cooking or the problems associated with rationing during the wars. At our long-stay unit we were able to produce a recipe book from the patients and staff discussing favourite menus. Books, newspapers and magazines have a fund of material to promote communication. Discussions about the changes in fashion over the years of development of do-it-yourself techniques can reveal insights to both patients and staff alike. Taking an interest on a regular basis can alter a patient's outlook on the prospect of long-term care.

For many people, going into a long-stay unit is like a prison sentence with the release being their death. It is never easy to adjust to dramatic change, and the onus is on caring staff to help ensure that the transition is as smooth as possible and that a positive attitude is maintained. There will be those patients, however, who will withdraw and plateau presenting carers with a difficult challenge, especially as one must always have respect for the individual. Unfailing optimism can sometimes have the opposite effect and cause greater retreat and depression. Ensuring that physical comfort and peace is maintained, and showing a quiet concern, may provide the reassurance.

The treatment of a patient in the ward environment can present problems to the speech therapist. It is important that the patient can see the therapist and the materials presented. This may involve ensuring that there is proper support for sitting or being propped up in bed. Hospital wards are busy, often noisy places and it is important to give the patient quietness and privacy to assist reduced attention and memory spans. Whilst shielding the patient from all activity and interest is not encouraged, most dysphasic patients cannot compete with television, radio, traffic noise and general background distractions (Rolnick and Hoops, 1969).

For individual speech therapy treatment it is best to have a separate room that is sound treated, involving carpeting, double glazed windows, acoustic tiles on the ceiling and acoustic tape round the door jamb to reduce outside noise.

THERAPY

After assessments have been completed and a profile of the patient's abilities and problems has been identified, therapy will begin *at the level at which the patient is just able to make a successful response.*

Progress will depend upon many factors – such as severity of the lesion, motivation, associated deficits, health during recovery. However, the patient will be helped considerably if both relatives and staff are aware of, and understand, the techniques being used by the speech therapist to improve communication. For example, if the patient has a severe dysphasia resulting in negligible verbal communication and limited residual abilities, a communication system such as Amer-Ind Gestural Code may be introduced (Skelly, 1979). This enables patients to convey basic concepts via manual signals. Successful acquisition relies heavily on everyone in the patient's environment reinforcing and promoting their use.

Every patient will experience varying levels of difficulty and will require a different therapeutic approach. It is therefore vital that there is close liaison between the speech therapist and other care staff so that communication can be encouraged 24 hours a day and not simply during the therapy session.

Group therapy

Groups are as much a part of therapy as individual treatment because of the encouragement patients can give each other to communicate and the stimulation of competition with peers. Depending on the various levels of communication difficulty present, it may be beneficial to have mixed groups of those people who have specific communication difficulty and those who are able to converse freely. This is particularly helpful in social groups but selection of participants is important and must be carefully considered.

The appendix gives some of the activities used by the speech therapist at our long-stay unit. These activities are used in a large group of patients who attend the Roxbourne Activities Centre (see Chapter 16). This group has mixed abilities in communication skills and is run by the speech therapist with the help of a physiotherapy aid and an occupational therapy helper as well as a volunteer. Dividing into teams can promote lively competition and it is the residents who keep a close eye on the scoreboard! For those residents who are not able to attend the centre or who choose to remain on their ward but enjoy smaller groups of three or four participants, many of these activities can be adapted to promote communication in discussion.

General guidelines to consider when communicating with patients with speech/comprehension deficits

If there are problems understanding language:

1. Make sure that you have the patient's attention. Many dysphasic patients have difficulty concentrating. Touch and eye contact can be helpful in gaining and holding someone's concentration.
2. Remove any distractions such as the TV.
3. The patient may respond better if the speaker uses clear slower speech within a well defined context. (Gardner, Albert, Weintraub, 1975).
4. Use short sentences, but not childish language.
5. Unless deafness was present before the onset of communication problems, it is unnecessary to shout. It is unusual for sudden acquisition of hearing loss unless specifically linked to disease.
6. Ask simple questions requiring a yes/no answer rather than a choice, e.g., 'Do you want to go to bed?' is easier to respond to than 'Do you want to go to bed or watch television?'.
7. Use of gesture, pointing and facial expression may reinforce what you are saying.

If the problem is with expression:

1. Give the patient lots of time to respond.
2. If they cannot say what they want, can they:
   (a) point to it or show you
   (b) gesture
   (c) write it down (one or two letters may be enough of a clue)
   (d) draw it
3. If the patient has a chart or communication aid, make sure it is at hand, and encourage them to use it.
4. Do not pretend you have understood if you have not, as this only heightens frustration – especially if the patient has no receptive deficit.

5. Try simple questions needing a yes/no response to get you onto the correct topic.

CARE OF THE INDIVIDUAL BY THE TEAM

The word 'communication' has been used many times in this chapter, but an important factor in the treatment and management of patients is good communication amongst all members of the caring team. In hospital the patient may come into contact with nurses, doctors, paramedical staff, social workers, porters and ward clerks as well as visitors during the course of a day. All wish to spend time with the patient and this has to be fitted into the routine of meals, baths and some much-needed rest and sleep. It is important that all members of the team know who else is scheduled to see the patient so that a balanced timetable for the day can be planned. It is vitally important that each member of the team knows what the other members are doing for the patient so that the care does not become fragmented and the patient treated as anything less than an individual. Regular meetings are necessary to co-ordinate the care and to encourage team members to support each other and where possible reinforce the work of colleagues. All the people concerned are aiming for the same target which is the comfort and well-being of the patient.

Relatives of patients are among the most important members of the caring team. Carefully explaining problems the patient has and advising on the best ways of dealing with the difficulties that arise is time well spent. The family may be just as devastated by the realization that their relative can no longer be looked after at home and now requires residential care. Explanations may need to be repeated on several occasions, and in different ways, before the implications can be absorbed. Relatives and close friends are the key to providing the vital background information for professional staff. Knowledge of the patient's interests, occupation, personality and general communicative level can help staff ease the transition from independent living to residential care. A depth of understanding will allow staff to encourage the patient to adapt and to motivate the patient to make the most of the new lifestyle.

CONCLUSION

Helping people to communicate is not the sole prerogative of a speech therapist. Communication goes on at all times, not just when a speech therapist visits. For many old people, loneliness and isolation are the destructive feature in their lives and while many crave a time of peace and quiet, for many more there is nothing so fearful as the sound of silence.

We live in a far from perfect world and our National Health Service resources are already sorely stretched. It is often very difficult for professional staff to fulfil the communication needs of patients because staff shortages result in tremendous stresses and often there is not time for a nurse, for example, to sit and just have a chat. In many long-stay hospitals there are no speech therapists employed to help in developing communication skills or even assess and advise on management of new patients with acquired speech and language difficulties. Volunteers can be of great help in promoting communication (Meikle *et al.*, 1979) but certainly in the first instance they, too, need help and guidance when faced with a dysphasic stroke patient. There is a need to develop inter-disciplinary education. Short courses and study days can achieve much, but support and education needs to be regular and continuing. The speech therapist is not available 24 hours a day, and cannot hope to achieve her aims by working in isolation. Being a good communicator is not simply a skill limited to the speech therapist, and patients can be greatly helped by educating those caring for the patient. It is important to remember that 'Remediating the communication problems of elderly patients without working with significant others in the patients environment may be futile, inefficient and inappropriate.' (Lubinski, 1988). This is not to say that our roles are interchangeable, but care must be taken to consider the total patient and not be fragmentary. Everyone must share a combined positive approach.

In recent years we have become more aware of the potential benefits that can be available for the elderly in long-term care. Even though the current philosophy is moving more towards community care, we must ensure that resources are balanced and that those elderly people who need long-term care continue to receive a high standard quality service. After all, none of us have any guarantees where we will end up.

REFERENCES

Barnett-Douglass, H. (1986) Communication needs of the elderly in the community. *Coll. Speech Therap. Bull.*, 409.

Gardner, H., Albert, M.L. and Weintraub, S. (1975) Comprehending a word. The influence of speed and redundancy on auditory comprehension in aphasia. *Cortex*, **II**, 155–62.

Helm-Estabrooks, N. and Ramsberger, G. (1986) Treatment of agrammatism in long-term Broca's aphasia. *Br. J. Disord. Commun.*, **21**, number 1.

Logemann, J. (1983) *The Evaluation and Treatment of Swallowing Disorders*, College Hill Press, San Diego.

Lubinski, R. (1981) Speech, language and audiology programs in home health care agencies and nursing homes, Chapter 20 in *Aging* (eds D.S. Beesley *et al.*), Grune and Stratton, New York.

Lubinski, R. (1988) Foreword *Communication Problems in Elderly People*, Rosemary Gravell Croom Helm, Beckenham, Kent.

Meikle, M., Wechsler, E., Tupper, A. *et al.*, (1979) Comparative trial of volunteer and professional treatments of dysphasia after stroke.' *Br. Med. J.* **2**, 87–9.

Porch, B.E. (1971) *Porch Index of Communicative Ability.* Consulting Psychologists' Press, Palo Alto, California.

Rolnick, M. and Hoops, H.R. (1969) Aphasia as seen by the Aphasic. *J. Speech Hearing Disord.,* **34**, 49–53.

Skelly, M. (1979) *Amer-Ind Gestural Code Based on Universal American Indian Hand Talk.* Elsevier Science Publishing, New York.

APPENDIX

Activities for communication group at Roxbourne Hospital

Many of these activities were linked to a particular theme, e.g., shopping, weather, clothes, famous people.

1. *Auditory*
   Quizzes

General knowledge	Proverbs, sayings etc.
Geography	20 Questions
History	'Who am I?' } games
Famous people	'Guess my occupation?'
Television, films theatre	

   Singing
   To tapes/piano
   Carol concert at Christmas

   Sound lotto
   Identifying everyday noises

   Discussion
   Current events (a) local
   (b) worldwide
   Specific topics, e.g.   money   cooking
   politics   teenagers
   childhood   memories, etc., etc.

   Daily time and place orientation

2. *Visual*

Newspapers	Headlines
	Reading selected articles
	Spotting specific articles/advertisements
Maps	England and world, capital quizzes
	Following directions
	Treasure hunt
	Map of the area/Roxbourne Hospital
Crosswords	General
	Specific
Anagrams	
Bingo	
Miming	Occupation
	'In the manner of the word'
Library Books	London
	Fashion
	Animals, etc.

Memory Games	Remembering objects on table
	Selecting an object to describe

Reading out quiz questions to each other

Drawing Competition
    Directing therapist to draw an item
    Guessing partly drawn items

3. *Tactile*	Feeling and guessing objects in bags
	Naming different coins by touch
4. *Smell*	Guessing textures – sandpaper, cotton, wood, etc.
	Guessing various smells, e.g., lemon juice, vinegar etc.

Chapter 10

Education and life in the long-stay ward

The use of purposeful activity in the long-stay ward is now increasingly common. Education has been shown to be a most effective medium for this, as it is the structuring of experience which leads to the development of human capacity. The essence of this kind of experience is that it is intended, is purposeful, and is adjusted to the changing abilities of the learner. At each step in the process the learner is motivated to respond to specific stimuli. It is the nature of the response which develops capacity. This development enables the learner to experience even more widely, to acquire more knowledge or more skill: it can lead to profound change.

There is practically no limit to the range of subjects which can be studied by many of the patients in long-stay wards. The main determinant is the availability of the right teacher. The subject most commonly found is art, in various forms, while French, current affairs, cookery (in a psycho-geriatric hospital), music and drama, poetry and play-reading, and local history have been instituted with various degrees of success. All programmes have features which are instructive.

THE EDUCATIONAL EXPERIMENT

Poetry writing has been initiated in both a New York nursing home, and in England, at Redhills, a 104-bed hospital for the elderly in Exeter, Devon. The hospital supplements art and music therapy with poetry-writing initiated by Margaret Valk (1980) who uses the methods of Kenneth Koch (1977)

A group of four to nine patients aged between 70 and 90, all in wheelchairs, meets once a week for an hour. Mrs Valk and another volunteer set a theme – perhaps 'wishes' or 'sleep', and those patients who can, use notebooks to record their poems, while others dictate to one of the volunteers. One essential part of the procedure is to read aloud what each has written, and for a volunteer to comment on some aspect. The results are of great interest. A selection of the poems has been published by Redhills Hospital (1980) and they show simplicity, beauty and sincerity. The poetry activity caused an occupational therapist to comment: 'People in this group feel able to talk about things they wouldn't otherwise talk about. The atmosphere is right for them to open up . . . It is also of immense value to staff because it gives us insight into their personalities and helps us to relate to them . . . back on the ward.' (Kirkham, 1981).

Mrs Valk suggests that the use of poetic language can 'enable people to look at things around them in a fresh light' (Kirkham, 1981). The importance of this, in the restricted circumstances of the long-stay ward and for a disabled person in a wheelchair, cannot be over-estimated.

Koch himself (Koch, 1977; Valk, 1980) initiated a group of similar age in a New York nursing home, though here the number in the group was much larger – twenty-five – and inspired projects in other settings of elderly disabled people. There were usually four people acting as facilitators for each group. He notes that his aged poetry-writers seemed to have more animation and more confidence; they had more to say to others and they spoke more clearly. Their eagerness to express their thoughts replaced vagueness and, for some, even silence.

A class in French conversation was begun in a hospital for the elderly in East Anglia, England, and although it continued for only three months it produced some interesting comments from the participants. The group met twice a week for about an hour, with an experienced secondary-school teacher of French. The six participants were chosen by the consultant mainly because they were likely to benefit. One of these students, Mr H (who was 83, suffering from osteoporosis, degenerative joint disease, postural hypotension, and a past history of diabetes controlled by diet) said, when interviewed:

> I am alone in the world. Very grateful to be here. I enjoy being with other class mates – look forward to the break in the routine. The class has gone well. I enjoy most the gradual build up from the beginning of the book. Like the feeling of learning more and more. Between lessons I read the book again. We (the members of the class) use phrases in passing one another in the ward.

Another student, Mrs L (aged 72, with spastic paraplegia, mitral valve disease, and bilateral cataracts), said:

> I enjoy the class very much. Would like to get on quicker, have a lesson every day. I can't see, so I don't see the right place, but I am getting used to it now. Wish I could make notes on the lessons. The teacher brings a tape-recorder, and that's very good. We look forward to the lessons. We'll be sorry when the holidays come. I would like a lesson on something else on the other days. It gives our brains something to do.

A programme of teaching local geography and history was instituted by an occupational therapist with elderly patients in a large urban hospital. The choice of subjects was determined by the educational background of the therapist. Again, this was a small group, and only one session a week could be provided because of pressure on the therapist's time. Her comment after several weeks indicated that 'the project . . . showed up the great need to provide stimulation and help to a specific group of patients who tend to sink into the shadows on an acute ward and become institutionalized'. This is reported in detail in Jones (1983).

There is a continual need for more systematic evaluation of the outcome of educational programmes in long–stay wards. A brief account of such an assessment is given in Jones (1980a). Six patients who participated in an art class in an outer London elderly patient hospital were re–assessed by the medical staff three months after classes began. The participants had previously had two classes a week in drawing, painting and modelling in a room separate from their wards, the teacher being a local education authority tutor of the community education service. One lady in this class, Mrs H of 83 years, was completely chairbound suffering from severe arthritis and a slight stroke and was accordingly in a very poor state before the art class began. She was indifferent to her surroundings, had difficulty in propelling her wheelchair, and was frequently incontinent by day as well as by night. She scored 5 out of 10 on Hodkinson's (1972) mental test; she knew neither the name of the hospital nor that of the Queen. Three months into the classes medical staff reported:

> Marked physical improvement. Where previously needed two nurses to propel her wheelchair, now wheels herself about unaided. She is still chairbound, but now only requires minimal help with dressing and feeding, and is much more co–operative with staff. Washes herself, cleaner in her habits, completely continent . . . Brighter mentally. Most dramatic improvement noticed by all staff, and her daughter, who says she is brighter and easier to talk to. Mental test score 7 out of 10.

Of course one swallow does not make a summer, and it is well known that there can be many reasons for improvement. The classes might just have coincided with a spontaneous uplift in the patient's condition, and may not have been a principal contribution to it. It happens that every single one of the patients in that art class showed significant improvement in their physical and psychological states, though none as striking as that of Mrs H.

A larger -scale programme, in music and movement, was evaluated (Jones, 1983) in two hospitals where very severely deteriorated patients were cared for in wards for the elderly. There were two periods of activity each week conducted by a trained and able teacher, provided by SHAPE.

Reports were made at intervals, over four months, by senior nurses and paramedical staff. Some of the patients showed sustained improvements in cognition or information-process in emotional state or feeling-tone and interaction, in self-care, or activities of daily-living and mobility; and in a few – striking – cases, in continence, single and double. One lady of 95 demonstrated some of these features. She had had a cerebro-vascular accident, and suffered severe dysphasia. Before the educational programme began she had never sat up; after it, she always did, and swung her legs out of bed. She had never washed her hands or face herself; now she sometimes did. She now always fed herself, a previously rare event, and was more sociable and co-operative.

If a new drug were to achieve such results we should urgently want to investigate its use and effects. Does educational intervention show enough promise to warrant such serious attention? Suffice it to say that every educational experiment in a ward or hospital for the elderly, which has been reported, has shown positive outcomes (Naylor and Harwood, 1973).

These positive outcomes compel attention. They demonstrate much about the truly educational process, 'the development of human capacity', which was referred to earlier. They go much further, however, in the way that they illuminate the nature of experience in wards for the elderly, and what has brought patients to them. Jones (1980b) includes a short account of some of the classes and their outcomes.

TEACHING AND THE HOSPITAL CONTEXT

Education is not a panacea – there is no magic. It is really a question of augmenting, and in some cases changing, the nature of the patient's experience. In so doing we seem somehow to change the quality of life for the elderly patient. By virtue of the extent that this can be achieved, the process warrants consideration. Jones (1977) described how educational programmes can be instituted. A revised and shortened version of this essentially practical guide is given in the Appendix to this chapter.

There are two features which a teacher needs in order to succeed in the elderly patient setting: a deep knowledge of his or her subject, and a commitment to sharing that knowledge with older and often disabled men and women. The methods are not peculiar to this student body, though there must be some modification to meet the special circumstances. The most important condition, the absolute *sine qua non*, is that an educational programme must be taken seriously by all concerned. It is not another occupation, a pastime, a token dose of stimulation, a pleasant interlude, a disturbance of ward routines. Where it is treated in any of these ways, it is doomed. The most successful programmes are those where the most senior staff – consultants, nursing officers, and administrators – understand what is in process, and give it their full support.

The seriousness with which an educational programme is viewed is evidenced by the choice of time and place, the commitment of senior staff, the selection of, and encouragement given to, the teacher. Whether the teacher comes from within the hospital, an occupational therapist perhaps, or from outside, they must be given every consideration in their demanding task. Where the experiment fails, it is often because the teaching involved is regarded as yet another 'treatment' to be given.

Education is not something the patient has done to him in the style of the 'medical model': it is something the patient does. It is the opportunity to be, to act, to express, to manipulate, to rehearse, to listen, to participate, to practise, to perform. The patient is not here the object of attention, the dependant, but increasingly the chooser, the mover, the doer.

The psychological effects of a lack of stimulation in unvarying surroundings are well known, as are the physical and psychological effects of lack of exercise, because there is nothing which tempts patients to move. It is not difficult to understand why many wards for the elderly have had an aura of hopelessness, helplessness, apathy and their accompaniments. Where there has been no attempt at positive active intervention, it is extraordinarily difficult for staff to secure job satisfaction and sustain morale.

INDIVIDUALS AND CHANGE

There are many ways of changing such a situation positively. The whole-hearted adoption of education programmes is but one. As a generalization, one could argue that the whole ethos and routine of the long-stay ward require radical transformation if it is to become an environment where ordinary people can maximize satisfaction, or indeed sustain any personal goals other than sheer survival with the minimum of pain and discomfort.

It is essential that we note that every patient has a history, a previous series of experiences which have resulted in the present situation, and which are in some degree responsible for the tendency to become a passive recipient of care. If this tendency is paralleled by a desire, and indeed a duty, on the part of staff to provide care, then the formula that results in inertia is an overwhelmingly powerful one.

It is essential, too, that some recognition be given to the patient's mental condition, however inadequate and partial that recognition is, so that remedial action in the long-stay ward will be based in a broader context than has been usual. Patients should be regarded in a whole sense, as persons with a biography, and with individual needs, expectations, goals and desires, however frail or disabled they may have become.

We can take as a starting point the broad sweep of human needs set out so comprehensively and lucidly by Maslow (1970), familiar to most people in the caring professions. He postulated a hierarchy of needs, viz.:

1. Physiological
2. Safety
3. Love and belongingness
4. Esteem (for the self, and from others)
5. Self-actualization

Shared with other animals are the physiological needs for air, water, food, warmth, sexual satisfaction, and so on. Deprivation of these vital needs leads to the death of the individual, and in the case of sex, of the species. In Maslow's classic statement: 'Man does not live by bread alone except when there is no bread'. In other words, survival, and therefore effort, depends on our seeking the satisfaction of these needs. When deprived of food or warmth nothing else engages our attention. However, when these basic survival needs are met we are impelled to move to the next level.

The safety needs replace the physiological, and become as vital and as pressing. Our whole social and community life can be seen as ensuring that these needs are met. Briefly, our needs for safety are satisfied by the removal of threats to our existence and security. Where this is not the case (as in emergencies such as war, famine or civil commotion) our attention, our drives, are devoted to the attainment of safety to the exclusion of all else.

The need for love and belongingness becomes imperative for our survival as human beings; it becomes a dominant drive or force when deprivation is experienced. We all need to feel accepted by a group, wanted and needed. This governs much of our social behaviour; indeed it provides the driving force that makes us social beings, not only willing but in general desirous of behaving in socially accepted ways. When these physiological, safety, and love needs are broadly met, Maslow suggests that the need for esteem, to have a healthy and positive view of ourselves, and to have the good opinion of others, becomes foremost.

It is the highest, most distinctively human need – for self-actualization – that makes us most individual, most truly ourselves as persons, and which gives the greatest satisfaction, that is worthy of close attention. In Maslow's powerful phrase: 'What a man can be, he must be'. The deprivation of this need, to become what we are capable of becoming, whether to paint, write, cook, garden, create, care for others, or to appreciate music, can give rise to profound frustration. When we are not doing what we are fitted for we become restless and dissatisfied. When we do what we are not fitted for we become resentful and anxious.

This is the supreme importance of satisfying the need for self-actualization.

It is not necessary to accept Maslow's scheme without question. It is extremely worthwhile, however, to consider how the distinctively human needs may be met in the long-stay ward, difficult though this is. The long-stay ward is the constant environment and the arena of life for its residents. How may the vital needs be met? It is in this consideration that we can assess the purposes and effects of interventions in ward life, and these include the evaluation of educational programmes.

The ward regime which greets the new patient is of great significance. Whenever we enter a new environment or social situation we explore it and observe, learning what the 'rules' are, what expectations are held of us and our behaviour, before we relax and adopt a posture which represents an equilibrium between what is expected of us and what we need. In this way we learn how to achieve the satisfaction of our needs by observation, and by trial and error. If acquiescence and a quiet, passive attitude are expected, there will be heavy pressure on us to adopt such a style of living in order to 'earn' the rewards of such behaviour. If, on the other hand, we discover that initiative, activity, and participation in the life of the group are the order of the day, we will be encouraged to act accordingly.

The importance of the initial set of responses is that as long as the régime is regular, predictable and persistent our behaviour will persist. 'Caring' in every aspect of life induces dependence, with its attendant apathy and inertia. Seligman (1975) shows how, when our needs are met without our having to exert ourselves, this very quickly induces subjective awareness of helplessness and the danger of a lapse into depression.

THE EFFECTS OF EDUCATION

The introduction of an educational programme in the form of regular classes in a hospital for elderly patients can be expected to have a number of effects. There are obvious changes in the patients who take part and, perhaps not so obvious, changes in staff attitudes and behaviour. Very little systematic observation has been carried out in such situations, so what follows must be regarded as very tentative, providing the basis for hypothesis rather than definitive guidelines for action. On the other hand, bearing in mind the need for tentativeness, we should without doubt be encouraged to initiate such programmes where feasible.

The physical outcomes

The physical outcomes are various. At a basic level there is the sheer encouragement to move parts of the body, such as the arms and hands in painting, or the motor co-ordination of a cortical kind which is called for when we handle an object. All these are of great importance in restoring and maintaining the health of the body, its joints and muscles, to the extent which is physically possible. There is the added and vital factor of locomotion.

Educational activity requires the use of the body for manipulation, even to turn the pages of a book, or to use a pencil or, in the case of poetry-speaking or playing the recorder, the use of the facial muscles and vocal chords, as well as the respiratory organs (rib-cage, diaphragm etc). The activity also invites the person to take part, to get to the scene of action, and to alter posture from time to time. There is nothing like the incentive of enjoyment and interest to tempt the person to move – to make an effort. The key is motivation. The activity is satisfying, whether it is poetry-speaking or painting, and the person participates in this by using the body. Such participation is use, and it is lack of use which destroys.

One finding which has been reported in at least one of the educational programmes (Mulford, 1979) is that the participants' eyes are brighter. This is certainly not a trivial outcome. While its significance is not at all certain, it may well be that the eyes are an indicator of health. Eyes can reflect the interest in the surrounding world (if it is worth looking at and participating in) and can easily become dull through disuse. Thus the eye brightness which accompanies educational programmes, though a small detail, is not without considerable significance. When considering the physical outcomes which have been reported as concomitants of educational activity, the effects on continence are also worthy of consideration (see p. 175).

The social outcomes

The social outcomes are extremely interesting. There is not much social life in the average ward for elderly patients. The casual visitor often encounters silence and lack of movement. Conversation after meals and toileting is fairly unusual. Why do people not talk in such a circumstance? First of all, the patients in a ward have not normally chosen their location or their companions. It can be reasonably argued that they are in much the same circumstance, of disability, of needing care, and are so much of an age as to give them a good deal in common. Consequently interaction should flourish, but it does not. In this silent setting one is driven to the conclusion that what can be said in the midst of routine, in the absence of variety and stimulation, has been said, and that it is very little. A second factor is lack of privacy. After all, the tradition of keeping yourself to yourself for fear of getting involved or one's personal privacy being invaded by the people next door, is a tenacious feature of domestic life for many. The reality of the ward is to be surrounded by strangers who are daily and hourly witnesses to one's physical frailties, and to social exchanges with family and friends where these exist; where there is no wall, no front door and often not even a curtain to separate patient from patient. Under such circumstances there must be some new agent, some extra factor which will penetrate the wall of silence that replaces the physical partitions we all need from time to time, and which the majority of us have in our homes.

Any event which breaks the routine can act as a catalyst. The significant factors in the educational, as opposed to other similar events, are that the patient must respond, move, give attention, act, and more particularly, respond in the company of others who are doing likewise. The experience is satisfying, and it is *shared*. In the learning situation the events are (a) under the control of the participants, freely-chosen and controlled, and (b) shared physically and psychologically. It is often the case that there is the need, and frequently the opportunity to communicate with the teacher, and the fellow-student. It is important to note the change of role from *patient*, the dependant, to *student*, the active person.

In such a new psychological, and if possible, different physical environment, social interaction is not only possible and encouraged, but necessary, as when students co-operate in a group activity. Through co-operation, the sharing, the absorption and concentration which feature, and which these inspire, and which can only be described as *joy*, there is an overflow of energy, the very need to communicate, to comment, to observe. As an accompaniment to sharing an activity there is the strong tendency to identify with one's fellows, and thus to converse.

This social interaction need not remain confined to the class. The fellow students have had, and are continuing to have, a common experience. They have something to say when they meet between classes. They have something to relate to their fellow-patients, and to the staff, when they return from the class. They very often have some continuing activity, and material to work on when they are in their wards; some paper and pencil activity, a small craft, a poem to read, a story to create. The activity which is satisfying to the 'student' may well prove of interest to other patients. It is something different: differences that are worthy of comment, attract interest and provide the spur to interaction and communication. Thus the educational activity can initiate social activity in the ward.

Ernst *et al.* (1978) have shown that physical, social and emotional isolation are key intervening variables which 'disclose functional symptoms of disorders'. They argue that 'treatment . . . . . countering isolation will alleviate or reverse symptomatic disorders whether or not brain pathologies . . . . are present'.

It is not only communication and instruction which are encouraged by a shared activity. A small but significant change to a neater appearance has been noticed in many participants. So much in our everyday lives depends on our meeting with others whose opinion we value. It is only when we are separated from their company that we notice the tendency to let ourselves go, e.g. a man perhaps does not shave every day, or does not dress till late. While long-stay patients are rarely alone, the improvement in their appearance and self-care when they engage in a shared satisfying activity probably indicates that they are then in a group which is perceived as different from being in the average ward.

The psychological outcomes

The psychological outcomes are of the very greatest importance and may be divided into those of two kinds – the cognitive and the affective. The division is one of convenience, made for the sake of analysis. It must not be forgotten that people will act and react as a whole, not as a collection of parts.

Cognitive change The cognitive changes which accompany educational activity as reported include improved memory, alertness, sense of identity, concentration, and a better grasp on reality (Jones, 1980a, 1980b). Even the most superficial acquaintance with a ward for elderly patients indicates that these changes are of the very greatest significance. So often the opposites are observed: forgetfulness in various degrees, lack of interest in surroundings, a lack of self-initiated activity, concentration or conversation. All these features may of course be described as symptoms of 'dementia' or of other disorders, some of which may be treated. They are, on the other hand, common in long-stay wards and may indeed therefore come to characterize it. Besdine (1978) points out that many of these symptoms, often described as 'dementia', are treatable, if properly investigated. What is interesting is the extent to which these symptoms in some patients may be alleviated by the opportunity to participate in a satisfying and progressive activity, not merely being 'stimulated' but being expected to respond.

Improvement in memory is a main feature of learning, because learning something of interest holds the attention. Most poor remembering, and this applies to all of us, is the outcome of poor attention. What we attend to we recall. We are equipped to notice differences, and to become immune to sameness – the bases of a theory of boredom. Engaging in a novel activity, noticing, giving attention, adjusting our responses to the changing stimuli, whether visual, aural, kinaesthetic or proprioceptive, these are manifestations of attention to something outside ourselves which tempt us to remember the acts and sensations involved. Practice in remembering assists the recovery or at least the maintenance of memory. It is the reverse, having nothing worthy of our attention, which causes the damage. Remembering and attending are closely intertwined. Thus, education can help in this attempt to normalize the life of a long-stay patient.

There is a big difference between lack of contact with the outside world as a temporary withdrawal, and the almost continual daydream or inertness so common in the long-stay ward. Reverie, the opportunity to fantasize, to erect a barrier between one's consciousness and a dull or irritating environment filled with companions who find the environment of similar character, may be protective. All then conspire, however silently and unwittingly, to make a grey, predictable and routine setting for those in it. It may be an adaptive response which leads to its own form of disorder which it becomes habitual. This lack of contact with reality and its very frequent accompaniment, incontinence, comes to characterize the ward for elderly patients, however false the picture may be in individual terms.

The educational enterprise directly attacks this syndrome. When successful, and this varies greatly between individuals and settings, the results can be dramatic, as in the case of Mrs. H. (Jones, 1980a) above. Having something interesting to attend to, interacting with other patients and the teacher, producing a tangible end-product, communicating with others, a communication needing thought, having an enjoyable and satisfying event to anticipate, all this makes inroads into the drift from reality, from one's fellows, and indeed from one's self. No wonder the patients' ability to remember is prone to improvement when they re-learn the satisfaction of concentration, and improve their grasp on reality, when reality itself becomes worthy of attention, when above all, stimulation is met by self-initiated response.

A word about stimulation is perhaps appropriate at this point. Many hospital staff members, noting the boredom, the routine, the dullness of many patients in the long-stay wards, move to the conclusion that stimulation is lacking. In a sense this is absolutely correct. However, the results of providing this stimulation are often disappointing. This is because, beyond a temporary flurry of excitement, the patient seems to be no more stimulated or lively than before. I refer to the 'conversations' which staff or visitors may initiate, the sing-song a visiting pianist attempts to start, the youngsters from a local school who provide a lively entertainment, the floor games which a well-meaning occupational therapist's aide may inaugurate. None of these activities are to be decried. They are worthy attempts to divert, to occupy, and to stimulate. What these situations lack, in my opinion, is the opportunity to respond in a meaningful, constructive, distinctly human way.

To respond in this human sense is to go beyond reflex, or reaction; it is to act, to recognize, to become conscious of sensation, to become aware of one's own contribution, of one's participation. When we talk of patients needing stimulation, what we should really be describing is the need for responding.

It is obvious that not all patients will want or be able to respond in the degree described. Raphael and Mandeville (1979) surveyed 143 old people in six hospitals for the elderly. When asked what they liked best about their lives only three patients (out of a list of 180 responses) replied that they liked the activities and entertainments which were provided, while among the things they liked least (out of 65 responses) 14 commented on the lack of activities and entertainments. It is significant that more comments were made about occupations than on any other topic.

Admission to the long-stay ward is a social–medical matter, and as such is not a matter for specific consideration here, except in so far as it governs or affects the régime within the ward. That the reasons for admission do have effects on the régime is exemplified in the Royal College of Physicians of London (RCP) Committee report of 1981, which shows that 'memory loss', incapacity and loss of control are seen by many physicians as characteristic of elderly patients. In hospital and institutional populations such a view is understandable. If not the reasons for admission such symptoms are accepted as very common in wards for the elderly. With such expectations prevalent among doctors it is unsurprising that hospital regimes have been constituted in ways which expect little response from patients. Such lack of expectation, as in schools, can rapidly become self-fulfilling prophecy when little is expected and little is forthcoming. If we treat people as incapable of appropriate response the result can fully support our diagnosis whether with children or the elderly.

The RCP report defines dementia, a syndrome commonly found in wards for the elderly as:

> . . .the global impairment of higher cortical . . . functions including memory . . . the capacity to solve the problems of day-to-day living, the performance of learned perceptuo-motor skills, the correct use of social skills and control of emotional reactions, in the absence of gross clouding of consciousness. The condition is often irreversible and progressive.

It very diplomatically hints at the difficulties of diagnosis, and, by implication, at the dangers of incorrect diagnosis. This is re-iterated by Roberts (1988). He reports on the 'difficulties of diagnosis in early cases of dementia and the lack of precise knowledge about the natural history of the disease'. Considering that stage 1 of Alzheimer's disease, involving memory loss and disorientation can last up to seven years (Roberts, 1988), there is a clear need, as the RCP Report emphasizes, for the education of all concerned, whether professionally or otherwise, with the elderly.

On the subject of treatment, the RCP Report points out that 'there is need for research into fundamental causes and also into agents which are effective in symptomatic control'. The provision of an *appropriately stimulating environment* may prove to be among those agents effective in symptom control. Such provision may even affect those defects in cholinergic neurotransmission and the cerebral blood supply which can accompany and result in cortical deterioration and intellectual decrement.

Routtenberg (1978) has suggested that 'the pathways of brain reward may function as the pathways of memory consolidation . . . . When something is learned actively in the brain, reward pathways facilitate the formation of memory'. The reward pathways of which he speaks involve the transmission of the catecholamines, dopamine and norepinephrine. Learning, therefore, which invariably involves memory consolidation must stimulate the passage of the neurotransmitters. It may be then, that in place of or in addition to the application of cholinergic drugs, the encouragement and stimulation to learn can enhance or restore neurotransmitter action directly. While cholinergic deficiency may reduce memory, it could be that more occasion for use of memory could induce cholinergic activity.

Livesley (1978) has argued that 'if we exclude depression . . . (which) can mimic the symptoms of brain failure due to many other causes . . . initial acute cerebral ischaemia has been for some years . . . the most common unidentified cause of brain failure'. Whatever improves blood flow, then, may militate against brain failure. The reason for this is that the brain uses oxygen transported by the blood, and that reductions in blood flow reduce oxygen supply and impair cortical function; indeed, severe and sustained reduction will destroy neurons. However, neuronal function itself can aid blood flow. Ingvar (1976) provides abundant evidence that in non-anoxic brain tissue the blood flow is controlled mainly by the functional activity of the neuron. Davison (1978) has it that problem-solving increases the blood supply to the premotor and frontal regions of the brain. Thus education, by increasing cortical exercise, may postpone its deterioration, and this not only in verbal or symbolic activity, as in literature or mathematics, but in the problem-solving involved in physical games. Games with a soft ball, or aiming at targets, involve motor co-ordination and attentional processes which exercise appropriate areas of cortex and nervous system. Physical activity of a purposeful kind involves the brain as well as the rest of the body.

Affective change. While most people would agree that education has a great deal to do with the cognitive aspects of life, with learning, thinking, knowing, remembering, understanding and information-processing in general, it is possibly not so obvious that it has much to do with the affective, emotional, motivational facets of persons. To be stimulated in such a way that we respond constructively, creatively, with interest, with curiosity, with the motivation to repeat or to continue the process, as in the act of true learning, has emotional affective concomitants worthy of analysis. So many levels of emotional, motivational response may be involved that we need to particularize.

When we learn we change; that is a basic fact. However, we do not only change in the sense that we now know something we did not know before, e.g. studying Spanish, or can do something that we could not do before, e.g., learning to knit. To learn anything is to demonstrate to ourselves, and often to others, that we are *capable* of learning, that we have the capacity. We see ourselves in a new way. our self-concept changes to include this component: 'I am capable of speaking Spanish, or knitting a jumper, or mending a fuse'. The recognition of our own ability is reassuring. Thus depression born of the perception of help-lessness (Schulz, 1976, 1980) can be held at bay. Csikszentmihalyi (1975) has demonstrated the joy derived from the exercise of skill which extends us but does not over-extend us (which latter he suggests causes anxiety) and which is the opposite of a constant diet of activity or non-activity which makes no call on our potential skilfulness. The lack of demand on our abilities, he suggests, is at the root of boredom.

The prompting of outside interests is another of the potential benefits of education, and by no means the least important. This appeals at any age, but the burden of physical constraint that, for example, follows a stroke, and the sameness of surroundings which often accompany such constraint can very easily precipitate a pre-occupation with one's own ruminations, and quite understandably, with one's bodily processes. When we talk of 'occupation' or 'diversion' it is these as remedies for such a pre-occupation with the self which we are seeking. Educational activity offers a very great deal to encourage expansiveness. The awakening of curiosity; the temptation to manipulate; the need to hear and understand questions and instructions; being drawn to experi-ment or play; the recognition of situations, objects, words, which have brought pleasure in the past; the revival of memory, the use *par excellence*, of the senses, in touching and listening, the reflexiveness of speech, the kinaesthetic awareness in movement, the feedback to the motor brain of proprioception from the muscles; all operate to channel the stream of consciousness outside the barrenness of an internal pre-occupation.

The healthy and productive diversions from the self seem to occur when a person is active, mentally and physically, in contemplation, appreciation, or attending to a scene or event outside. In particular it also occurs when they themselves are participating in an activity which literally takes them out of themselves; when they lose their egocentric self-absorption and become, if only momentarily, at one with the world, when they act and re-act in harmony with it.

The outward orientation can explain the fascination of creative activity, whether the exercise of a craft, or writing; it certainly underlies the passion which many people put into acting, producing and other make-believe situations. Even conversation with a peer can so divert, as can reading. Many of our 'escape' pursuits, such as watching television, or seeking the novel sights and sounds of foreign travel, can be seen as attempts to escape the constant demands of the self for attention. So can the consumption of tranquillizers. To become involved in an outside activity in which one participates fully is the best cure for the disorders engendered by self-preoccupation, and such absorption lies at the root of the therapeutic uses of educational activity.

Incontinent behaviour

The restoration of continence as the by-product of an educational activity is an intriguing possibility. Mulford (1979) reports on the outcome of a large-scale programme in a psychogeriatric hospital in the North-West which initiated art, craft, drama, music and communication studies, with a number of different classes. She says of the participants, 'they have become more alert (and) . . . . there has also been some improvement in continence during the day-time . . . . personal appearance (has) become more important' (pp. 1–2). While the observations about alertness, continence and appearance are, as we shall see, fairly certainly related to each other, let us concentrate on the note regarding continence. This is consistent with the experience of Mrs H. (mentioned earlier in this chapter) who became 'completely continent' having been frequently incontinent by day as well as by night.

In the study reported in Jones (1983), eight weeks into the educational programme, four patients out of twenty-eight showed an improvement in continence of urine, while two of these showed a similar improvement in continence of faeces. After a further eleven weeks, three of the four had sustained this amelioration, and six further patients enjoyed a restoration of continence. Thus, 9 out of 28 participants had improved, and six had become more continent of faeces. Full details are set out in the 1983 work. It is of great importance to those planning an education programme to note that a much more significant improvement in the state of patients became apparent after nineteen weeks than occurred after eight weeks. The longer period was much more pronounced in its effects than the shorter one.

In his very important paper on the psychology of incontinence, Sutherland (1976) lists eight mechanisms: repression; symptom selection; disturbance of conditioned reflexes; dependency; rebellion; insecurity; attention-seeking; and sensory deprivation. The educational experience seems to have some influence on many of these causes, and this may be why some patients achieve a measure of relief from incontinence. A full discussion of this effect is to be found in Jones (1983).

CHANGING THE PERSPECTIVE OF THE LONG-STAY WARD

If education and other purposeful and satisfying activity were to be central to the life of the long-stay ward, with medical, caring, and domestic services provided in support of this, we would then see fulfilled the transformation in the later lives of people who needed care, which would benefit all of us, young and old. An account of how this could be achieved in the case of the residential home for the elderly is given by Jones (1978).

Initiating education or similar activity in a long-stay ward has powerful effects if carried out whole-heartedly and with the support of all concerned – porters as well as consultants. It is certainly beneficial to the patients; it inspires staff. That prospect offers promise to us all.

REFERENCES

Besdine, R.W. (1978) *Treatable Dementia in the Elderly.* Mimeographed. Hebrew Rehabilitation Center. Rosindale, Mass.

Csikszentmihalyi, M. (1975) *Beyond Boredom and Anxiety*, Jossey-Bass, London.

Davison, A.N. (1978) Biochemical aspects of the ageing brain. *Age Ageing*, **7**, Supplement 7–11.

Ernst, P., Beran, B., Safford, F. and Kleinhauz, M. (1978) Isolation and the symptoms of chronic brain syndrome. *Gerontologist*, **18**, 468–74.

Hodkinson, H.M. (1972) Evaluation of a mental test score for assessment of mental impairment in the elderly. *Age Ageing*, **1**, 233–8.

Ingvar, D.H. (1976) Functional landscapes of the dominant hemisphere. *Brain Res.*, **107**, 181–97.

Jones, S. (1977) Teaching the elderly, in *The Quality of Life of the Elderly in Residential Homes and Hospitals* (ed. F. Glendenning), Beth Johnson Foundation and Department of Adult Education, University of Keele.

Jones, S. (1978) A Residential College for the Elders, *Heads and Hearts*, Residential Care Association, Ossett, near Wakefield, W. Yorkshire.

Jones, S. (1980a) The educational experience in homes and hospitals in *Outreach Education and the Elders: Theory and Practice* (ed. F. Glendenning), Beth Johnson Foundation in association with Department of Adult Education, University of Keele.

Jones, S. (1980b) Education for the second half of life, in *Living in the 80s* (ed. N. Dickson), Age Concern, London.

Jones, S. (1983) *Learning and Meta-Learning with special reference to Education for the Elders.* Unpublished PhD thesis, University of London Library.

Kirkham, C. (1981) Poetry at Redhills Hospital, *Involve* (Volunteer Centre) 14, Spring.

Koch, K. (1977) *I Never Told Anybody: Teaching Poetry Writing in a Nursing Home,* Random House, New York.

Livesley, B. (1978) The treatment and prevention of brain failure. *Age Ageing*, **1**, Supplement, 27–34.

Macdonald, E.M. (1970) *Occupational Therapy in Rehabilitation,* 3rd edn., Ballière, Tindall and Cassell, London.

Maslow, A.H. (1970) *Motivation and Personality,* Harper and Row, New York.

Mulford, J. (1979) *Hospital Job Creation Programme,* Unpublished report, Newton-le-Willows College of Further Education, Lancashire.

Naylor, G.F.K. and Harwood, E. (1973) Action research: music for the elderly. *Proc. Aust. Assoc. Geront.*, **2**, 26.

Raphael, W. and Mandeville, J. (1979) *Old People in Hospital,* King Edward's Hospital Fund, London.

RCP Report (1981) Organic mental impairment in the elderly. Implications for research, education and the provision of services. A report of the Royal College of Physicians by the College Committee on Geriatrics. Reprinted from *J. Roy. Coll. Physicians London*, **15**, 141–67.

Redhills Hospital (1980) *Poetry,* League of Friends of Redhills Hospital, Exeter.

Roberts, G.W. (1988) All quiet on the Southern front. A summary of the conference on Alzheimer's Disease. *J. Roy. Coll. Physicians London*, **22**, 101–4.

Routtenberg, A. (1978) The reward system of the brain. *Scient. Am.*, **239**, 121–31.

Schulz, R. (1976) Effects of control and predictability on the physical and psychological well-being of the institutionalised aged. *J. Person. Soc. Psychol.*, **33**, 563–73.

Schulz, R. (1980) Ageing and control, in *Human Helplessness. Theory and Applications* (eds J. Garber and M.E.P. Seligman), Academic Press, London.

Seligman, M.E.P. (1975) *Helplessness: on Depression, Development and Death,* W.H. Freeman, San Francisco.

Sutherland, S.S. (1976) The psychology of incontinence, in *Incontinence in the elderly* (ed. F.L. Willington), Academic Press, London.

Tobin, S.E. and Lieberman, M.A. (1976) *Last Homes for the Aged,* Jossey-Bass, London.

Valk, M. (1980) Poetry can help: the work of Kenneth Koch. *Br. J. Soc. Work*, **9**, 501–7.

APPENDIX

Requirements of educational programmes in the long-stay ward

Preliminaries. As with the initiation of any innovatory feature in the life of patients the utmost care must be taken in preparing the ground for an educational programme. The socio-professional structure of even the smallest ward is so complex and interlocking that no change can be made in any part of ward life without affecting the whole in some degree. The patients are very vulnerable to action which can affect them. It is not always possible to consult them fully before a new venture is begun; sometimes it is only by making a start that the patients concerned understand what is involved. For these reasons it is essential that the greatest degree of understanding and support is sought beforehand. Whatever the source of the idea that education classes should be tried, two things, I believe, are essential: the full understanding and support of the consultant geriatrician responsible, and full consultation with, and briefing of, all those professionals who are in regular contact with the patients. Where the consultant is committed then all else can flow from this: the co-operation of nursing staff, the interest and help of the other professionals such as occupational therapists, social workers and physiotherapists. Nobody should underestimate the need for unequivocal leadership and for the utmost measure of co-operation that is possible in regard to innovation of any substance. In a hospital with little experience of such innovation it can be taken for granted that the consequences will be far reaching, and if wisely handled, of the greatest benefit to all concerned. Conversely, without the strong support of the persons responsible for the patients' welfare no programme can be successful.

So many people who are concerned with the patient are affected by innovatory features of his daily life – doctors, nurses, paramedicals, domestics, administrators – that their questions and concerns must be considered at an early stage. The work of the occupational therapist is most closely concerned with the nature of the educational programme; in many ways it parallels her own tasks, though differing in some aspects. The authoritative work of Macdonald (1970) indicates the relationship. In talking about 'Intellectual and Educational Activities' she suggests that for the occupational therapist 'a knowledge of . . . . library facilities available is necessary, as is a readiness to seek the help of other experts or enthusiasts in subjects outside the range of the occupational therapist herself or her staff' (p. 26), and 'for older patients courses can sometimes be arranged with local teachers, who may be willing to volunteer to help an individual, or through classes arranged with a local education authority for which, if the group is large enough, instructors can be provided'.

In some institutions the occupations taught by the occupational therapy (O.T.) staff are approached in the educational modes already described in this chapter; they are progressive and approached in a positive, enlightened spirit. Occupational therapists are however very much in demand in providing instruction in the activities of daily living as part of the preparation of patients for discharge to their own homes. Their possible deployment in the long-stay ward is not, as a result, exploited to the extent which would be desirable. Even in such circumstances of lack of time, however, consultation with the occupational therapists is of great importance. Whether or not O.T. staff do the actual teaching, securing the right teacher is obviously the prime task of any educational programme.

The teachers. If occupational therapy staff are not available, or are not committed to this kind of programme, there are various other sources.

The local education authority should be approached first. They will often have a community education service which can provide tutors in a variety of fields and with experience of teaching adults. No charge is made for this service in England but there may well be limits on the extent of provision because of reduced funds and other competing calls.

Volunteers may be sought from among those able and willing to give a few hours each week. Willingness, though vital, is not enough. As has been emphasized earlier in this chapter, the quality of the teaching is all-important. Whoever undertakes it must be well-qualified in their subject, and preferably experienced in adult education. The teaching is demanding because much ingenuity and adaptability will be required. Individual patients will vary widely in aptitude, previous experience and the type and extent of their disabilities, which are often multiple. If a volunteer tutor is sought, thought must be given to the need for commitment and continuity. The tutor will need to work in consultation with a senior member of hospital staff, whether a nursing or senior occupational therapist, on a day-to-day basis, and must be given the full support and recognition of the consultant geriatrician.

The tutor will need to be briefed fully by the staff concerned, and to meet the patients before the programme is planned in detail. The space to be assigned to teaching, and any equipment necessary, will have to be arranged well in advance, and staff who may be involved with patients who are to have the class should be fully briefed on what is planned and what the purposes are. There is no question of some strange person arriving one day and being assigned to a group of patients who are to be taught. This is a serious exercise and must be taken seriously by all concerned.

The subject matter. No mention has yet been made of the subject matter which will be taught, and there are two reasons for this. First, the right person is of the utmost importance, and if available, he or she can teach whatever they feel enthusiastic about. Secondly, there is really no constraint on the subject matter which a hospital programme employs.

Although art and craft have traditionally been the commonest activities found in long-stay hospital wards there is no reason for them to be the staple diet. Both are admirable, but there are many other alternatives. The choice is confined by the abilities and interests of the tutor, and by the physical disabilities of the patients.

An example: nature study. A ward for elderly people in a hospital in outer London, where the virtues of an educational programme were recently revealed, discovered that a lady volunteer, who had been assisting the domestic staff by serving the patients at meal times, was a qualifed teacher of biology who had retired early from a secondary school teaching post. She was now asked to consider the scene from a different perspective. What kind of education programme would be appropriate (a) to a setting of a score of old, disabled ladies and (b) to her qualifications and interests? The teacher's enthusiasm and initiative were quickly aroused.

At this stage a senior nursing officer, the geriatrician, and the ward sister were involved, together with the writer (an 'outside' educationalist) who had been invited to advise. The programme would be based on nature study both in and out of the ward. Six to eight of the more alert patients would comprise the first class, which was to meet twice a week, in the mornings, for an hour or so. The ward routine was altered and furniture was rearranged willingly, with the full co-operation of nursing and domestic staff. The pathology department produced some disused beakers and other glassware, and a hunt was started for an old microscope. A scientific supplier's catalogue was secured by the tutor, and simple equipment ordered. Formica-topped benches were installed in the ward, and arrangements to supply gas for bunsen-burners were discussed.

As part of the planning for educational experience, flower-beds outside the ward were surveyed for possible exploitation. A large glass tank having been discovered, it was decided that the first live samples of nature would be fish of various kinds, to be followed by small birds in cages, and insects where these could be suitably housed. This meant that class members and others would be able to take an interest in growing, live specimens of plant and animal life between classes, and would, above all, provide an interest of a very productive and continuing kind, and a reason for purposeful activity. It was likely to be an infectious interest too, with non-members of the class, it was thought, rapidly beginning to participate in caring, observing, and joining in the instructional periods.

The class has not yet started for organizational reasons, but there is much to be learned from what was planned and how. The teacher, well-qualified and highly committed, was already in contact with the hospital. The decision to offer nature-study was not based on what might or might not be suitable for long-stay patients; it arose quite naturally from the abilities and interests of the teacher who was available. She was not only consulted about the requirements for the class but was given a very free hand, and the willing co-operation of nearly everyone involved. Once the subject had been settled, the ways in which it would be taught took full account of the opportunities and, in the degree necessary, the special circumstances of patients.

The ability of the patients. The group of patients which it is easiest to teach, and this applies to any potential class, whether of children or adults, is obviously the most able and alert. They will understand best what is required, and will respond soonest. It is of the utmost importance that the most able enjoy the opportunities for education as well as other activity in order to reduce or possibly combat deterioration, mental and physical. Nevertheless, we very much need to involve the patients of lesser ability, including those who are inert and apathetic, as well as the intermittently confused. Of course it takes great patience, persistence and skill to secure response, but if this can be achieved it may be the best service that the education programme can render.

If the explanation of the need for stimulus to thought and action is at all valid, then those who are least capable of connected thought and co-ordinated action are those who are in most need of such stimulus, so long as any response is at all possible. Such response should not be ruled out unless and until the stimulation has been provided, under optimum conditions, and not abandoned unless there is quite obviously no response. It may be, I put it no higher, that persistence and imagination, if applied to these problematical patients, will prove to be rewarding. This applies to every kind of stimulation – psychotherapy, occupational therapy, conversation with nursing staff – as well as educational activity. Unrewarding in its early stages, it may yield returns of great significance.

There is no doubt that prevention is much more useful than attempts to cure, but we have to deal with the world as it is, and the world of the long-stay patient is very often a sad, silent, and dull one. Transformation of this world, the only one the patient has beyond fantasy and endless rumination, is an urgent priority.

We know little about methods in teaching the less able patient. I suspect that the methods are very similar to those used with backward children, based on patience, imagination, experience, and, above all, commitment to the needs of the individuals. We know little about the methods for two reasons. The first is that very little has been done that is directed specifically to this group; the second is that very little has been reported about any teaching experiments, regardless of ability. We urgently need the most successful practitioners to report their experiences. They will prove to be of the utmost value to all who are concerned – a growing number.

There is no doubt that, as with the poetry-writing class in Exeter, and the nature study project described above, the less-able would be reached as a result of the main thrust of the teaching. Numerous helpers were employed in the poetry teaching. Many of the patients were physically unable to write, and each normally had an amanuensis. In such circumstances even the slightest response of a verbal kind would have been recorded, with subsequent encouragement for the speaker. It is not difficult to imagine that the less-able speakers may have found a new channel of communication by such means, and thus have been enabled to join in. The nature programme would inevitably have attracted the attention, and fairly certainly the interest of nearly everyone in the ward. The flowers, birds, and fish would ensure such attention. It would not be long before many, other than those recruited to the first class, would have been spurred into curiosity and active attention.

The teaching space. A room separate from the ward is of the greatest importance for teaching, and certainly in arts and craft, as well as in many other subjects. There are two solid advantages in such separation (Chapters 8 and 9). First, the use of a separate room or studio is a great asset when it comes to the use of space, specialized equipment, storage, and the lack of interruption from uninvolved persons. Secondly, the transfer of patients from their wards to another location, while it presents problems with wheelchair movement, has desirable side-effects in that it heightens the stimulation of the occasion for the patient, making a welcome break from an over-familiar environment.

It sometimes happens, however, that with the best will in the world no location other than the ward can be found: – nowhere, that is, that approaches suitability, or where porterage is available for moving a number of patients within a short space of time. Wheelchairs take up a great deal of space, and no room that can hold say six people in wheelchairs, and a teacher, may be found within easy reach. In such circumstances the class will have to be provided in the ward, or no class will be held at all. Almost every ward has a space which can at least be made available for a few hours each week, if the activity is taken seriously, by moving some beds and armchairs. This is what we planned for the nature-study class.

Some teachers believe that using the ward for the class may not be entirely disadvantageous. Although less convenient, it is true, it does have the quite likely outcome that patients who are not initially involved in the class, far from interfering with its operation, may become so interested that they will want to join in. Further, the domestic, nursing, and other staff will have a chance to see and hear what is going on, and this can be a very positive exposure. The teacher can be present only for a few hours each week, and for the other staff to know what has been taught or demonstrated means that they will be able to provide encouragement and possibly supplement the instruction when needed, between classes. Once again, we need the reports of experienced teachers, and other observers.

Chapter 11

Art education

INTRODUCTION

A successful experiment carried out between 1970 and 1975 showed clearly that people in advanced years, even while living in long-term wards in elderly patient departments of hospitals, welcome the opportunity to learn something new. Awakened interest developed, and concentration improved, particularly when a suitable room was set aside away from the wards – creating a space for quiet and study for the introduction of the subject.

Whenever people are segregated away because of calendar age, preconceived ideas can be created as to what 'they' want or do not want to do. Many interesting aspects were revealed from the comments of those on the receiving end of the project. The following are some brief details of the history of the research and of its interesting recent developments. Included are ideas for the benefit of staff wishing to extend the interest of their residents in all types of residential care institutions, particularly elderly patient departments of hospitals.

THE PROJECT

History

In January, 1970, the King Edward's Hospital Fund for London gave a grant for the development of a project: 'Art for the Elderly in Hospitals'. This was later also supported by a grant from The Centre for Policy on Ageing (then the National Corporation for the Care of Old People). The project lasted for five years. The purpose was to provide opportunities for the serious study of art on an equal footing with that already provided for able-bodied adults in the community. The classes were presented with, as near as possible, the same facilities as those provided for adults of all ages attending the local adult education institute art classes. In order that equal opportunities could genuinely be said to be provided for these elderly people living in the hospital context, the research emphasized the importance of the following three development areas:

1. *Suitable accommodation*. This involved persuading the elderly patient departments of ten hospitals in the London area to provide a room away from the long-term wards suitable for use as a studio.
2. *From their point of view*. Opinions of the elderly students and of the hospital staff were monitored as each new class was introduced and developed in these ten different studios.
3. *Training courses*. These were designed and organized specifically for specialist art tutors interested in extending their teaching to elderly people living in residential care, and in particular, elderly patient departments of hospitals. Courses now extend to care staff themselves interested in introducing creative interests to their residents. (This is discussed further in this chapter under 'New Developments').

The students selected for this educational provision were of course the most important people involved. The average age of students in this project was 80 years. The students were confined to wheelchairs, and the majority could use only one hand. Most of them had been in hospital for at least five years. For these people, formal education finished at an early age, and none had had any previous instruction in art.

We were dealing with an age group we ourselves had not yet reached so that it was not easy to imagine with any accuracy what life was really like looking out onto the world through the eyes of an elderly person living in these wards, trapped physically, yet with a sensible and alert mind. Therefore, their comments were vital throughout the project, and formed the guidelines for its development.

Emphasis was placed on the classes being as much for art appreciation as for active participation, bearing in mind that the patients may not necessarily choose to study the subject of art if a wider choice were presented. Once it had been really emphasized that they did not have to paint or draw if they did not want to, opinions and interest came readily within the quiet atmosphere of the studios. Some showed a desire to look at art and other reference books while others examined natural objects, often through a magnifying glass, which later could become the inspiration for practical work.

The ten hospitals concerned included, in one case, the building of a purpose-built art studio with a kiln provided by the League of Friends. All the studios contained, as well as painting and drawing materials, the nucleus of a small library with art and other books for reference, opportunities for examining natural objects, and facilities for film and slide projection. Of the original ten hospitals involved, three were closed as part of the Department of Health and Social Security's spending cuts in 1979. The remaining seven continued to have flourishing studios and to form the pattern for classes elsewhere. Six of these studios have progressed from their original room to superior accommodation.

Each of the new classes, after the first four months, settled down to a steady group of between 10 and 14 students, with a nucleus of approximately six students who developed a sustained interest. All the classes had some people who came regularly for at least two years. All the tutors reported considerable improvement in the skill and understanding of the subject by their elderly, often very physically disabled, regular students. An increase in their visual observation and ability to concentrate after the first six months, was also noted.

They were learning. Among the opinions most readily repeated by a variety of elderly students, as the classes progressed in the ten different hospital studios, was an appreciation of a room set aside from the wards, especially for the work in hand 'somewhere quiet where we can concentrate'.

Here, in addition to the often existing bingo and sing-song, was an activity introduced with a serious element of learning.

In the past, many hospital staff had failed to recognize that there are people in their long-term wards who had the potential for study of any kind. Nursing staff were often surprised to see their elderly charges studiously concentrating on a painting or completely absorbed as they looked at colour reproductions in a well-illustrated book on art.

Media and studies included drawing and painting, fabric printing, calligraphy, and in some studios, pottery. Three studios eventually bought their own kilns. Here, the elderly people have, in addition, the opportunity to gain first-hand knowledge of pottery (Figure 11.1), and to observe and take part in the exciting process from biscuit firing to glazing of their own pots. All of these activities were experienced by the elderly people concerned, in most cases for the first time. Skills were developed and successfully carried out by these 80-year-old-plus students while living in long-term care in the elderly patient departments of their hospitals.

As classes progressed, sketching out of doors and visits to galleries were arranged, as well as slide-shows within the individual studios. These were all very much appreciated; as one lady of 82 years, living in the elderly patient department of a hospital, said: 'I had always wanted to visit a gallery, but my husband was never interested in such things, and I had a big family to bring up. I never thought I would ever have this opportunity'.

Exhibitions of the elderly students' work took place in all the hospitals concerned. These have generally been held in the studios, and linked with the annual hospital fetes.

Good mounting and presentation will enhance any art work, and the paintings by the elderly students are no exception. Framing and mounting of their pictures for the hospital exhibitions gave added dignity and

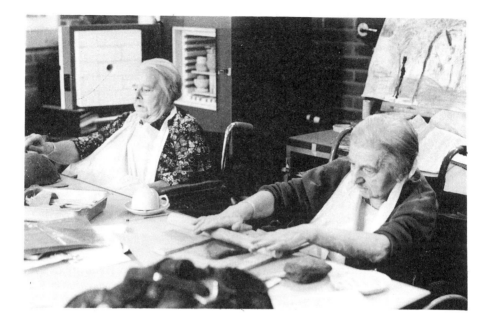

Figure 11.1   An opportunity to gain first-hand knowledge of pottery.

quality to the exhibits, which delighted the artists and was appreciated by staff and relatives of all generations.

Two major exhibitions, representing the work produced in the ten hospital studios have taken place since the project began. One exhibition in December, 1975, was held at County Hall, Westminster, with the support of the Inner London Education Authority, and the second was held at the Royal Festival Hall, London, with the support of the Counsel and Care for the Elderly in March, 1979. The aim of both these exhibitions was to promote the idea of the project. It was also an opportunity to show selected works of a high standard produced by the elderly students, not just for the interest in the unique background of the artists who had produced them, but as paintings in their own right, giving pleasure to all generations. In most cases, it was arranged for the exhibiting artists to visit these major exhibitions to see their work in a professional setting.

The tutors were all qualified art specialists. They had also been trained on a course especially designed for those tutors interested in extending their teaching to elderly people living in residential care. Presenting an art class in the setting of a hospital or residential home is very different from the atmosphere of school or college, to which most of the tutors were accustomed. It was important, therefore, that they had a prior understanding of the role of hospital and other residential care staff, in order to slot in to this particular environment successfully. An insight into the lives of their prospective students when they were not attending the class, as well as knowledge of specific methods, materials and approaches are all of great value to a tutor before embarking on this type of teaching.

The first of these courses took place in 1972 at the University of London Goldsmith's College and was called 'Teaching Art to the 80-year-Olds'. The course continued in London annually under the title of 'Art for the Elderly in Residential Care'. Two national courses also took place, one of which was directed by the Department of Education and Science.

The trained tutors, having completed the course, are salaried by their local education authority and attached to the appropriate adult education centre or institute while taking the classes in the hospital studios.

The majority of the tutors, as well as being trained on the course mentioned, also often had considerable experience in creating an enthusiasm for art in school-children of all ages and interests. These same tutors successfully created a similar enthusiasm with their students within the hospital studios. All the elderly people selected for the project eventually developed an interest in the subject, either through art appreciation or through practical experience in one medium or another provided in the hospital studio classes.

Before giving further details of interesting recent developments, here are hints gathered from the project worth mentioning for the benefit of those in other hospitals or residential care institutions who may be interested in making this provision in art for their elderly residents.

Establishing an art class

The importance in hospitals, in particular, of early meetings between all interested members of staff cannot be over-emphasized when introducing new classes in residential care institutions. This is necessary to gain interest and to make sure everyone is adequately informed beforehand. At these preliminary meetings, the staff must first decide whether there exists a nucleus of older people who have already expressed a positive inclination towards new ideas and who may benefit from joining the classes.

Suitable accommodation for the future classes is of prime importance. All institutions are short of space and it is, therefore, essential to discuss these matters right from the beginning. The variety of type of space and accommodation provided by hospitals and residential homes for this type of interest is unlimited in its originality as each new class is established. It is amazing what accommodation can be discovered when it is inspired by interest and enthusiasm of the staff to get the class going successfully.

Although every situation is different, the following are basic essentials for those considering setting up studio facilities for their residents.

1. An internal telephone should be in the room, or very nearby, in the hospital. Tutors are seldom trained in first-aid or other nursing skills, and it is essential that they can reach trained nursing staff in an emergency.
2. Toilet facilities should be within easy reach of the studio.
3. The room should have adequate heating, be reasonably soundproof, with good light – daylight where possible.
4. A water supply and sink, ideally in the room or close by, is essential. If pottery is envisaged, plenty of shelf space and a sink, especially for this purpose with a built-in sediment tank beneath it within the working area, would be needed.
5. A wall area for the display of students' work and teaching aids.
6. Some sturdy tables high enough for wheelchairs to be pushed under.
7. One or more cupboards for storage, large enough to contain A.1 paper (594 mm × 841 mm), as well as other art materials.
8. The room should be large enough to accommodate six to eight people in wheelchairs at a table or tables for painting, clay modelling or pottery and, in addition, to enable two or three students to sit quietly examining natural objects, reference or art books, or observing the others working.
9. If possible, the room should have access to a garden.

The above are the essential basic needs for a studio which can be extended and added to as money and other considerations permit.

Every effort should be made for the area or room allocated to be exclusively for the use of the art classes so that it truly becomes 'the studio' in which art paraphernalia can be left, and in which an atmosphere of quiet study can be created (Figure 11.2).

Having decided provisionally on an appropriate room for the classes, a formal meeting can take place. This should include all hospital or residential-care heads of departments concerned with the elderly people who may be involved, as well as representatives from the local education authority should a tutor be invited. The meeting would be arranged to:

1. Check again that the proposed room is not planned for other uses. It is important that both students and tutor feel secure in establishing the classes and building up an atmosphere for learning in a stable situation.
2. Make sure that the room really is geographically in a suitable position – unhampered, for example, by difficult stairways.
3. Choose a suitable day and time for the class.

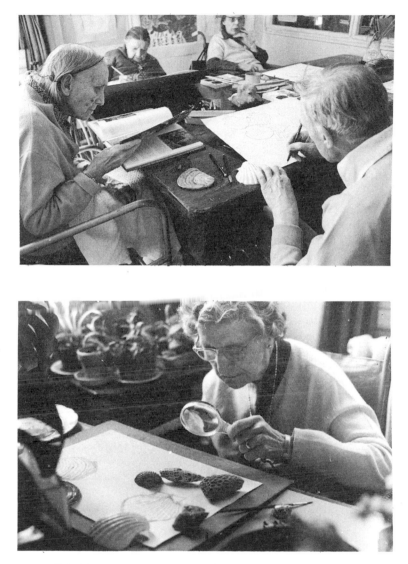

Figure 11.2 'We like somewhere quiet where we can concentrate'.

4. Discuss availability of porters if the class is being introduced in a hospital.
5. Ensure that all are adequately informed of the educational nature of the classes, including the art appreciation element, and of the type of elderly person most likely to benefit from attending the classes.

6. Discuss financial matters — for example, cost of materials and payment of students' fees.

On the success of these first meetings rests the establishment of successful smooth-running classes for the next few years. Their importance cannot be too highly emphasized.

Materials

From the allocation of money agreed upon during the first meetings,
materials can be ordered for the new classes. The following were used
successfully in the project, and are suggested as basic requirements. A
variety of tempera block paints, 1½ inches in diameter, arranged in plastic
containers, each holding six blocks. These were found to be ideal and
were provided in the classes in this project (see details of suppliers at the
end of the chapter). These six-block containers are heavy and make a
steady base for those students with the use of only one arm. The colours
can be mixed boldly, adding white for an opaque effect and water for trans-
parencies. The six colours suggested are: red, orange, blue, yellow, black
and white – Ostwald colours where possible. This palette of predominantly
primary colours gives wide scope for mixing. Opportunities to discover
that blue and yellow make green, that red, yellow and blue equals brown,
and that red and blue become violet, is very much enjoyed by those being
introduced to the delights of colour-mixing for the first time.

   Brushes should be of good quality and include both bristle and sable.
Suggested sizes are: bristle, sizes 3, 6 and 4; sable, sizes 2, 4 and 6. A
selection of both white cartridge and grey sugar paper should be sufficient in the early stages. Water pots should be heavy to avoid spilling
by unsteady hands. White china plates are heavier, therefore steadier,
than plastic, and are a good substitute for expensive artists palettes.
Charcoal, a variety of felt-tipped pens and other sundry items would
be purchased at the discretion of the tutor. If pottery is to be introduced
be sure to use only non-toxic glazes. An extractor fan should be fitted
in the room in which the kiln is housed.

   It is better to purchase a few good-quality materials than a large amount
of substandard equipment. Do not be tempted to accept poor-quality
materials for your class because it is 'only for beginners'. Students
learning new skills need every encouragement. Good-quality paper,
especially, is important, since it is not likely to disintegrate with water
and pressure of the brush.

   If money permits, it is well-worthwhile purchasing some art and
natural history books containing first-class prints, with the hope that
these will form the nucleus of a small library. One or two large magnifying glasses should also be available.

In most of the hospitals concerned in the project, arrangements were made for the local library to supply books on art and related subjects at regular intervals, adding variety to the small permanent studio collection. The volunteer organizer in a hospital or the matron of a residential home may wish to organize this with the local library before classes commence. This could be followed by volunteers and others sharing the interest of the books with the prospective students during their general visits and conversations.

Plants can enhance the appearance of the new room. Choose varieties that will not be affected by central heating and can successfully survive the tutor's holiday periods. Tradescantia, small palms and cacti have proved sturdy plants in this respect, and can form the basis of a larger collection. The art tutor would of course be very much involved in setting the scene of the studio and making the room inviting for that very important first visit of the students. The aim should always be for the room to become a focus – attractive to both staff and patients alike.

In the meantime, staff may wish to talk to the elderly people about the classes, in which case they must be sure to explain to prospective students that they do not have to paint if they do not want to, emphasizing that the classes are as much for art-appreciation as for participation, explaining that they have a choice and may come to visit the new studio 'only to look' if they wish. Many an item has been bought on the initial understanding that you do not have to buy.

It is important also for the tutor to give as much time as possible before the classes begin to visiting the wards from which students are to be selected. These visits will give the tutor a valuable insight into the environment in which the prospective students are living when they are not attending the art class. Getting to know the staff and hearing their opinions of the patients is also very valuable to the tutor. Chatting informally with the elderly people themselves in the ward gives both tutor and prospective students a chance to understand each other's point of view before the idea of the art class is delicately explained. The final selection of elderly people to join the first class should always be the result of a joint agreement between staff, patients and tutor.

The introduction of the classes to the elderly people should never be hurried, so that they feel always that it is in their time and as they choose. They should always feel free just to visit, or participate on a regular basis if they wish.

After the classes have taken place for a few weeks, and are becoming established, further follow-up meetings should be arranged. These should be, as before, with the appropriate heads of departments from the hospital or residential home and representatives of the local education authority. They should be held at regular intervals of approximately three months. Their aim would be to monitor the progress of the classes and to

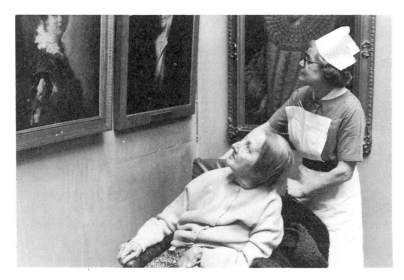

Figure 11.3 'I had always wanted to visit a gallery, but my husband was never interested in such things'.

overcome initial problems, or perhaps to organize the first visit to a local gallery (Figure 11.3), sketching out of doors or plan a future exhibition of work.

NEW DEVELOPMENTS

A decade later, that is, since the project was completed, many hospitals throughout the UK are introducing educational opportunities and creative interests for the benefit of their physically disabled patients. The basic essentials still apply, that is:

1. The importance of a room suitable for use as a studio, attractive to both staff and elderly students alike.
2. Continued enquiry as to the needs of the students with development guided by their wishes.
3. Tutors, volunteers and care staff prepared by courses and/or meetings beforehand.

Among the elderly people concerned a sustained interest in art has continued, not just for weeks or months, but for years as their knowledge and interest of the subject continues to evolve.

Some consultants may well say that the need is now different and that the elderly people in elderly patient departments of hospitals today would not benefit from a learning situation as they did in 1978. Yet new classes continue to begin in hospitals where rooms are provided for use as studios with elderly people benefitting and appreciating opportunities to study art seriously. An art tutor who has had considerable experience in teaching elderly people in hospitals and other residential institutions said: 'Through the practice of art they evolve a sense of worth and confidence, and discover that their point of view matters'.

In the elderly patient department of one hospital in south-east London, as well as painting and drawing, the elderly students have begun a new interest as they work in their studio with stained glass. One lady in her 70s, who has been in hospital for at least five years, has produced to her own design a crucifix in coloured glass which now hangs in the hospital chapel in a position which she chose herself above the door. Working with glass could be dangerous, particularly for a disabled person, yet with the guidance of a trained tutor and suitable working facilities this is made possible.

Integration not segregation

In one residential home for the elderly, a resident said: 'It is very nice here and we have beautiful grounds, but we are cut off from the mainstream of life'. Also, in elderly patient departments of hospitals people, because of calendar age, are segregated from other generations. Where the pursuit of the knowledge of art has led to the classes going out on visits or other generations invited in, the stimulated comments from the elderly students involved show clearly the need for a wider involvement with the outside world. Effort to enhance mobility and transport for such visits is truly rewarded.

In a hospital in the south-west area of London where new classes have recently begun, the extension of art appreciation has led to a contact with the Courtauld Institute of Art. The elderly students visit this fine exclusive gallery in London. Young student lecturers attached to the gallery, with prior consultation, come to the hospital or residential home and give talks with slides, giving those unable to visit the gallery an opportunity of a professional lecture.

After observing her patients attending the new art class and enlightened by their development, an assistant senior nursing officer said: 'There is nothing to compare to seeing a patient blossom into discussion and laughter from a new interest'.

At a residential home for elderly peple, after regular visits to the adult education centre art class, residents said: 'We like to see the young people and to listen to their conversations, especially at tea break in the canteen when they come down from the other classes in other subjects'.

Sketching out of doors, including the hospital grounds, also brings contact with other generations. Passing members of staff and visitors are enlightened to see what the elderly long-term patients are doing, as well as heightening the overall awareness of the students concerned as they concentrate on their work.

New training courses

Trained tutors who completed the courses designed and organized for the project previously mentioned are teaching in all parts of the country, not only to those of advanced years living in hospitals, but also in a similar manner to elderly people living in all types of residential care accommodation, including residential homes and sheltered housing, day centres and clubs.

These courses have since extended to advanced courses for the previously trained tutors, and courses for course organizers, to encourage continuity.

The trained tutors themselves have now formed a national organization, ASNAT, 'Association of Special Need Arts Tutors' (details are given in the Appendix).

Where a tutor is not available

In some areas of the country it has not always been possible to obtain a tutor. For this reason, courses have also been designed for managers of homes, care staff and volunteers interested themselves in extending the interest of the elderly people in their care in a variety of residential care accommodation, day centres and clubs. In Surrey, England, in particular, courses in creative interests and educational opportunities have been popular among care staff and certainly prove to fulfil a need among the elderly people concerned. Enthusiasm for a subject by amateur as well as professional can interest others around. The courses have given the opportunity for staff to learn successful ways of introducing their interests and building a sustained interest among their residents. As a result of these courses, rooms have been successfully set aside and in them ideas have been introduced.

Subjects have varied from art to wine-making, history of kings and queens, computer uses and nature studies. As subjects have progressed, more knowledge and study is needed by staff and residents alike. In order to extend their interests further, members of local clubs, wine-making and history groups are being invited to visit and exchange ideas with residents and occasional return visits are arranged. In addition to the existing programme of light entertainment there are now opportunities for serious progressive learning.

Although much success can be achieved by care staff volunteers and other members of the community, the aim should always be to invite an adult education specialist tutor in the subject to the group whenever possible at some point – maybe for a limited number of sessions in order to widen the perspective of the chosen interest for everyone.

The tutors' fees are paid by their local education authority. The students concerned, through their appropriate hospital or residential home, pay the old age pensioners' students' fees in the same way as they would if they could get along to an adult education institute. In some areas of the country these fees are financially assisted further by their local borough.

Conclusion

The provision of educational opportunities in art for elderly people living in hospital care, residential homes, sheltered housing, day centres and clubs, has proved successful in the project described. Here, suitable accommodation and trained tutors were provided on a scale equal to facilities offered to adults of all ages attending mainstream classes in local adult education institutions. Education authorities should, therefore, heed the early pioneers of adult education and continue to make tutors available to this segregated area of the adult community.

Further, planners of the future should include a space for quiet study in their designs for all buildings where elderly people are expected to live in residential care or spend time in day centres.

Those of us working in residential care with people of advanced years are almost always dealing with an age group beyond our own. It is of prime importance, therefore, that we bother to ask their opinions before deciding what is best for them. Every one of us is an individual and has a different attitude to life, and the 'elderly' are no exception

Each successive generation of older people will have different needs. We must make sure, therefore, that the opinions of the elders of the future continue to be considered by successive younger generations regarding educational opportunities, or for that matter, anything else.

REFERENCES

ASNAT (Association of Special Needs Art Tutors), 15, Streetfield Mews, Blackheath Park, London, SE3 OER, England.

APPENDIX: SUPPLIERS OF ART MATERIALS

George Rowney & Co. Ltd, 12 Percy Street, London W1.
New York Central Supply Co. (suppliers for George Rowney & Co. Ltd), 62 Third Avenue, New York, 10003, USA.
Pentalic Corporation, (suppliers for George Rowney & Co. Ltd), 132 West 22nd Street, New York, USA.

Oswald Sealy (Australia) Pty Ltd, (suppliers for George Rowney & Co. Ltd), 4 George Place, Artarmon, NSW 2064, Australia.

NB George Rowney & Co. Ltd stock Ostwald colours among their opaque colour block range, as well as fitted palettes.

Winsor & Newton, London Showroom, 51/52 Rathbone Place, London W1TP 1AB. Head Office: Wealdstone, Harrow, Middlesex HA3 5RH.

Winsor & Newton Incorporated, 555 Winsor Drive, Secaucus, New Jersey 07094, USA.

Winsor & Newton Pty Ltd, 102/104 Reserve Road, Artarmon, NSW 2064, Australia.

NB Winsor & Newton also stock Ostwald standard colours in poster blocks in round cakes of three different sizes with polystyrene palettes to contain them.

Reeves Dryad, 178 Kensington High Street, London W8.

Educational Colours Pty Ltd, 25 Clarice Road, Box Hill, Victoria, Australia.

NB Reeves Dryad supply Tempera Block colours in polystyrene palettes to contain them.

All the above firms stock brushes, paper and a variety of other art materials.

Kiln – suitable for use in hospital studios: Electric kiln – Thermo-save range, T50–12'' × 15'' × 18'' obtainable from: Fulham Pottery Limited, 184 New Kings Road, London SW6.

Diamond Ceramics Limited, (suppliers for Fulham Pottery Limited), 52 Geddes Street, Mulgrave, Victoria 3170, Australia.

Ferro Industrial Products, (suppliers for Fulham Pottery Limited), PO Box 108, Brakpan 1540, South Africa.

Chapter 12

Dramatherapy

INTRODUCTION

This chapter will consider dramatherapy under three main headings: firstly, 'What is dramatherapy?', secondly, 'Why is it useful in the practice of extended hospital care?', and thirdly, 'How may it be undertaken in this setting?'.

WHAT IS DRAMATHERAPY?

Professional dramatherapists are relatively new, having developed in the UK as a body since the early 1960s. They evolved along with the new wave therapies. Peter Slade had established the use of dramatic play as essential to child development, and has paved the way for drama in education. Brian Way extended its use into personal development, and Sue Jennings and her colleagues pioneered remedial drama and its progression into the field of therapy. 'Sesame', a branch of the Religious Drama Group, took volunteer actors into institutions to perform and to involve patients in their performance. From these varied sources, a new profession has emerged.

The therapeutic use of drama is, however, as ancient as man. Its roots lie in the rituals, dances and actions of our ancestors which were used to promote the welfare of their communities over a wide range of experience. Each community had a councillor, confidante and leader of rituals called the shaman, who in time became particularly associated with the rituals of healing. The fact that he was consulted about both personal and community problems illustrates that the links between social organization and health were recognized long before they were re-discovered in more recent times.

Considering drama, *per se*, will help one to understand dramatherapy and its application. The word 'drama' is derived from the Greek *dran* – a thing done. So it is about action. However, nothing dramatic can be achieved without the vital addition of creativity. Drama is also about imagination, feeling, symbol and metaphor, the latter representing the 'as if' quality of drama.

Landy (1986) writes of the interactive meaning of drama for the individuals: 'For drama to occur it is necessary for the actor, one who acts in everyday life, to distinguish between either one aspect of the self and another or between self and non-self'.

Drama can be seen as a continuum, the components of which are: Ritual – Play – Movement – Mime – Dance – Games – Role play – Theatre. The dramatherapist can use components at all levels of the patient's ability, the activities suggested below being adaptable to all levels of individual need.

Ritual

Ritual has already been referred to. There is a tendency to relate it only to primitive societies and magic. However, there are many rituals in the present which we cannot disregard, both personal – that people create for themselves – and cultural.

Children often have a bed-time ritual of bath, story, and to bed with a good-night kiss. Without their ritual, they feel unhappy and fear disaster. Adults have similar rituals of going to bed and getting up in the morning, completing chores, etc. They are often referred to as routines, but can become embued with a sense of security.

Cultural rituals are accepted as the norm – particularly the religious ones around birth, death and marriage. They may not be highly valued as such in our society, but they have their uses. The rituals around death, for example, allow for expression of sympathy to the mourners, help them to come to terms with bereavement and facilitate the grieving process.

Play

Drama is an extension of play. It is accepted that children learn through play, but all can learn from the play element in drama. The 'make-believe' involvement of acting 'as if' it were real allows for a detached objectivity which promotes a sense of security. The action is not real, but once removed, and therefore safe for experiment.

Play is a part of drama only if it is used to some purpose and deliberately undertaken for dramatic action to take place.

Movement/dance

These elements are all basic to life. Infants move instinctively. Finding a joy in the movement itself they experiment with more movement. The more active they are the more they discover, thus strengthening muscles, learning co-ordination and balance, and gaining confidence in their bodies. Repeated movement develops rhythm and continuity, and enters the realm of dance.

Adults tend to lose this facility to enjoy movement for its own sake and spontaneous dance. Schooling teaches that there is a 'right way' to do things, and an appropriate time and place. Yet movement as part of dramatherapy can still be a medium for learning or re-learning – for example, balancing skills or coordination after a stroke.

Movement is important at all ages, but particularly to older people. If limbs are not exercised regularly, they become stiff and painful and finally cease to be of use at all. Exercises, unless enjoyable, can be a bore. Motivation will then fade and action suffer. Exercise that is built into an enjoyable dramatic context is more liable to be undertaken.

Mime

Mime is a word that can be misleading. Mime artists are highly trained and skilled people with muscular control and expertise beyond the capabilities of the untrained. Perhaps a more useful term is 'non-verbal communication'. Most professionals are aware of the need to understand and co-ordinate body language and speech as an important component of social skills training.

Games

Organized games can be simply a recreation, but if used with a specific purpose in mind, can form part of a therapeutic programme. Games are basic drama that can be used either creatively on their own, or as a 'warm-up' to other dramatic activities

Role play

Each individual has many roles in society (Moreno, 1946). As people grow older roles change and often diminish. Practice is often needed to expand present roles, and rehearse new ones. There may be grief and bereavement over lost or diminished roles. Moreno writes: 'Working with the "role" as a point of reference appears to be a methodical advantage as compared with "personality" or "ego"'.

The word 'role' is taken from the name given to the written part an actor played in Greek theatre. It was written on a 'roll'. Modern actors research the role of the characters they are playing, the role being the feeling and attitudes the character will have in the situation in which he is depicted.

Real life roles are about a place in society, be it family, professional or social. There is an expectation of accepted behaviour in this role. Role play as therapy often concentrates on behaviour. Dramatherapy pays heed to the theatrical source of role, emphasizing feelings and attitudes as of equal, and sometimes greater, importance.

Theatre

Theatre is the presentation of a story, mime or sequence of events by one person, or a group, to another person or group. It is a good medium for allowing people to become more aware and understanding of experiences so far unknown to them. The audience identifies with characters on stage, and they 'live' the events portrayed 'as if' audience and players were one. As well as being a means of escaping from the reality of everyday, this is also an opportunity to view experiences 'once removed'. This exchange of experiences between audience and actor – be they painful, pleasant, amusing or desired – allows for acceptable access to feelings that are normally hidden. The therapist then has an opportunity to discuss personal issues and feelings with patients either individually or in a group.

Theatre is the communication of experience, and the higher the standard of the actor's performance the more clear is the communication. In all other aspects of drama, the therapy is in the doing, and not in the standard of performance. Involvement in performance is the only time when the patient is concerned with the standard at which he works.

For a patient, the experience of being part of an audience allows:

(a)   Involvement in make-believe by 'the willing suspension of disbelief' (Esslin, 1976).
(b)   An opportunity to view life experiences through metaphor.
(c)   A sense of being part of a corporate body with the other members of the audience.
(d)   Interaction with other members of the audience.
(e)   An opportunity to escape from reality.

The experience of being a performer can be equally rewarding by:

(a)   Encouraging creativity and imagination.
(b)   Creating a new social role.
(c)   Creating self-confidence and enhancing self-esteem.
(d)   Accepting the discipline of theatre by setting boundaries.
(e)   Relating to other members of the group in a different way, and learning to work as a team.

THE USE OF DRAMA

The dramatherapist can call on any or all of these components of the continuum to meet the needs of the individual or group with whom he/she is working.

Depending on the needs and abilities of the group, the dramatherapist may take them through activities either in a planned programme of experiences selected from the continuum, or use issues as they arise and select action spontaneously. Either method constitutes a dramatic process in which the flexibility of movement within the continuum is a response to the needs of the participants.

Patients are admitted to hospital because they are sick, and because the ensuing disabilities cannot be accommodated at home. This may be a continuing state or a temporary one. Dramatherapy is rooted in action and creativity, so the dramatherapist, whilst acknowledging disability, works with the preserved ability of the patient towards the goal or rehabilitation (discussed later in this chapter) or healing.

WHY DRAMATHERAPY?

Now that the nature of dramatherapy has been described, it is necessary to consider why it is needed and what it may contribute to the life of someone confined to residence in hospital.

A hospital ward offering extended care is a community of twenty or more residents and, overall, maybe as many staff. Those involved, be they residents or staff, will possess very different abilities and will come from very different backgrounds, yet all, in their own way, personal or professional, are trying to come to terms with the challenge of living or working, over long periods of time, with illness or disability.

Each patient, within himself, and by the use of his remaining attributes, physical or mental, has to adjust to his disability and meet and express his personal needs. Additionally, he has to make social adjustments. These will have commenced at the time when hospital life was forseen but not implemented, and will continue through transfer to extended care and the subsequent learning about and coping with new patients and staff. Illness notoriously turns us in upon ourselves (consider trying to be sociable with a raging toothache) and enforced social adjustments at this time will be particularly taxing and potentially overwhelming.

The social adjustments are in two directions. Towards fellow patients there may, out of anxiety, be either identification ('I shall get like that') and/or a distancing ('I'm not like these other people'). Anxiety may also be felt towards caring staff, in or out of uniform, who will carry authority to impose strange and uncomfortable clinical procedures. Furthermore, professionals, even if only in the quest for objectivity, will distance themselves in terms of human relations. The closeness of patients to ward orderlies and cleaners, more so than to doctors and nurses, is well known. In a ward most relationships are short-lived;

staff do their jobs and go home. Social mobility, at least for staff, and maybe for patients, is high with all that that means for lack of social cohesion.

Staff are part of the ward community and also have their own groupings. They have professional standards and import personal values from their home life. They will have to cope with the projected fantasies that patients have about them and get on with each other in a multi-disciplinary team. Their needs also bear attention.

It is common experience that the diversity of illness and personality seen on any one ward is enormous, even when attempts at strat-ification have been made into, say, psychiatric or elderly communities, or into medium and extended care. A stroke may, to a greater or lesser extent, impair physical autonomy; depression may impair drive; or confusion (in either the short or long term) may impair mental autonomy. There are many more variations when the subtleties are considered. Disability may not be total, or multiple disabilities may be present in different combinations, so one patient may be physically active and optimistic (but totally confused) while another is physically depen-dent but mentally sharp, with a third being depressed in a way that augments physical disability. A naturally anxious person shows more distress than someone who is more phlegmatic. Some will conduct an aggressive search for aid while others will be unnaturally sub-servient.

Then there may be premorbid personal problems without direct connection with the illness, but still of great relevance to the indi-vidual; personal issues such as variations in mental and physical aptitude may influence the presentation of illness; or social issues such as poverty, lack of, or problematic family supporters, burdensome family responsibilities, no home, or the necessities and chores of giving up a home.

Finally, in any long-term hospital ward there is an element of terminal care. Facing death oneself as a patient or in others as a relative or staff member includes coming to terms with both the anxiety of anticipation and the management, afterwards, of bereavement and mourning.

This attempt to understand the mind of a disabled patient and the nature of the community in which he lives in a broader context illustrates the complexity of the task of those responsible for treatment and life in an extended care hospital ward. A patient will want to feel understood as a person, and the provision of extended care does not stop once strictly professional/technical needs are met. There is a 'well' side to his existence based on a rich individual experience of life, as well as a 'sick' or dependent side. The broader view does not invalidate the need for pro-fessionals to diagnose, classify and care for the types of physical and mental disabilities seen, but to stop there is premature. An individual treatment plan in extended care requires that all facets of life are considered.

Some regard permanent hospitalization (or residental care) as the interval between social and physical death. Need it be so? Clinical staff are well trained in making traditional diagnoses or assessment but are not so well trained in looking beyond strictly bio-medical/nursing needs (this is discussed later under 'The role of staff in providing quality of life').

What is there over the strictly bio-technical horizon? There are many models by which human nature and needs can be classified, but some that seem of particular value in making the task of extended care more meaningful and easier to understand are described below.

MASLOW'S HIERARCHY OF HUMAN NEEDS

Maslow (1943) looked at human motivation by arranging goals in rank order: from those that are primitive and the most demanding, particularly if unsatisfied, to those that are complex and creative but which are also vulnerable in the face of challenge. There are various cultural paths to each goal.

Table 12.1 Maslow's motivational goals (after Maslow, 1943)

1. Physiological	Homeostatsis for e.g. food, fluids, heat
2. Safety	Particularly in the face of unfamiliarity
3. Love	Affectionate relationships
4. Esteem	For self and from others
5. Self-actualization	Creative self expression

Maslow described the most primitive and demanding needs as those for physiological stability, e.g., food, warmth and fluids. At this level needs must be met, even in the face of hazard to higher order needs. This is survival.

Next in turn comes safety: protection from threat and physical danger.

Safety, once assured, is followed by the social need to belong: to be able to give and receive friendship and love.

Then, in turn, there is a need for esteem, autonomy, self respect, achievement, and the appreciation and respect of others.

Finally, there is self-fulfilment of a creative kind: self actualization.

As the most primitive of these needs are the most demanding it is only when they are met that the individual feels free to indulge needs of a higher order, but once biology and safety are assured then interest can turn to social and creative needs. However, these, being tender plants, need nurturing.

The environment of a conventional hospital ward, in Maslow's terms, provides food, warmth, and reasonable safety (but accidents and cross infections too). A sense of belonging may be actively discouraged if resettlement is the aim: autonomy is often eroded, (but need it be excessively so?), respect may come more from professional rather than from individual concern, and the opportunities to create and contribute are minimal. Wards like this don't do very well beyond Maslow's second level. However, there are models of rehabilitation which, if implemented, may help towards a better way of life.

SOCIAL REHABILITATION

The dangers of institutional care are now too well known to require more than brief mention. It is only too easy for the patient to fall into the 'sick role' and accept, enjoy and even exaggerate the dependency that this brings.

Rehabilitation attempts to offset these tendencies by maximizing role performance in the individual patient, by making him the principal determinants of, and actor in, his own life. Physical rehabilitation maximizes accomplishments in a physical world; psycho-social rehabilitation develops role performance in a social world.

The gains from rehabilitation may be large or modest but are appropriate even when small. In any case the valuation of 'gains' is relative; not everyone aspires to the heights, and in difficult circumstances there can be job satisfaction for the carer even when gains are small. It is important for all staff whether professionally trained or not, to understand the value of apparently simple daily activities in rehabilitation. Sharing a photograph, or a story from the past, or the physical contact of an arm round a shoulder or a held hand can be important professional as well as human activities and should be appreciated as such. Resettlement, i.e., the placement of a patient outside hospital may be one, and perhaps in hospital care the ultimate aim of rehabilitation, but it is not the sole aim.

Social rehabilitation is achieved by defining, in collaboration with the patient, appropriate roles as personal targets for growth and change, small or large. Understanding and motivation will need to be conveyed by explanation; the patient needs to know what is expected of him. Appropriate skills will need to be learned, strengthened, or re-learned, so that the roles may be undertaken. For example, assessment and discussion with the patient may reveal that he wants to make friends with other patients but lacks the necessary social skills. The defining of the task may have motivated him to learn how, say, to find an opening to a conversation, something that has never been easy for him, and is now more difficult because of dysarthria following a stroke. He is then helped to learn the necessary skills and is given sufficient practice to make them acceptably easy and free from anxiety. Note that in social terms it is facilitating the role 'friend' and not just offering, say, speech therapy.

Rehabilitation theory (Bennet, 1977) tells us that roles are always multiple and changing with e.g. age and work status. What roles are available in an extended care ward? Which can we create? The very fact of admission to such a ward suggests that the condition is more than transitional and that some degree of pre-admission role failure (or of role imbalance, because of failure by others to attenuate role demands) has occurred. Confidence in any or every role performance may have been eroded, so keeping roles 'open' is vital to self esteem. The role of 'patient' may, to some degree, have to be accepted, but not to an excessive or disabling degree, and the patient may need help to strike a balance.

The role of 'decider' should be open to all, although the complexity of the decision may need to be matched to the clinical disability. Some may be very able at financial affairs; others, because of memory or cognitive loss, may be capable of little more than deciding what to eat or wear at that moment in time.

THE ROLE OF STAFF IN PROVIDING QUALITY OF LIFE

What can be achieved in practice? Staff are hard pressed and orientated towards the professional rather than the expressive side of patient care. Nevertheless, however, even if not competent in some of the broader roles of total patient 'care' (the word sounds too passive in this context), they can help to provide an acceptable milieu by involving others, such as dramatherapists, who do have the necessary skills. Patients may reach the outside world by outings, but something of its quality can also be imported into the ward. So a patient may expect more of a doctor than a prescription, more of a nurse than a facility with bathing, and more of a dramatherapist than physical exercise, etc., etc.

Staff time is always precious, and its allocation raises the question of priorities. How is time and effort apportioned between the demands of heavy nursing and the need for quality of life. There is here an opportunity for conflict, which can be either creative or destructive depending upon the way that it is handled. The potential for conflict in extended care, and how it may be handled, is well illustrated in a study of residential care of the physically disabled conducted by Miller and Gwynne (1972). It has lessons for all those engaged in long-term care. Initially the authors set out to investigate low staff morale in a residential care home. In the process they identified, in staff, two conflicting ideologies of care. On the one hand there was a traditional, humanitarian strategy in which patients, seen as sick, passive and compliant, were subject to active intervention by others. This was called

Table 12.2 Systems in the care of the physically disabled (after Miller and Gwynne, 1972)

Humanitarian	*Liberal*
Preserve life	'Really normal'
Offer care	Promote autonomy
Problems	*Problems*
Dependency	Failure/Exclusion
'Warehousing'	'Horticultural'
Not either/or but 'Which approach at which time?'	

the 'Warehousing' model. On the other hand, there was a liberal strategy that respected individuality and independence and called for effort and a contribution on the part of the client. Because it emphasized growth it was called 'Horticultural'. This was excellent for those who could cope, but inability to meet expectation lead to a sense of failure, scapegoating and exclusion. Balanced decisions were needed: when, in the face of true dependency, to offer care, and when to switch to the 'DIY' growth model, perhaps in the same patient, when the task was within his reach.

Individuals, in real life, present with a mixture of autonomy and dependence. A single strategy aimed at only one, say dependence, will always be inappropriate when autonomy is present, and vice versa. Any one strategy, if used exclusively, will always be wrong some of the time. Inappropriate strategies will lead to unnecessary suffering for both the patient and staff. The art is to know when to use which strategy, and that *is* an art which requires much and constant thought, some experiment and rehearsal and a lot of experience; it is not easy. For this reason Miller considered that the best way of maintaining a balance was to make 'supervision' available to staff so that problems can be analysed and solutions debated and, if necessary, rehearsed. It does not necessarily involve a line manager. Indeed, there may be disadvantages in exploring some of the complex human reactions to caring within a professional hierarchy. Rather it means an opportunity to share and be helped to understand one's personal and professional reactions with others who are in the same boat. It is a psychotherapeutic or counselling model which should allow the ventilation of personal feelings, and understanding of the feelings and roles of others. It gives an opportunity for problem-solving and, perhaps, rehearsal of responses.

BRINGING IT ALL TOGETHER

Attention has been drawn to the multiple problems that a patient may bring with him to a long-stay ward. The carer must find a middle path between essential and excessive support for not only the individual but for the group, and tension may arise in both patients and staff that need to be attended to if the community is to prosper. A case has been made for exploring personal and group issues and for setting realistic goals for both clinical and social rehabilitation in which some of the higher aspects of human expression are given consideration and outlet. Whenever possible it is a matter of sharing between patient and professional; it is participative rather than prescriptive.

The very words of social rehabilitation form a bridge between clinical practice and drama; there are so many in common, role, performance or role play, rehearsal, which is analogous to repeating rehabilitative tasks under supervision, and dialogue (over conflicts).

There is also the enriching and sensitizing effect of artistic apprecia- tion or expression, the exploration of self through role play and reversal, and the use of dramatherapy for getting the patient out of the sick role, both for assessment and therapy. For staff, although dramatherapy is not the only tool for 'supervision' and the exploration of the interaction of professional and person, it is one such tool which can help to promote understanding and cohesion. These contributions are summarized in Table 12.3

Table 12.3 The contribution of dramatherapy

Dramatherapy can contribute to the life of the long-stay ward in a number of ways.

For the patient
1. Helps to enrich life and contribute to self-esteem and creative expression.
2. Helps to explore emotional problems of disability and to rehearse coping strategies.
3. Helps to develop personality and skills that may be needed in a new way of life.

For the member of staff
1. Increases job satisfaction from the enriched life of the ward community.
2. Helps in sharing with other professionals and in developing solutions to the problems aned conflicts of care.
3. Helps in assessment by seeing the patient in a different social context.
4. Helps in formulating broad treatment plans.

HOW MAY DRAMATHERAPY BE PRACTISED IN EXTENDED CARE?

Reference has already been made to the value of the play element of drama, and the metaphoric 'as if' quality of its application. This section will demonstrate some specific ways in which dramatherapy can contribute to life and work in a ward offering extended care.

Quality of life

Drama should be enjoyable, and games, play readings and improvized plays can contribute to creating a friendly, relaxed and stimulating environment.

Inviting a theatre group into the ward makes a social occasion, and a trip to the theatre, if that is possible, widens horizons and is an event in itself. Drama used with the overall goal of improving quality of life is therapy in its broadest sense.

Social adjustment

With other patients. The anxiety caused by unfamiliarity can be mitigated in the dramatherapy group. If there is a regular group session, newcomers can be helped to find their own place in the ward community. There is usually a ritual of introducing new patients to the group. It may be simply a formal introduction, or group members may introduce themselves adding three personal statements they would like the newcomer to know. Some other introductory games are:

(1) Throw a ball around the group, each person giving his/her name as they catch it.
(2) When people are aware of some names, they can call the name of the person to whom they are throwing.
(3) Find three things you have in common with your partner. These may be very obvious things like both having blue eyes or wearing spectacles. It does not matter how simple they are, the sharing will move to a more personal level when the group is ready.
(4) Tell your partner about your favourite TV star/actor/sportsman/piece of music/book/painting.

These simple games can help to ease the anxieties of being 'the new patient'. If offered in isolation, the individual may wonder what is happening. So it makes sense to use the games within the security of a group session, where the content of dramatherapy is explained and accepted. The relationships formed in the group, and the discussion commencing there, will be developed outside it.

With members of staff. Patients usually relate to staff, particularly those in uniform, in a fairly passive manner. The staff are authority figures who will tell the patients what to do, or will minister to them if they are disabled. This attitude fosters dependancy, and whilst that may sometimes be necessary, it is important to encourage personal choice and independence as far as possible in order to avoid the negative effects of being in an institution. Some methods of encouraging alternative ways of relating are:

(1) Available staff join the dramatherapy group *as ordinary members* entering into the games and activities with enthusiasm; the shared experience can become a bond which helps to create a different kind of relationship.

(2) A ward notice-board show photographs of staff and patients, both as they are seen on the ward, and with their families. This may be part of reality orientation, either in specific sessions or informally, and it is available at any time.

(3) Trust exercises can be a means of creating a trusting, cohesive group. They can encourage trust in oneself, and also hold a measure of responsibility for others. If staff are prepared to join the dramatherapy group it is possible to promote a different quality of trust. Also, when a patient finds himself or herself responsible for the well-being of a staff member, opportunities for a more reciprocal relationship occur. Some simple trust exercises are: (a) Close your eyes and allow a partner to take your hand. Discuss your feelings. (b) Close your eyes and allow a partner to lead you across the room. It is important to stress that the leader is totally responsible for his or her welfare, and must avoid bumping into furniture. Discuss your feelings. (c) For the more able: stand in a circle and with each supporting the other, by joining arms; stand on one leg. This can also be done in pairs. Discuss your feelings. It is particularly necessary to discuss each trust exercise because some people find them very threatening.

(4) Touch is a very important means of communication which can be explored openly in the dramatherapy group. Some people enjoy physical contact, others do not; staff may feel it is not professional to use touch as a means of communication. It is important to be aware of the feelings of each individual, in both the group and ward. An elderly patient may appear endearing, or perhaps be distressed, and the impulse may be to offer comfort with close physical contact. This may be just what the patient needs and wants, in which case it is appropriate. However, if the individual is one who finds touch difficult, staff should restrain their impulse and consider the needs of the receiver. Indiscriminate use of physical contact can be seen as patronizing.

It is not only important to consider touch while socializing. It is easy, when under pressure in a busy ward, to communicate stress to patients by the manner of touching them whilst carrying out routine procedures, thus communicating staff problems to patients.

REHABILITATION

Physical rehabilitation

The need for movement after illness or surgery needs no emphasis.

Elderly people who have pain or difficulty in moving are at risk of further permanent disability if they do not exercise. Encouragement and motivation are often necessary to get people on their feet. Physiotherapists may visit regularly, but their work can be complemented in dramatherapy groups. It is essential to consult the physiotherapist in selecting the group members and finding suitable exercises, to avoid undoing the good work done by them. Here are a few suggestions for keeping patients mobile.

(a) Throwing and catching a soft ball whilst sitting in a circle.
(b) Kicking the ball across the circle, still seated.
(c) Playing 'balloon football'. The group face each other in two lines. The aim is to keep the balloon(s) in the air. If a balloon reaches the floor behind a team, then the team sitting opposite, who have patted the balloon, score a point.
(d) Walking in time to music, especially marches, helps a rhythmical step, co-ordination and balance. Try singing 'Onward Christian Soldiers' as the group walk around the room.
(e) Swing arms to a waltz tune. If possible, waltz with the more able.
(f) Those who are more mobile hold hands in a circle for support, and then gently rise onto tip-toe.

Wheelchairs

Most games and exercises can be modified for people confined to wheelchairs. Given sufficient helpers, the group can create 'wheelchair dances'; these are fun, giving a sense of movement and skill to people with limited mobility.

Adapting to being confined to a wheelchair is a process that is not always given much attention. In fact, the chair can become part of the body image. Time needed to get from one place to another is different. Work around personal perceptions of the chair as part of the body image: how big is it? how long does it take to do things? This is particularly useful for people in self-propelled chairs. Here are some ideas of the kind of games one can invent:

(a) Place obstacles around the room and see if people can complete the course without bumping into things.
(b) Guess how long it will take each individual to complete the course. Then check it out.
(c) Place furniture with varying gaps. Speculate on whether a wheelchair will pass between without touching. Check it out.
(d) Ask the patient 'What would you like to say to your wheelchair?'

Then, 'If the wheelchair could talk, what do you think it would say?' This is a useful way of helping people express their feelings about their lack of mobility.

Social rehabilitation

Rehabilitation, at its best, aids patients to return to their usual way of life. For most of the patients in continuing-care wards, this is unrealistic, and rehabilitation has to be about making the best possible use of the abilities left to the patient after illness. In the social sense, this may mean learning to live with relatives, in a residential home, or permanently in hospital. For people who have lived alone or with only a partner for several years, this adjustment can be difficult. Dramatherapy can be valuable in learning to adapt to role changes and learning (or re-learning) social skills.

Social skills training. (a) Games which encourage eye contact, such as ball games, name games, and games of exchanging chairs with others. (b) Pass on object around the circle, feeling its texture and sharing reactions. (c) Tell your partner about a book you've read, or a TV programme you've enjoyed. (d) Describe a place you know well to a partner. (e) Describe an outfit that would be suitable for your partner to wear to a wedding/trip to the seaside/visit to the theatre etc.

Role exploration and training. (a) See how many roles you have in common with a partner. (b) Mime an action associated with a favourite working/social role. This should promote considerable discussion and sharing. (c) Tell a story of some interesting event in which you played a leading role. (d) If a patient is to move into other accommodation, it would be possible to set up a simulated situation to 'try out' in fantasy, experimenting with different approaches. (e) If a difficult interview (perhaps with a relative or prospective residential home staff) is pending, rehearsal in a role simulation can be helpful.

Emotional rehabilitation

It is important to remember that a variety of strong and possibly conflicting feelings will have been aroused by admission to hospital. Unless these emotions are acknowledged and allowed expression, the patient will have difficulty coming to terms with the new situation. There is an administrative ritual for admission to hospital, taking details of next of kin, personal property and a medical/social history, but there is no accepted ritual to ease the transition for the patient.

There may well be a sense of bereavement if a patient has to give up independent living. Actual bereavement, the death of a carer, may be the reason for admission. Loss of roles may be felt acutely, with a feeling of having 'come to the end of the road'. There may be mourning over lost social life and a feeling of social death. Patients may be facing up to the prospect of physical deterioration and death. There may be anger towards the family who have allowed hospitalization, or towards the illness or disability itself. Frustration at restricted mobility is common. There may also be a feeling of relief at being cared for, and for no longer being responsible for day-to-day chores. All or any of these feelings may exist at the same time, leaving the patient disturbed and confused.

Dramatherapy is an excellent medium for exploring feelings and coming to terms with life events. If people are not aware of their individual feelings, but are tense and upset, it is possible to work metaphorically, perhaps starting with appropriate stories and myths. Working on a fantasy level allows people to enter into situations that engender the same feelings being experienced in real life. This 'once removed' method of looking at emotions, creates a secure environment, and encourages objective appraisal. Some ideas for encouraging expression of feelings are:

(a) Find an individual body posture showing how people are feeling this moment. Discuss similarities in the group.

(b) An individual places objects, (cushions, buttons, pieces of cloth etc.) to represent feelings, noting the size, weight and colour (sculpting). The patient can then debate the importance of each feeling and differentiate between them.

(c) Patients draw a picture of themselves depicting their emotional state. It doesn't have to be a work of art – pin men/women can be very expressive.

(d) Individuals write a 'secret' fear or anxiety on pieces of paper that are then shuffled and distributed at random. Each person is then asked to speak about the subject on his/her new paper, as if it were his/her own fear or anxiety. Anonymity breaks through shyness and fear of being exposed.

Patients often feel that they are alone in their emotional response. Opening up subjects for discussion allows people to share their feelings. It is a great comfort to discover one is not alone, particularly with 'bad' feelings.

RELATIVES

Patients are not alone with their mixed feelings. Relatives may have the same sense of loss and separation, fear disability and death, be angry with the patient for being ill and at the same time relieved to hand over the caring to professionals, yet feel guilty as well.

Dramatherapy support groups for relatives could help them to express and cope with these feelings. This would ultimately benefit the patient by improved and – hopefully – more honest relationships. Techniques similar to those suggested for patient groups could be used.

Many people suffering from dementia are admitted to extended-care wards. Visiting friends and relatives are often at a loss for means of communication. They can be encouraged to join the 'enrichment' groups. A shared experience, even if it is a simple game or sing-song, can be a means of communication.

STAFF

Support

Hospital staff are frequently under presure. Most disciplines are understaffed, and individuals feel they are working at full capacity. There is often a failure to realize the emotional strain put upon them. Apart from feeling overburdened, staff have to come to terms with their own feelings aroused by contact with patients.

Working with elderly, often terminally ill patients is, for staff, a constant reminder of their own ageing and mortality. Inevitably, staff grow fond of people in long-term care, and the death of a patient can be a source of bereavement. Equally, staff can dislike patients, particularly if the patient is disagreeable or difficult. There is a widely held view that staff should like all their patients, so feelings of guilt may arise.

Lack of opportunity to express and share feelings creates yet another burden, and increases the risk of 'burn-out'. Dramatherapy staff support groups could help to resolve the problems of individual members of staff. Similar techniques to those suggested for patients can be used, along with role play and role reversal.

Supervision

It has already been noted that Miller and Gwynne recommend staff supervision to look at group processes within teams. 'Process' super-vision is not about management, but about psychodynamics. The team sets aside a regular time for meeting with an external supervisor to look at what is happening in the relationship between staff and patients, and the interpersonal relationships within the staff team. This method of analysing interaction is accepted in the field of psycho-therapy, and is becoming more common in the helping professions in general. Sculpting, role play, role reversal, projective techniques and many other elements of dramatherapy are invaluable in supervision groups.

SUMMARY

Dramatherapy is a process of artistic involvement with a therapeutic intent. It can be applied to improve the quality of life of people in continuing care. More specifically it can enable patients, relatives and staff to express and explore emotions and come to some resolution of conflict. Given some training and stimulation of ideas, most staff members could work at the 'quality of life' level. Further training is necessary to work psychotherapeutically. As most staff are already working to their full capacity, a dramatherapist included as a member of the team would be invaluable.

REFERENCES

Bailey, C.H. (1981) Drama in health education. *J. Brit. Assn. Dramath.*, **5**, 1–9.
Bennet, D.H. (1977) Psychiatric rehabilitation, in *Rehabilitation Today* (ed. S. Mattingly), Update Books, London.
Esslin, M. (1976) *Anatomy of Drama*, Abacus, London.
Fairclough, J. *et al.* (1977) Drama for the blind. *J. Brit. Assn. Dramath.*, **1**, 14–16.
Grainger, R. (1987) Evaluation in dramatherapy. *J. Brit. Assn. Dramath.*, **10**, 17–22.
Jones, L. (1984) Dramatherapy and research work. *J. Brit. Assn. Dramath.*, **8**, 11–18.
Landy, J. (1986) *Drama Therapy*, Charles C. Thomas, Springfield Illinois, USA.
Langley, G.E. (1983) Dramatherapy with the elderly. *J. Brit. Assn. Dramath.*, **7**, 13–19.
Langley, D.M. (1981) Dramatherapy in the training of psychiatric nurses. *J. Brit. Assn. Dramath.*, **5**, 19–20.
Maslow, A.H. (1943) A theory of human motivation. *Psychol. Rev.*, **50**, 370–396.
McLuskie, M. (1983) Dramatherapy in a psychiatric hospital. *J. Brit. Assn. Dramath.*, **6**, 20–25.
Miller, E.J. and Gwynne, G.V. (1972) *A Life Apart*, Tavistock Publications, London.
Moreno, J.L. (1946) *Psychodrama* (first volume), Beacon House, Beacon, New York, USA. (Fifth edition 1976).

FURTHER READING

Langley, D.M. (1987) Dramatherapy with elderly people, in *Dramatherapy, Theory and Practice*, (ed. S. Jennings), Croom Helm, London.
Langley, G.E. (1982) Quality of life in extended care, in Conference Report: Quality of Life in Extended Care, Royal College of Psychiatrists, London.
Langley, G.E. and Kershaw, B. (1982) Reminiscence Theatre, Theatre Paper No. 6, Dartington College, Totnes, Devon.
Langley, D.M. and Langley, G.L. (1983) *Dramatherapy in Psychiatry*, Croom Helm, London.

APPENDIX 1

1. *Some physical requirements for the practice of dramatherapy*

1. A pleasant, uncluttered, well-lit room with a carpeted or smooth wooden floor, depending on the activities to be undertaken.
2. Assured freedom from interruption, for a defined period, from phones, catering trolleys, and 'Oh I'm sorry I didn't know'!
3. Preferably freedom from uninvolved observers; join in by all means, or stay away.
4. Record/tape reproduction.
5. Props such as: balls, photographs of old haunts or recent activities, things to hold, touch, reminisce or talk about, percussion instruments, objects such as cushions to represent feelings in projective games, simple drawing materials, lengths of fabric.
6. Reasonable access to toilets.
7. Appropriate seating for all.
8. Comfortable casual clothes for all.
9. Extra lights, such as coloured or spot-lights, are not essential, but can be a useful adjunct.

2. *Reports of applications and evaluation*

'Dramatherapy' the Journal of the British Association for Dramatherapists (from the Association address as listed) contains many articles on work in progress. Evaluation to date is mostly at the descriptive level but this is not inappropriate (Langley, 1983). A 'cross over' trial of dramatherapy with patients suffering from schizophrenia sets a model for a more rigorous approach (Grainger, 1987), while others have used dramatherapy techniques as a research tool (Jones, 1984), in training nurses (Langley, 1981) or as a health education tool (Bailey, 1981). It has also been used with the blind (Fairclough *et al.*, 1977) and in psychiatric hospitals (e.g. McLuskie, 1983).

APPENDIX 2

For advice/information

The British Association for Dramatherapy PO Box 98, Kirbymoorside, York, YO6 6EX. The British Association for Dramatherapy publishes a membership list of names and addresses.

Qualifing in dramatherapy

Three Colleges offer a two-year post-professional course leading to a Diploma in Dramatherapy:

1. The Hertfordshire College of Art and Design, 7, Hatfield Road, St. Albans, Herts., AL1 8RX.
2. The College of Ripon and York St John, Department of Drama, Film and Television, Lord Mayor's Walk, York, YO3 7EX.
3. The South Devon College of Arts and Technology, Department of Music and Theatre Arts, Newton Road, Torquay, TQ2 5BY.

Other people/organizations

1. Manchester and Salford Dramatherapy Group, 13, Milwain Road, Levenshulme, Manchester, 19.
2. The Course Secretary, Creative Therapies Research Department, Prestwich Hospital, Bury New Road, Prestwich, Manchester, M25 7BL.
3. Dramatherapy Consultants, 6, Nelsons Ave., St. Albans, Herts.
4. Dramatherapy North West, c/o John Casson, Brindle House, 34, Church Street, Hyde, Tameside, SK14 1JJ.

Chapter 13

The value of music to the long-term patient

Music is a many-splendoured thing. We can find it everywhere in our environment as an enrichment, an entertainment or a recreation which affects our mind, body and emotions. The evocative power of music is immense. It can bring to our imagination stories, places, people – in the past and the present. At many different levels music brings a message to each of us, irrespective of education, age or physical state. Van de Wall advocated as early as 1936 that:

> The hospitalized patients should enjoy music as a cultural and social interest and occupation that is entirely divorced in their minds from concepts of illness. The sheer contact with efficient and sensible musicians and with an art that, like fresh air, sunshine and flowers introduces in the ward elements of joyful cultural and social living, has value in improving the quality of his life and pervades it with ideas, feelings and events which are part of normal social life at its best.

HOSPITALIZATION

The words 'long-term hospitalization' or 'continuing-care patient' call to mind a number of ideas, images and feelings. They mean to the patient a complete change in lifestyle with loss of independence, of familiar environment and accustomed way of life. The patient is separated from people and objects which have been part of his surroundings and have provided a sense of security. This feeling of security may be replaced by the expectation of services, competent medical and physical care, food, warmth, light and in most cases, devoted attention – in short the essentials of material life. Even so, many patients become frustrated and are in danger of leading an uninteresting, monotonous existence.

Usually long-term hospitalization is necessary when, little by little, the patient loses the ability to cope with life and to organize himself. It may be due to a gradual decline or to a sudden traumatic deterioration of mind and body following a stroke or accident. Continuing-care wards therefore have not only those people who have gradually physically and mentally deteriorated, but also orthopaedic cases, brain damage or stroke patients, and accidents or surgery cases who can be rehabilitated and whose minds are still receptive. There may also be subnormal patients unable to live independently, but able to function socially at their own level. Although this last group of patients is condemned to be in hospital throughout life, they can enjoy, and even sometimes make, music at their own level of mental achievement. For them the perception of sound and the pleasure they derive from it may stay at the level of a sensation without an intellectual structure. It can be apprehended at low brain level and remembered. The result is that musical experience with subnormal individuals can be undertaken at very different levels without hindrance to the pleasure they derive from it. Music helps them to develop their auditory perception, their awareness of sound and their memory of patterns of melody and rhythm. We can improve their handling of simple instruments, develop their social sense as members of a music making group. These remarks can also apply to continuing-care patients whose minds are deteriorating.

I believe that any human being should be given at any time a chance to lead a dignified life and enjoy what gives value to the environment. He should be helped to retain or regain his identity. There are many instances in which a patient has found in music a chance of asserting personality and of finding a sense of purpose within the hospital environment. I have never met a patient who did not have any feeling for music, but it has to be discovered in order to help him to assert himself musically, both with dignity and a sense of purpose and enjoyment.

New experiences can stimulate progress. They should be guided expertly by the therapist in order to be continuous and to renew the interest of the patient. Many of them have never seen or handled an auto-harp, a ukelele or a bongo drum, instruments easy to understand and to handle. The origin and the making of musical instruments are interesting; they bring new knowledge to many people, irrespective of their intelligence and education, if the objects are there to be touched and to be heard as a concrete reality.

The musician who trusts a person with the handling of an instrument shows them respect. I experience this feeling when I let a patient handle the cello on which I have myself just performed. The link between the patient and me is often memorable; it means mutual enjoyment, respect and sharing an experience with the instrument as intermediary.

In a well-known subnormality hospital employing three music therapists, the number of musical activities is rewarding and has changed the outlook of the patients towards the hospital and the outlook of the staff towards the patients. There, the musical activities begin at a most elementary stage, for instance playing loud or soft, quickly or slowly, imitating very simple rhythms or tunes, part of a dance or melody by

Haydn or Mozart. Subnormal patients can be put in contact with great music, and some of them seem to be reached by it. I remember having attended a concert given by several groups at that hospital. Their care for and love of music was obvious. A patient who had been hospitalized for 15 years and was half blind, performed on the flute a simple melody by Mozart with the most spiritual and sensitive style. I also heard a lively percussion band playing extracts from Swan Lake and Carmen to the delight of staff and patients alike. Such achievements may completely change the patient's quality of life.

COMMUNICATION

A person develops throughout life within his own community, matures from the environment, communicates, gives and takes. Perhaps the urgent, immediate need for the material necessities of life makes us forget that human beings do not live by bread alone. They have many other needs, including those for beauty and harmony. They are gregarious creatures in need of means of communication of different kinds, at different levels, and not necessarily utilitarian. People can make things of beauty and create harmony. They need to express themselves and to find an outlet for emotions and creative impulses, wherever they are. They have created their own means of communication and self-expression, not necessarily based on verbal processes. Music has been, and is, a universal means of communication at all periods of history, and is one of our most precious inheritances, irrespective of the form or the meaning it has taken.

MUSIC

What do we mean when we say the word 'music'? What images, feelings and memories does it evoke? If we think of the use of music, we relate it to our own individual contact, to religious, ceremonial or public occasions that would be barren without it. When we think of introducing music in a long-stay hospital, do we believe that it would bring a better quality of life to the hospital community, as it does to the community outside the hospital? The benefits that could result are all due to the attributes of music and basically to the nature of sound of which music is made. The evocative nature of sound gives music a special power over us because the power of sound itself is irresistible. It penetrates and we absorb it at different levels of consciousness. It may stay there, buried, still associated to past events, ready to be revived.

This characteristic of music exists in each of us. It binds the past to the present, the real to the unreal, and may create a link between people quite dissimilar in taste or education. Music binds listeners together irrespective of the unspoken feelings it evokes in each of them; it can unite players together through the rules of music that every player is meant to follow. Music in all these occasions is the common denominator which can bind together, for a while, a great diversity of people, different in their way of life, age, in education and memories, in mental and emotional state. So, while music has its place for all of us as a solitary and passive experience, its great worth is in sharing and communicating feelings which may be difficult to express in words (Warwick, 1988).

Listening to music

The audience in a concert hall is composed of hundreds of different people, each of them responding, listening and being reached in a different way. Music is a common inheritance related to family, school, social occasions and for which no basic study or training is necessary, although study and training give it another dimension and significance. The fact is that everyone possesses a wealth of musical memories which can unite vastly different kinds of people such as you would find in a hospital, not only among the patients but among staff as well. Wedding and military marches, popular melodies, folklore songs, dancing tunes, operatic favourites, negro spirituals, hymns, war songs, activity songs, exist in everyone's memories ready to be called back and are part of the patient's former life and identity. The loss of identity is often a result of hospitalization which increases the effect of the illness.

Throughout life, people mature and acquire an identity often attached to their function and to the part they play in the community. A person develops a sense of purpose and responsibility. Moreover, up to middle age, people are adaptable. However, when someone begins to lose his mental and physical flexibility he may find it increasingly difficult to adapt to change and to find new fields of interest. This can apply to music but its immense versatility can be adapted to any situation and fulfil the patients' needs. Listening to music is a complex process not easy to analyse and its results are not always predictable. Attention and perception form the auditory basis of musical enjoyment. Music is a continuity in time which includes an awareness of sounds and silences, and the anticipation of sounds to follow one another. The process produces imagery which binds the real and unreal, memories of places, people and events. Silence around the listeners can help them become deeply involved in the music. Although silence may be a rare commodity in a hospital, it is a condition to the enjoyment of music, whether as an individual or as a group experience. Some people prefer listening by themselves and when music is on records, earphones should be provided for the sake of privacy. The choice of music should be left to the listener.

Background music

The use of background music in hospitals is controversial. Unobtrusive music may bring pleasant feelings of a relaxing or stimulating kind, and fill the emptiness of a ward, but it should be kept under control, lest it should bring irritation or lethargy. The benefit of listening to such music may not be obvious because it is the inner response of the patient which matters – a response mixed up with personal memories and feelings, which do not always show, and which the patient does not always wish to share.

Musical activities

Music can offer a new field of activities at the time when doors seem to be closing on former pursuits; a new field, or one which can be revived and extended. The feeling that one can learn new things is rejuvenating and stimulating. It creates a forward-looking attitude in the individual and in the group. I remember a lively old lady of 92 who told us one Thursday, 'Do not worry, I will hold on until you come again next week.' She did.

The music room

The aim of a music group in a hospital is to unite people who may have little in common except disability and age – to give them a common goal, opportunities to enjoy and learn new things, and to revive pleasant memories. It may produce recreation, enjoyment, deep experiences or a community feeling, according to the aim of the music therapist in charge. The group can include a small or large number of people who listen to or make music together, experiences based on auditory attention and memory, leading to enjoyment.

The meeting place for the group should be considered as 'musical territory' belonging to the group. It must be acoustically suitable and away from outside noises. Special or adapted lighting may be required, especially if some patients suffer from poor sight. Seating arrangements should contribute to the feeling of unity and comfort. The seats, which should not be too high, should be placed at an easy distance from one another. One has to consider the elbow room required for playing certain instruments. A crowded orchestra will never function happily.

Whatever its size and wherever the venue, the music group should be arranged in a circle or a semi-circle, each member being able to see and hear the others. The semi-circle can consist of two or more rows. This arrangement is necessary for the integration of the group. It can be used in a ward with patients in or out of bed, in the garden of the hospital, on a terrace or, even better, in the day room or the art room. If a special room is available, musical activities become more dignified, can be better planned and make a deeper effect.

Care of the instruments is most important. They should be kept in good repair, stored in a spacious cupboard and transported on a trolley. The piano and auto-harp should be regularly tuned and cleaned. In some hospitals the care of the instruments is left in charge of an able-bodied, responsible patient. Thus the music group may become a kind of music club belonging to the hospital, but run by patients.

The hospital library can be helpful in providing books on music, sheet music and recordings on cassettes. Books can include biographies of musicians and composers, history, the making of instruments, and so on. There are some beautifully illustrated books. 'Speaking books' on cassettes and the larger-print books for patients with failing sight are also available.

Two kinds of groups

Patients involved in music can be divided into two categories: the music-making and the listening groups. An experienced music therapist should be able to form suitable groups with very diverse patients, which can make the undertaking difficult when one aims at a reasonable musical standard, without which there cannot be satisfaction. Each patient should have a function in the group. His satisfaction depends on how well he can fulfil it.

Singing groups. Community singing is the most simple form of music-making group. It demands no high level of performance – even patients who have lost their voice may be able to join in unconsciously. The group, in spite of its musical shortcomings, may be one of the most beneficial social activities. It works on the patients' memory of songs and tunes absorbed over the years and for which no special ability is needed, not even the ability to read music. All this would rest on a low musical denominator, but one should aim at higher standards, for instance, in part singing where the singing can be more ambitious and individual. It is then possible to study new songs and aim at improvement by making more demands on the singers. Even a madrigal ensemble might be attempted with its sophisticated music. However, it should not be forgotten that folk music always makes a direct appeal and is easy to remember because of its repetitive elements. Whatever its nature, a good choir is an asset to any organization. It can contribute to any event, gathering or celebration which unites all those taking part.

Instruments and instrument groups. Musical instruments are an extension of the human body. The shape, size and make of instruments is intriguing. It usually provokes stimulating comments and questions. Music can open the door to history, acoustics and ethnography, even at an elementary level. An exotic or primitive instrument can provoke interest and stir up the imagination.

There is a wide range of musical instruments suitable for group or individual work (Figure 13.1). The main recommendation is that they should be of good quality with a clear resonant tone. The tuned ones should all be perfectly tuned to the same pitch. Some of these instruments can be adapted to physical disability, for instance by inserting the stick of a drum in a rubber tube, which enables the fingers to grasp it solidly. Some techniques aim at provoking specific movements of the fingers or wrists to which small bells are attached. Each movement becomes a sound that provokes awareness and enjoyment. Other instruments, such as pipes, melodica, mouth organ and recorder, improve breath control. There are shakers, maracas and tambourines which stimulate movements of the arms in space; chime bars and xylophones which demand visual accuracy in the hitting movements, all kinds of tambours and drums which develop the rhythmical movements of hands and fingers; brass cymbals on which the control of physical strength can be practiced, and many others. Instruments such as combo drums, cymbals or xylophones can be shared, creating one-to-one relationships between members of the group.

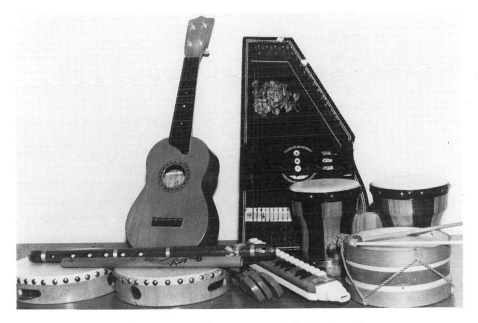

Figure 13.1 Musical instruments for group or individual work.

The most basic playing group is one formed with percussion instruments (Figure 13.2). It may be outside the experience of some of the patients, and as such open a new field of sounds, activities and interest. Even without using manufactured instruments, the ready-made percussion of hands and feet can express a number of feelings, especially in a group. A percussion band may be a new experience to many patients if it is not taken at the level of a kindergarten. A collection of drums, African or Latin American, is intriguing to handle, and in their shape and sound can open a new world to patients and excite their curiosity.

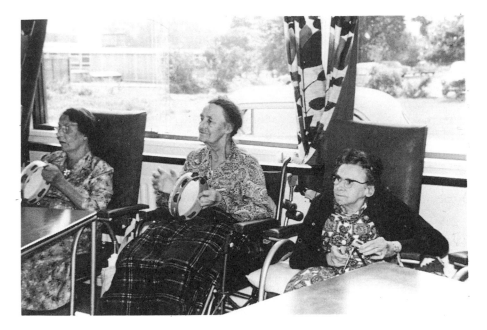

Figure 13.2 Three patients with percussion instruments.

Most people are interested in sound-creating objects; they want to touch them and make them sound. The motivation seems to be just curiosity, but often it is the primitive urge of bringing life to an inanimate object and making it speak, an instinct which exists in each of us, irrespective of age or education. We may consider the sound as a voice expressing an actual feeling. There is a close relationship between the sound, the player and the movement in time and space. The use of a musical instrument develops physical awareness and control which benefits the whole person regardless of the musical result. It should improve the rhythmical quality of the body in an activity that unites body, mind and expression. A player without previous experience should be offered a choice as wide as possible among instruments he can handle easily. This gives him a better chance to identify with the instrument of his choice, in the same way as other patients identify with a tune or a song.

The patient's satisfaction depends on how well he can fulfil his function within a group. We may find among the patients a violinist or a pianist or a singer able to perform well who should be given a chance to use this talent, to give pleasure and accept responsibility within the group, the choir, the band or the orchestra. A number of books can be helpful and give advice in order to get the best results in an unconventional situation. Even the general posture of the players can improve and becomes more dignified when playing or singing, the head is lifted or shoulders straightened. The music therapist should work towards these signs of physical and emotional liberation which show the quality of the experience.

Recording and playback. All techniques with people whose attention is limited should lead to immediate gratification, followed by some progress in the individual or in the group. The playback of the recording of a patient's performance provokes immediate attention and awareness, as it works on immediate recall. In the playback the identity of a voice or the sound of an instrument is easily recognizable. It gives a sense of reality and actuality to a past event and carries the personality of the players taking part. The listeners can discuss, praise or criticize the individual performance. Remarks made by the listeners show their awareness of the musical personalities in action. They notice, for instance, a very loud sudden sound on the cymbal, or a series of very rapid notes on a drum, or a long silence. In the technique of free improvization such characteristics are obvious and can become meaningful and revealing. The playback helps the group to take an identity. For instance, The Binfield Park Orchestra, the Leawood Singers, the Sound Revellers, are actual names chosen by the patients themselves.

Group improvization. Music exists in all of us. The sound produced by musical instruments may be perceived at the level of a pleasant resonance, while even single unorganized sounds can bring emotional relief to the player. They can express inner feelings spontaneously and carry anger, love, irritation, impatience, sadness or aggressiveness. This is why improvization techniques can be so effective as an emotional outlet. The aim of the improvization group is to give players the opportunity to express themselves freely on their instruments under the protection of the group. One can detect real musical communication taking place between the members as vivid and often more telling than in verbal communication.

This modern technique is widely and successfully used in many hospitals and rehabilitation centres. It does not require any previous musical training, as it bypasses the conventional rules of music. It is often called 'instant music'. The results are stimulating, unexpected and expressive. The improvization is performed on untuned instruments or on instruments tuned to a specific scale, usually the pentatonic, the sounds of which always blend in a harmonious way. In consequence players can follow their own impulses. A tape-recording of such sessions can lead to many comments and is revealing of the mental or emotional state of the player or the listener.

In another context the evocative power of music can provide many themes to an improvizing group, telling a story in music with imitative sounds, each of the players representing an element in the story. I remember vividly a concert in a hospital given by such a group to patients and staff. It included a birds' tea party at the top of the tree with lovely birds' songs, interrupted by a thunderstorm – and a solemn Chinese march with bells and gongs.

Listening groups. A listening group where the music is selected, enjoyed and commented on, can be a source of pleasure, information and learning since music is related to most human activities. It ranges from immature pleasures to aesthetic and intellectual pursuits. The use of music throughout history, in the village and at court, can be told and illustrated to different types of audiences by suitable speakers whose aim is not to teach but to interest and to entertain.

MOVEMENT

Musical activities can provoke other beneficial pursuits, especially those related to movement. They can enlarge the sense of space, give scope to the use of expressive movements and help physical activity through their rhythm and their continuity. They can help the patient to become aware of his lungs, throat and breathing processes, aware of a physical rhythm when moving in time. Exercises to music give a feeling of physical well being often used by physiotherapists, followed by an improvement in a limb, in the posture and in general appearance. Action songs are always a source of enjoyment and can be used in a more or less elaborate way.

Ruth Bright (1972) gives good advice on 'keep fit' work in which beneficial movements are related to specific musical pieces, from the Skye Boat Song to Tchaikovsky's Pathétique Symphony. A good music therapist working with a physiotherapist can formulate their own programme.

THREE GROUPS

In a hospital where I worked for several years, I had formed three musical groups. The first group functioned in a large ward with a few patients in bed and others out of bed. Our 'musical territory' was in the middle of the ward with enough space to hold three wheelchairs, four ordinary chairs, and a trolley for the instruments, which were small and easy to handle in bed. We planned for each patient to see and to hear well, and to communicate with others.

A number of patients were newcomers and not yet accustomed to their environment. We had to use versatile techniques to show varied sides of a music session. We used short pieces with instruments simple enough to use near a bed, with accompaniment of guitar or auto-harp. They were often accompanied by movement or dancing easily visible to everyone in the ward. We also played music on cassettes or gramophone which had been popular some 20 years ago. We might have ten to twelve patients in this group, which was popular.

The second group was a responsive and lively one, ready to verbalize, to exchange memories, usually happy ones, of places and people. The group responded well to rhythm, they were still physically active and learned the handling of percussion instruments to accompany dance music. We found in folk music an infinite source of material: songs from Spain, Hungary, Russia or Italy, with guitar or piano accompaniments. We also used extracts from light opera, the Merry Widow, the Blue Danube, Swan Lake, Gilbert and Sullivan operas, or easy-to-follow marches and polkas. All these require the patients' active participation on percussion instruments. Certain recordings of bird-song can create interest and imagery. Certain descriptive pieces, such as the storm in the Beethoven's Pastoral Symphony, La Mer by Debussy, Fingal's Cave by Mendelssohn, or My Country by Smetana, also aroused much interest.

Two of the most active members of this group, Mr Brown and Mr Palmer, attended every week. Their musical personality was strikingly different. Neither of them had had a proper musical education. Mr Brown, a hemiplegic confined to a wheelchair, was a 67-year-old widower and still a robust man in every way. He never spoke of his wife and had nowhere to go during the weekend. His only vistor was his elegant daughter, who came infrequently for short visits. He seemed to have very few friends. He had accepted hospitalization with fortitude and serenity and never complained. The music sessions and the art sessions meant everything to him and helped him to make friends with other patients. He was a natural leader, possessing a powerful voice and a strong sense of rhythm. He had a large repertoire of songs and contributed to our activities with enthusiasm. We entrusted him with a very large drum which he could hold in his lap. He learned quite quickly how to handle the two sticks, to vary his rhythm and to develop control over his hands. He enjoyed his special position of responsibility and leadership without imposing it or playing too loud. He was usually able to suggest a tune familiar to the rest of the group, who recognized his leadership and called him 'our drummer' – words which seemed to answer his need to be in charge. The other accomplished musician in the group was Mr Palmer, a stroke patient who had kept the use of his voice and limbs. He suffered from incontinence and was unable to exert himself. He had a quiet sense of humour, was reserved and extremely sensitive to beautiful music. He had kept his nice voice, through which he could express himself and give great pleasure to others when he was in the mood. He had a most devoted wife who visited him almost every day. Sometimes he was allowed to go home for a weekend. Perhaps this made hospitalization harder for him. He suffered from frequent attacks of depression during which he was unable to communicate. This sometimes happened on music day. However, he had a great sense of allegiance to the group and did not wish to let us down. His singing, so musical and sincere, created a deep impression on the group. He made a considerable effort to sing in spite of his depressed state and this we acknowledged.

I believe that in any group, however disparate, each member can make a personal contribution, not necessarily in playing, but in expressing a wish, a choice, or making a suggestion. Mr Gwilt, a Welshman, was always asking for Welsh tunes or songs and we tried to add to our Welsh repertoire and to make the auto-harp sound like a Celtic harp. Another patient, a retired sailor, enjoyed any music reminding him of the sea. Everyone in the group became familiar with Debussy's La Mer, Fingal's Cave by Mendelssohn and sea-shanties from Peter Grimes by Benjamin Britten.

The third group was formed from those who enjoyed listening to music without singing or playing an instrument. We played imaginative and colourful music for them such as the Storm from the Pastoral Symphony, My Country by Smetana, Night on a Bare Mountain by Mussorgsky, and others. Such music is likely to provoke verbal comments and to widen the group's musical range. We tried to encourage members to choose a piece among those they knew, or to find more new pieces. With that group, the incentive to play or sing was minimal and never insisted upon. Some patients played records of their own, others did not need the presence of the group to enjoy it. The need for privacy should be respected, and not intruded upon unless it becomes a pathological or obsessive need for isolation.

CONCLUSION

Music cannot always be a means of communication and projection. In certain cases of mental disorder, music may answer a morbid desire for isolation, introspection or escape from the environment. Some patients indulge in the vacuum created by repetitive and monotonous sounds which build a wall between the individual and the world of reality. The remedy is to bring awareness to the experience by using a positive concrete object such as a musical instrument or a movement directly associated with the music and which gives reality to the experience.

In a continuing-care hospital, musical activities can be as varied as required, at a standard suitable to the condition of patients and to their social and musical needs. How music has reached them, a patient may be unable to say, but if beauty is in the eye of the beholder, it may also be in the ear of the listener, whoever and wherever they may be. There lies the power and the magic of music.

Music involves the whole person, its application includes an infinite number of psychological, physiological and social factors. A situation such as described in this chapter cannot be dealt with successfully by a competent teacher or good amateur. It demands a deep knowledge of the effect of music on human behaviour, which is the essence of music therapy, and includes love of music and a desire to help people and to reach them.

Music therapists may be born, but they are now being trained in the profession (Webster, 1988). Such work as described in this chapter concerns the selection of patients, the kind of suitable activities and the choice of suitable music and instruments. Understanding and co-operation between the members of the therapeutic team are essential to the improvement of the way of life of long term patients. Several organizations mentioned in the appendix can give names and addresses of suitable music therapists.

REFERENCES AND FURTHER READING

Allen, D. (1977) Music therapy with geriatic patients, *Brit. J. Music Therapy*, **8**, 2–6.
Allen, D. (1981) An exploration into musical speech therapy. *Brit. J. Music Therapy*, **12**, 2–7.
Alvin, J. (1975) *Music Therapy*, Hutchinson, London.
Alvin, J. (1975) The identity of the music therapy group. *Brit. J. Music Therapy*, **6**, 10–14.
Bright, R. (1972) *Music in Geriatric Care*, Melville, New York.
Bright, R. (1972) An unusual facet of geriatric care. *Brit. J. Music Therapy*, **3**, 9–12.
British Society for Music Therapy, Conference Papers (1973) *Music Therapy in the Clinical Team*; (1976) *Music Therapy in the Community*; (1979) *Music Therapy for the Young and Aged*, British Society for Music Therapy, London.
Bunt, L.G.K. and Hoskyns, S.L. (1987) A perspective on music therapy research in Great Britain. *Brit. J. Music Therapy*, **1**, 3–6.
Byrne, M. (1971) On a geriatric ward. *Brit. J. Music Therapy*, **2**, 25–8.
Dinn, F. (1979) *The Observer's Book of Music*, 3rd edn, Warne, London & New York.
Priestley, M. (1975) *Music Therapy in Action*, Constable, London.
Van der Wall, W. (1936) *Music in Institutions*, Russel Sage Foundation, New York.

Warwick, A. (1988) Questions and reflections in research. *Brit. J. Music Therapy*, **2**, 5–8.
Webster, J. (1988) Music therapy training. A personal experience. Ibid., **2**, 18–20.

APPENDIX

Useful addresses

Suppliers of sheet music

Novello & Co. Ltd., 3 Upper Thames Street, London, W.1 (Hymns and Negro
    Spirituals)
Keith Prowse & Co., 138 Charing Cross Road, London, W.C.2. (Home Series of Great
    Masters)
Boosey & Hawkes Ltd., 295 Regent Street, London, W1R 3JH (Song Books and
    Albums. Folk Songs of Trinidad and Tobago with Guitar and Percussion)
Vevenscroft Large Print Books Ltd., The Green, Bradgate Road, Anstey, Leicester
    LE7 7EU (Large print song book. Large print song words)

Suppliers of instruments

Boosey & Hawkes Ltd., 295 Regent Street, London, W1R 3JH
Chappell & Co., 50 New Bond Street, London, W.1

Organizations concerned with music therapy

1. British Society for Music Therapy
   Guildhall School of Music and Drama, Barbican, London, EC2Y 8DT (provides
   information about music therapy and publishes British Journal of Music Therapy
   and various papers)
2. Association of Professional Music Therapists in Great Britain (Secretary: H. Odel,
   69 Broadway, Granchester, Cambridge)

Organizations providing performances and entertainments
in hospitals

Council for Music in Hospitals, 34D Lower Road, Little Bookham, Surrey
Shape, 9 Fitzroy Square, London, W1P 6AE
Live Music Now, 38 Wigmore Street, London, W1H 9DF

Instruments for individual and/or group work

If group work is contemplated the choice of instruments should be left to an expert.

* a good piano, guitar and auto-harp	triangle
large hanging cymbal	* Melodica
finger cymbals	recorder
* 12 chime bars, soprano	rosewood xylophone
* small tambours	marraca
* tambourine	combo drums

* *minimum for group work*

Unfortunately the author, Miss Alvin, died shortly after completing her manuscript.

Chapter 14

Continuing care for the elderly mentally infirm – an occupational therapy contribution

INTRODUCTION

This chapter will focus on the nursing home unit, which is part of the Thornhill Unit, Moorgreen Hospital, Southampton, and the contribution of the occupational therapy staff to the demented patients. The nursing home unit will be described. The conceptual framework for intervention will be presented. The occupational therapists' role with demented patients within the Thornhill Unit and how this relates to the residents of the nursing home will be explained.

THE NURSING HOME

The nursing home sector was opened in March, 1987. The wards were being upgraded, and the nursing officer grasped the opportunity to introduce changes to the philosophy and practices as well as the decor in the areas that would be home for up to forty persons.

The residents

The residents are patients who have deteriorated to a point at which care outside hospital (even with respite admissions) is no longer feasible. It is rare for a nursing home admission to take place without a final period of assessment in one of the short stay wards. The placement is generally a deliberate and consultative process, involving the community psychiatric nurse, the family, the psychogeriatrician, the hospital staff, and the matron of the nursing home. Almost all of the patients are suffering from dementia, though many have other psychiatric and physical infirmities as well. A study (Warren, 1985) found that the demented residents (*n.* 20) on one ward were rated on the CAPE (survey version) as high-dependency with a mean score of −06.06 (Table 5, page 50). They were also all incontinent of urine at night (p. 32). One or two are persons with other psychiatric conditions and attempts at living in alternative accommodation have failed several times.

The decor

The decor reflects the determination to make this as homely as possible. Shiny walls have been covered with softly coloured figured wallpaper, complemented by matching or toning curtains. Floor coverings are matt and non-slip, and the lounge areas and dining areas are carpeted. Many wall light fixtures supplement and soften the main central source of artificial light. Ornaments, pictures, and plants are in evidence. A hearth graces each sitting area. Many types of seating are available, including 'beanbags', two-seater settees, and wooden 'Captain's' chairs.

Key workers

As part of the emphasis on domestic scale and style, staff members are designated as 'key workers' for two to four residents. Each key worker has been asked to submit a pen-portrait of the residents for whom they are particularly responsible. The exercise involves finding out autobiographical details as well as current observations of abilities and preferences.

Meetings with relatives

The nursing-home staff, residents, and relatives meet regularly to become better acquainted and to discuss goals, issues, and problems. A clergyman and the psychologist also attend the group. From this gathering, a group was selected to plan the Christmas party, and joint decisions have been made about spending for amenities for the nursing home. Discussions about how best to meet the spiritual needs of the residents have resulted in regular attendance at this meeting by a pastor who endeavours to know the relatives and the residents well and to hold a short religious service at intervals. A questionnaire was devised and circulated to relatives and staff members by the psychologists to discover how they felt about the nursing home and various aspects of care.

More choice

Modifications to the hospital routine have been made as a result of observations by the staff and a greater appreciation of individual's preferences. For instance, getting up and going to bed times are generally later than they were. If someone seems inclined to stay in bed all morning, or indeed, all day, this is usually accommodated. Mealtimes are much more flexible; because people tend to get up later, breakfast is later so that lunch has been moved back to an hour after it is served in the other wards in the hospital.

Less medication

One of the stated objectives of the nursing home is to cut down on the amount of medication used. Closer observation of the resident's pattern of sleep, exercise, and response to the approaches and personalities of the staff and other patients mean that a clearer picture of the resident's normal and disturbed behaviour is established and therefore, a clearer indication of when medication is a necessity. Also the use of walks outdoors for the restless or cups of tea and a seat in the lounge for the insomniac during the night are examples of techniques that may lessen the amount of medication required.

THREE IMPORTANT IDEAS

Reality orientation has provided a model for staff to use when attempting to communicate with confused people. It seems that validation theory emphasizes the acceptance of what the confused person is trying to convey. Life planning promises to be particularly valuable for coordinating multi-disciplinary care over a period of time.

Reality orientation

Reality orientation was originally developed by Folsom, (1968) for the long-stay patients under his care in the Veteran's Administration Hospitals in the United States. Dr Folsom observed that although the physical care was excellent, the interaction between the patients and between the patients and the staff was minimal. He asked the nursing auxillaries, who had the most contact with the patients, to converse with the patients by using their names and referring to the weather, the ward, and the next meal, etc. He requested that they answer patients' questions honestly and as simply as possible, using short sentences. He asked that they speak distinctly and slowly rather than loudly. He listened and supported the nursing auxillaries attempts and gradually the scope widened, other grades of staff and other disciplines became involved, and eventually the classroom sessions of reality orientation became established.

In this country, the first published account of reality orientation was an evaluation of a programme at Warley Hospital in 1975 (Brook *et al.*, 1975). Since then, psychologists such as Hanley, Holden and Woods have contributed greatly to the understanding and application of the principles of reality orientation in this context.

Ian Hanley's emphasis has been on developing an environment that would enable the cognitively impaired person to function better. He has described methods of signposting the wards and training the patients to utilize the signs. (Hanley *et al.*, 1981). He has also described ways that the principles of reality orientation may be used to develop individual behavioural programmes to help overcome problems. (Hanley, 1986).

Una Holden has emphasized the need for increased sensory input, and, with Woods, she has produced a book (Holden and Woods, 1982) that describes ways of introducing this into classroom sessions of reality orientation. She has also developed a sensitive scale, the Holden Communication Scale, for evaluating interventions with this clientele group (Holden and Woods, 1982, pp. 258–9).

Perhaps Woods' most memorable contribution in this field is his oft-quoted response to the query of how to deal with rambling and confused speech, i.e., 'Do not agree: (1) tactfully disagree (on less-sensitive topics), or (2) change the subject – discuss something concrete, or (3) acknowledge the feelings expressed – ignore the content' (Holden and Woods, 1982 p. 161). (A fuller discussion of the application of these strategies is given on pages 161–2 of Holden and Woods' book.)

Validation theory

It would appear that further development of these strategies constitutes validation theory. Validation theory strives to accept the contribution that the (cognitively impaired or demented) person has made and to incorporate it into the interaction (i.e., to *validate* it) (Jones, 1985; Morton and Bleathman, 1988). This is probably a necessary corrective to the interpretation of reality orientation that implies that there is 'a right answer' and one must insist that the confused person gives 'the right answer'.

Life planning

One way of including as many of these good ideas as possible and of centring them on each patient is to use life plans developed by Chamberlain (1985) originally for mentally handicapped clients. Our psychologists are in the process of introducing this philosophy and method of viewing the resident, working out a plan that encompasses the 'whole range of life needs' (p. 4), and 'specifying the actions required to meet each need in such a way that achievement can be monitored.' (p. 11).

THE OCCUPATIONAL THERAPIST'S CONTRIBUTION

The remit of occupational therapists is to use activity to allow disabled people to live in as meaningful a way as possible. With progressively deteriorating conditions such as dementia, continuous adaptations to the environment and task simplification are necessary to allow the demented person to participate and function effectively. For each individual, this process must be paced to their particular pattern of impairment (Rogers, 1986, gives a more detailed discussion).

Possibilities and limitations

As implied above, there is an enormous contribution that occupational therapists with their particular blend of skills could make to the care of dementing persons as they progress through the course of their disease. The difficulty, of course, is that there is such a shortfall of qualifed therapists and other areas of work often appear to be much more rewarding. Speaking as a working therapist, if one has enough experience to feel ready to specialize, then working with demented patients, *throughout the course of the demented person's involvement with the psychogeriatric service,* can be personally very satisfying.

The involvement of the OT staff with the demented person

A brief resumé of the involvement of the occupational therapy staff with the demented patients in our unit may help to put our association with the nursing home patients into perspective. This discussion is limited to the demented patients, who constitute about half of the 900 admissions per year to the hospital sector of the unit.

First encounter

The person may be an attender at one of the day centres to which one of our occupational therapists is an advisor. The occupational therapy staff may first encounter a demented person at one of our (two) day hospitals. Hospital or day hospital OTs may be asked to visit a dementing person at home because of difficulties getting in and out of the bath, or some other problem associated with Activities of Daily Living. Alternatively, the person may be admitted to hospital because of an incident of physical illness, an acute confusional state, or for their first relief admission for the carer. Except in the first example, the community psychiatric nurses would probably be responsible for arranging the admission to the day hospital, the hospital, or for requesting a visit from the OT.

The relief admission patients

During the demented person's first two relief admissions the occupational therapy staff would complete a battery of assessments. They would attempt to involve the person in appropriate sessions and complete written reports for the ward and community staff. In addition, if we were not acquainted with the person's home situation, after consulting our community colleagues, we would arrange an interview with the carers and the demented person in their home. The purpose of the interview is fourfold:

1. To acquaint ourselves with the home situation.
2. To find out what the demented person does at home; the structure of their day; the activities (if any) that are shared by the carer and the demented person; the activities that were particularly enjoyed by the demented person and by the carer; and the limitations imposed by the patient's dementia.
3. To share the results of our assessments and observations in hospital and compare them with home; to discover how important the ADL tasks seem in the home.
4. To incorporate some features of the person's usual activities into the hospital routine, i.e., a walk, or a read of the newspaper.

The assessment battery would be repeated about every six months when patients are admitted at one-to three-monthly intervals. A repeat home visit would be suggested only about once a year, although contact with the relatives might be sustained when they visited the hospital, came to relatives' groups, or made contact by telephone.

Kindred groups

Through the use of the CAPE assessments and the evaluative research projects that have been carried out within the occupational therapy service, we have found that the regular relief patients and the nursing home patients, who are recommended for the activity sessions, are the same group; they are highly dependent people. We are trying to set up groups that will match the needs of these very impaired patients and include nursing home patients and relief admission patients in the groups determined by their needs and not according to where they live most of the time. From the manner in which our unit is organized one could argue that the nursing home patients are there simply because of their social circumstances, and not because their impairment is necessarily worse than that of those who are still living at home.

OT SERVICES FOR THE SEVERELY IMPAIRED

The activity sessions

The activity session, offered by the occupational therapy staff for selected residents of the nursing home, takes place every week-day morning. It is held in the occupational therapy department, a distance away from the nursing home. The nursing home residents arrive mid-morning and return upstairs before noon. There are usually 8–10 residents and three members of the occupational therapy staff.

The room most frequently used for the activity session is a semi-circular extension, with large windows affording an outlook on the grounds and the adjacent loading bay. The activity of a family of birds in a nearby tree, people walking in the grounds, and the traffic and noise caused by the loading bay, often occasion comment from the residents. A 'weather board', with the date, helps to elicit comments on the weather.

Generally, the residents sit around a large table, and the staff members move from person to person, spending a short time with each one. The activities include puzzles, paper and pencil/crayon/felt tip markers, reading the newspaper or looking at a book, singing, percussion, and listening to music, table games such as dominoes, lotto, and cards and rolling balls on the table or tossing balloons. Observation confirms that the presence and encouragement of the staff member fosters engagement by the patient; frequently, when the staff member moves away, the patient's involvement ceases. Nonetheless, although engagement may be only about 50% of the time, it is twice the level observed when encouragement, materials, and an appropriate space are not allocated (Conroy *et al.*, 1988).

Sensory integration

Sensory integration groups are being introduced into our work with the more severely impaired demented patients. They are based on the format suggested by Ross and Burdick (1981) in their manual *Sensory Integration: a Training Manual for Therapists and Teachers for Regressed, Psychiatric, and Geriatric Patient Groups*.

We plan to run the groups for four eight-week sessions and to ask the nursing home staff to nominate different residents for each eight-week block. We want people who come occasionally to the activity sessions but do not seem to respond very well. For the first eight-week session, two women were chosen from the nursing home unit. Both ladies had grave problems with communication; one because she could see and hear very little and the other because her first language was not English and she seemed to have lost all of her English. The other patients were relief admission patients, and again we particularly sought out those who were too severely impaired to include readily in other groups.

The groups are held twice weekly, and they last between 35 and 50 minutes each. There is a detailed agenda prepared for each group by the qualified OT, who also leads the group. The plan is to use each of the OT helpers in turn for a minimum of eight weeks until they are very well acquainted with the technique. We also request that other staff join us and that they are actively involved. A total of three or four members of staff for eight patients seems to be about right.

The activities are chosen to increase sensory stimulation in a structured manner, and emphasize touch, taste, and smell, large body movements and vestibular stimulation. A 'handout' is available for staff members and visitors. The leader of the group demonstrates each activity with a patient and then asks the other staff members to carry it out with the patients adjacent to them so that several individuals are being involved simultaneously. An example of an agenda would be:

Materials

Bell
Herbs, fresh if possible: mint, sage, thyme etc.
Two large balloons
Two metre length of elastic joined to make a circle
Feather
Heavy iron
Picture of a flat iron

Introduction

Shake hands; say names
Shake bell
Feel and smell herbs, e.g., mint, sage, thyme

Movement

Each patient is assisted to hold a large balloon with both hands, bring over head and lean forward and place near feet and then pass or throw the balloon to the next person.

A two-metre circle of 2.5 cm elastic is held by four patients and two staff members sitting in a circle. Everyone sways to the left and then to the right, then forward and back.

A staff member holds a patient's hand and gently pulls and then releases each finger in turn. They then turn the hand palm upwards and gently massage in a circular fashion each MCP joint.

Perception

(a) Place both hands on head (staff member demonstrates and assists, if necessary).
(b) Place both hands on head with eyes shut (again with assistance, if necessary).
c) Repeat with a few other parts of the body, e.g., ears, chin, neck, shoulders, legs, knees, ankles.

Cognition

Pass around a feather, a heavy iron, and a picture of a flat iron. Encourage comments about differences in weight and reminiscence.

Conclusion

Shake hands. Mention the day of the week, say which day the next group will be held on, and thank them for coming.

Assessments

The assessments we find most helpful are the Clifton Assessment Procedure for the Elderly (Survey Version) (Pattie and Gilleard, 1981), a local washing and dressing checklist, originally derived from the Functional Classification System (copyright 1980) Medical Center Rehabilitation Hospital, Grand Forks, North Dakota, USA, a unit form for recording help required with transfers and feeding, and the James Ward Questionnaire (Powell-Proctor *et al.*, 1981).

The Clifton Assessment Procedure for the Elderly (CAPE) is used throughout the unit to give us a dependency rating of the patients dealt with by the various sectors of the service. In the hospital, we use the information/orientation section most frequently on its own, and when the person is an in-patient we are able to supplement it with observations and assessments of washing and dressing, feeding and transfers.

The James Ward Questionnaire is an observational checklist developed for use on psychogeriatric long-stay wards. It proposes to focus on people's strengths and to assist the staff to set up small activity groups for people with similar assets; for example those who seem inclined to sit next to their neighbour and chat, and have good hearing, might enjoy a reminiscence-type discussion group, whereas those with good mobility and good eyesight might prefer to go on a walk. The graphical representation of the checklist does seem to make the person's profile of assets more apparent.

Activities of daily living

Much more work needs to be done on simplifying the tasks of ADL so that the demented person can continue to do as much as possible. In many instances we know how to simplify the task but somehow the opportunity gets lost. There is some ambivalence about the propriety of attempting to get demented people to continue to do things for themselves as opposed to doing it for them. It is probably quicker to do it for them, and there are so many patients and so many needs . . . Dementia is a deteriorating process so what is the point . . . These people, in the nursing home, are not going anywhere so why are we trying to use techniques employed in rehabilitation units to get people back home . . . This is their home so everything should look as homely as possible; feeding aids and upright chairs look like a hospital and not a home. These statements reflect staff misgivings, but for the much less articulate demented patient a statement about the importance of maintaining such skills can be elicited only *if the opportunity for making such choices exists.*

In the nursing home, if we assessed and offered all the options of feeding for those who have the knowledge and equipment to hand, it would be interesting to see whether the number of people being fed decreased. Getting food to your mouth can be a matter of choice and might well be a way of seeing whether severely demented people would persist in feeding themselves, as opposed to being fed, given the opportunity, support, equipment, and encouragement that might enable them to do so.

SUMMARY

Significant changes are occurring in continuing care for the mentally impaired elderly. There is a move towards more home-like surroundings and more attention to the needs of each person. Emphasis on knowing the person's autobiographical details, as well as their preferences, and including carers, whether relatives or health workers, who have been involved with the dementing person over a period of time, helps us to focus on the uniqueness of the individual.

The occupational therapy staff can contribute to this process by bringing with them their knowledge of the person's everyday activities and their assessments over a period of time. During the person's stay in the nursing home, they can help maintain the dementing person's active engagement by monitoring performance, offering and suggesting appropriate activities, and simplifying tasks as necessary.

ACKNOWLEDGEMENTS

Thanks to my husband, Ed Conroy, for his forbearance and for correcting my grammar. Many thanks also to Leslie Abraham, Sally Gore, Felicity Fincham, Colin Godber, and Laura Sutton for reading the draft, and for their comments and encouragement.

REFERENCES

Brook, P., Degun, G. and Mather, M. (1975) Reality orientation, a therapy for psychogeriatric patients: a controlled study. *Brit. J. Psychiat.*, **127**, 42–5.

Chamberlain, P. (1985) *Life Planning Manual*, The British Association for Behavioural Psychotherapy, Rossendale, Lancashire, UK.

Conroy, M.C., Fincham, F. and Agard-Evans, C. (1988) Can they do anything? Ten single-subject studies of the engagement level of hospitalized demented patients. *Brit. J. Occupat. Therapy*, **51**, 129–32.

Folsom, J.C. (1968) Reality orientation for the elderly mental patient. *J. Geriat. Psychiat.* **1**, 291–307.

Hanley, I. (1986) Reality orientation in the care of the elderly patient with dementia – three case studies, *Psychological Therapies for the Elderly* (eds I. Hanley and M. Gilhooly), Croom Helm, London, pp. 65–79.

Hanley, I.G. McGuire, R.J. and Boyd, W.D. (1981) Reality orientation and dementia: a controlled trial of two approaches. *Brit. J. Psychiat.*, **138**, 10–14.

Holden, U.P. and Woods, R.T. (1982) *Reality Orientation: Psychological Approaches to the 'confused' elderly*. Churchill Livingstone, Edinburgh.

Jones, G. (1985) Validation therapy: a companion to reality orientation. *Can. Nurse*, **81** March, 20–3.

Morton, I. and Bleathman, C. (1988) Does it matter whether it's Tuesday or Friday? *Nursing Times*, **84**, 25–7.

Pattie, A.H. and Gilleard, C.J. (1981) *Clifton Assessment Procedures for the Elderly (CAPE) Survey Version*. Hodder and Stoughton, Sevenoaks, Kent.

Powell-Proctor, L., Chege, N. and Savage, B. (1981) Creating and working with small groups in a psychogeriatric hospital ward. *Nursing Times*, **77** Sept 23, 1679–82.

Rogers, J.C. (1986) Occupational therapy services for Alzheimer's disease and related disorders (position paper). *Am. J. Occupat. Therapy*, **40**, 822–4.

Ross, M. and Burdick D. (1981) *Sensory Integration: a Training Manual for Therapists and Teachers for Regressed, Psychiatric and Geriatric Patient Groups*. Slack, Thorofare, New Jersey.

Warren, C.A. (1985) Assessment of Activities of Daily Living – a Comparative Study of Dementia in Older People. Unpublished M. Sc. (Rehabilitation Studies) dissertation, University of Southampton.

FURTHER READING

Allen, C.A. (1982) Independence through activity: the practice of occupational therapy (Psychiatry). *Am. J. Occupat. Therapy*, **36**, 731–9.

Allen, C.A. (1985) *Occupational Therapy for Psychiatric Diseases: Measurement and Management of Cognitive Disabilities*, Little, Brown and Company, Boston and Toronto.

Bailey, E.A., Brown, S., Goble, R.E.A. and Holden, U.P. (1986) Twenty-four hour

reality orientation: changes for staff and patients. *J. Adv. Nursing*, **11**, 145–51.
Bate, R., Weir, M. and Parker, C. (1984) Movement and growth patterns for the elderly and for those who care for them. Available from R. Bate, Moray House, Edinburgh, Scotland.
Feil, N. (1982) *Validation: The Feil Method*, Edward Feil Productions, Cleveland.
Levy, L.L. (1986) A practical guide to the care of the Alzheimer's disease victim: the cognitive disability perspective. *Top. Geriat. Rehabil.* **1**, 16–26.

Chapter 15

Continuing care for the elderly mentally infirm – a physiotherapy perspective

In describing life for elderly mentally ill people in a long-stay psychiatric ward it is not the intention to suggest that this is the most appropriate place for these patients to end their days. While these wards exist, it is important that efforts continue to be made to improve life for the remaining patients who reside in them.

THE LONG-STAY PSYCHIATRIC HOSPITAL

The typical psychiatric hospital, where the majority of continuing-care beds are still usually sited, is on the outskirts of a major city, often some miles from where many of the long-stay residents will have spent most of their earlier lives. It will probably be a Victorian Gothic 'Palace' with many pavilions, perhaps connected by open corridors. Some still have long-stay wards with 30 or more beds, often placed very close together, and perhaps without individual bed lights, lockers or individual cubicle curtains. The windows may be curtained, but these are not always drawn at night. In some units considerable efforts may have been made in the wards with bright wallpaper, bed covers, floor coverings and paintwork. The hospital grounds are usually extensive and well-kept but are not available to many residents who live in upstairs wards and who are unable to negotiate the stairs and for whom there are no lifts. The conditions in these wards are in stark contrast to those found in the majority of wards in most District General Hospitals.

THE PATIENTS

Some patients, having been admitted in their youth in the 1920s, have grown old in the institution; a few of them will have been admitted with mental handicap and have never been mentally ill. Others may have been admitted in middle age after repeated shorter-term admissions. They form the 'new' long-stay patients who, in spite of improvements in psychiatric care, are still being admitted. Some patients will have grown old in our special hospitals for the criminally insane and then have been

Patients Name: D.O.B. ....

Ward:

Diagnosis:

Date:

Activities	Scale 1 Time Date:-	Scale 2 Time Date:-	Details	Comments
1. Lying to sitting over edge of bed Bed height				
2. Bed to chair Chair height				
3. Sitting to standing				
4. Get to lavatory equipment/aids used Distance/time (measured in feet)				
5. Management of clothing to enable use of lavatory				
6. Gait equipment/aids				
7. Continent				
8. Incontinent Day Night				

Scale 1. Ability

0 Activity not achieved

1 Activity achieved with *maximum* physical assistance of *2* nursing staff or the use of a hoist

2 Activity achieved with *maximum* physical assistance of *1* nurse

3 Activity achieved with *limited* physical contact/assistance from *1* nurse (by handling not lifting)

4 Activity achieved by stand by supervision (verbal only)

5 Activity performed independently

Scale 2. Motivation/attitude

0 No response

1 Actively resists

2 Refuses

3 Responds to *repeated* requests (more than 4)

4 Needs encouragement to respond (up to 4)

5 Responds to first request

Figure 15.1 Assessment form used in a survey of long-stay wards in 1979.

transferred as they became too old and frail to remain there. Finally there is the group of elderly people who have been admitted for the first time with varying degrees of confusion and dementia, and who may have nobody in the community to care for them, or whose carers have been unable to provide the twenty-four-hour supervision people may need in the terminal phases of dementia. However, many elderly people with very similar problems and needs are still being cared for in their own home, or are supported in sheltered accommodation in homes for elderly people run by social services or, increasingly, in homes run by private or voluntary agencies.

A 1979 survey of two long-stay wards, using the assessment form shown in Figure 15.1, indicated that in one male ward of 31 patients, with an age range of 36–90 years, the diagnoses included 39 per cent chronic schizophrenia, 19 per cent dementia, 10 per cent epilepsy, 7 per cent mental handicap, 7 per cent alcoholic dementia, 7 per cent chronic depression and 3 per cent Huntingdon's Chorea. In another long-stay ward there were 32 female patients aged between 54 and 96 of whom 53 per cent were suffering from senile dementia and 25 per cent from chronic schizophrenia. When abilities were measured using the assessment form (Figure 15.1) 20 per cent of men and 25 per cent of women showed some signs of physical disability.

In 1988, in another hospital, a survey of two continuing-care wards showed that out of twenty elderly men who were aged from 72 to 92 years, all but one suffered from senile dementia and 17 had physical disabilities. In the other ward, with twenty elderly women aged from 65 to 90 years, 18 were suffering from dementia and had varying degrees of physical disability.

The patients' day

What is life like for the residents? In many units the patients' day begins early when they are woken up at 6 a.m. with a round of bed pans, washes and changes of bed linen. There is plenty of staff activity, but with very little social contact between staff and patients. Every patient is up for breakfast by 8 a.m. wearing clean clothes which may be their own or clothes taken from the clothing store. Breakfast is often associated with some bickering about places; patients sit at high tables on identical chairs, and there is seldom a choice of menu. Few clocks may have been provided to check the time, and there are few indications as to whether it is Monday, a Bank Holiday or Christmas. Everything is clean, protected and impersonal, and most risks and choices have been eliminated.

After breakfast another toileting round begins, and then many patients return to restrictive and inappropriate chairs. The toileting regime is a difficult time for both staff and patients; the distance separating day area from the toilets may make it hard for even the more able patients to manage independently, and there are probably no wall rails to assist the less mobile ones to get about. The routine is to put nearly all patients on commodes after meals without much effort to encourage those who could manage independently. Two nursing auxiliaries may lift a patient by the axillae and drag-lift or hoist him/her from sitting in a chair to the commode without the patient's legs touching the ground (Figures 15.2 and 15.3), so that even those with the ability to co-operate are not given the chance to assist with their feet or hands. This routine is repeated many times with patients often left in uncomfortable positions before being hauled back by the same lift to the chair from whence they were so recently raised. Occasionally patients who have just been lifted have been seen getting up and walking away, little attempt having been made to differentiate between those patients who are totally independent and those who, with suitable encouragement, can help themselves. The ward environment, with little space between the beds and inappropriate furniture, may make it difficult for the staff to assist patients appropriately or to use hoists. After all this action the staff may relax over coffee in the day areas. Useful physical or diversional activity for most residents is negligible or non-existent.

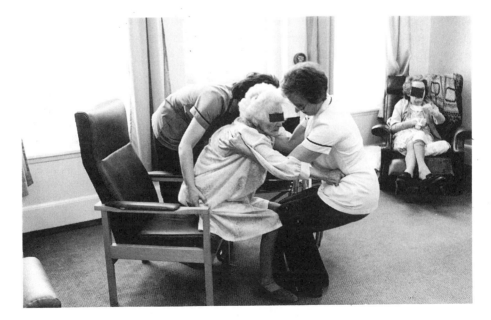

Figure 15.2 A patient being lifted from her chair.

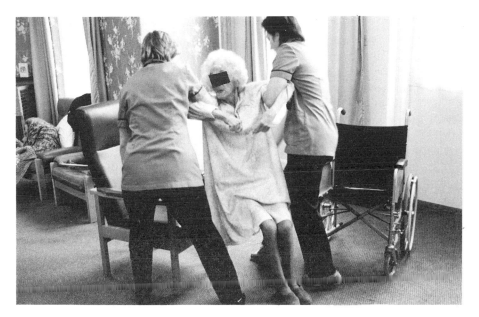

Figure 15.3 A patient being transferred to a commode.

STAFF

Nurses

Conditions for staff are usually poor, and although there are financial incentives to persuade nurses to work in these hospitals there is very little other encouragement to do so. The hospitals' comparative isolation from the rest of the health services, threats of closure and other uncertainties about the future may have lowered morale, reduced job satisfaction and affected recruitment. Nurses who have been psychiatrically trained have seldom had the benefit of training in the management of patients with physical problems. The introduction of the 'nursing process' should have led to a patient-centred approach, but in spite of its use much of the caring is fitted into a task-oriented organization. Training for nursing auxiliaries may be very limited, and in a psychiatric hospital the training may not have included much guidance on the management of physical problems, including effective and safe methods of lifting, handling, mobilizing, encouraging and communicating with dependent elderly people. The value of training shared with care assistants and others with similar needs is rarely available. Nursing auxiliaries may be imbued with low expectations, concerning their patients, early in their careers on the wards.

Medical staff

Medical and psychiatric care of long-stay patients varies. The consultant psychiatrists and their registrars are usually hard pressed to manage their large acute case loads, and may find it difficult to find time to visit these 'back' wards. Consultants from other specialities seldom, if ever, visit these wards at all, and those who need other medical opinions and skills are usually transferred to a general hospital – to be returned at the earliest opportunity with scant, if any, advice or follow-up. However, where patients have the benefit of a consultant with special interest in elderly people with mental illness, they are usually individually assessed, the multidisciplinary team involved, and realistic goals are set for each. In the past an annual physical examination might have been the only medical contact after admission but happily there is now usually increased medical cover for these wards, sometimes through general practitioners employed as clinical assistants.

Occupational therapists

Providing diversional therapy and rehabilitation for long-stay patients is both time-consuming and difficult. Qualified occupational therapists are in short supply and when they are available their priorities are usually the acutely ill where active rehabilitation can enable a percentage of these patients to return to the community and in some cases back to work. There may be only one or two qualified occupational therapists, and the service relies on large numbers of unqualified helpers. The organizational and philosophical separation between those therapists specializing in psychiatry and those working with physical disabilities can lead to a lack of sharing of ideas and expertise which could, if shared, be to the benefit of elderly mentally ill people with multiple problems.

Physiotherapists

The number of physiotherapists who work in psychiatry has increased but is still very small. There may be only one qualified physiotherapist in a psychiatric hospital with as many as 600 beds. The task may then seem so overwhelming, and the training so deficient in relation to work with elderly mentally ill people, that skills and expertise may be inappropriately spent providing a treatment service for the staff.

Speech therapists and dietitians

Posts for speech therapists and dietitians may not have been established. Where they have been provided the staff may be concentrating their slim resources elsewhere in the community. The isolation of many of these long-stay hospitals makes it particularly difficult for the smaller professions to be able to spare a few hours a week to provide even a limited advisory and teaching service for staff and patients. Frequently other hospital staff are unaware of the speech therapists' and dietitians' contributions, and so they make few demands for such services.

Chiropodists

Chiropodists are important members of the team. Patients mobility can be severely curtailed if their foot problems have gone unnoticed; often it is simply a lack of an effective toe-nail trimming service which is causing patients avoidable discomfort and hardship. As well as a specific chiropody service it is important that nurses and chiropodists have worked out a mutually satisfactory system to enable nursing assistants or foot-care assistants, with training from the chiropodists, to provide a toe-nail cutting service.

Students

If the service is to improve and develop, much depends on what students are taught in training. Student and pupil nurses may not have an attachment to continuing care, and clinical tutors and medical students may seldom if ever visit these wards. Very few occupational therapy/ physiotherapy/dietetic/speech therapy students are given the opportunity to discover the work that could be undertaken amongst this group of patients, and yet those who have had the opportunity are keen to continue. These factors clearly affect recruitment and attitudes to this work later on – qualified staff are less likely to apply to a type of unit in which the work is totally unknown.

WAYS TO IMPROVE THE SERVICE

Responses to the Rising Tide initiative (Developing Services for the Elderly Mentally Infirm, 1987) provide encouraging evidence that some imaginative community schemes are now being developed. 'Living Well into Old Age' (Kings Fund, 1986) suggests that long-stay care should be thought of as an alternative home and should be near the resident's original home, should be on a domestic scale, housing only small groups of people, should be preferably on the ground floor, having adequate grounds, and should provide individual bedrooms, sitting areas and toilet facilities. It should have a flexible input of services and have a lifestyle consistent with natural living. It should be possible to avoid many of the problems mentioned earlier, as continuing-care wards are closed and more appropriate provision, in small locally based residences, becomes available. Those elderly people who are likely to remain in continuing-care wards need to have a much improved quality of life for their remaining years. However, the service cannot be improved solely by the efforts of the staff working on the wards – a firm commitment and interest from senior managers in both Health and Social Services is essential to ensure that only patients who are appropriate are admitted. It is also vital to ensure that ward staff have adequate resources as well as the support and understanding of senior managers of all disciplines.

No one group can now tackle alone the numbers of elderly continuing-care patients. The situation can be alleviated only by collaboration and co-ordination of effort and by the realization that the multi-disciplinary team has to be prepared to assess and re-assess these patients on a planned regular basis so that slow progress or deterioration is detected and realistic goals are set for each individual, with management closely related to these goals. For any regime to be effective, staff attitudes to the expectation of inexorable deterioration have to be modified. If there is an expectation that most elderly people, as an inevitable result of ageing, become progressively immobile, then how much firmer is that belief when the elderly are also mentally frail. Much effort is wasted if staff are not convinced that it is possible to maintain and improve patients' functional capabilities.

The patients' day

Each event in the patients' day should be geared to encourage a response and lead to some active participation. Every morning there should be some flexibility within the regime to enable patients to get up, where feasible, at their own pace. Some should be allowed to have their breakfast in bed. Beds should be, if not of adjustable height, then at a level where patients can sit on the edge, rest their feet on the floor to make it easier for them to balance, and to dress themselves and, in some cases, to get up unaided. Where patients may need assistance then nurses should have received adequate theoretical and practical training. The Royal College of Nursing's advisory panel on back pain in nurses (1988) is doing much to promote good standards in lifting and handling patients. Its instructors' syllabus for handling and moving patients should do much to raise awareness of the hazards of injudicious lifting and assist instructors in teaching staff to stop, think then lift.

The importance of patients' clothing hardly needs emphasizing. Some clothes are obviously far easier to put on than others. The terylene dresses worn in so many of these units usually have zips which patients find difficult to manipulate. There should be an understanding that many ladies prefer to wear trousers and a choice of these should be available. The clothing display available on loan from the Disabled Living Foundation can give patients and nurses many ideas about suitable clothes, including the adaptations which allow for patients needing incontinence protection.

A variety of different designs in shoes should be available, and patients should be given a choice of footwear, with guidance where needed from chiropodists and therapists. Some 'travelling shoe shops' will willingly come to sell their products within the hospitals, and the choice that this service offers is appreciated by both staff and patients. Wherever possible arrangements should be made for staff or carers to escort patients to the local shops to choose their own clothes.

For patients who can wash themselves, every encouragement should be given to enable them to manage independently. The bathrooms should have basins at a height suitable for use in either a sitting or standing position, and with a mirror that can be used in either position. Baths and bath aids and showers should be adapted for use by patients using wheelchairs or other disability equipment, and should be supplied with rails and non-slip mats so that any unnecessary assistance from the nurses can be avoided and the patients can manage independently wherever possible and in privacy.

Entrances to the toilet facilities should be wide enough to enable hoists to be used. When facilities are upgraded, the DHSS design guidance (1986) is useful in illustrating the spaces required to enable disabled patients and assistants to manoeuvre easily. For patients who have to wash in bed, shallow-sided bowls on low tables are easier for the patient to manage. Lavatories should be adapted to be suitable for use by patients using wheelchairs or walking aids, and to allow room for their escorts to manoeuvre to assist them. Privacy whilst using the toilet must be ensured. There are many types of commode chairs on the market, and suitable ones should be selected for patients who can manage to transfer from either bed or chair to use them rather than bedpans or incontinence pads. Bathroom doors should be in a contrasting colour to other ward doors, and should be clearly labelled. Bathrooms should be fitted with an emergency call system. These basic adaptations should be provided in all continuing care wards. The distance from lavatories to the day and dormitory area is crucial, and it is important to remember that research by Doreen Norton (Norton, unpublished) indicated that elderly patients should never be more than 40 feet from a lavatory if accidents are to be avoided. However, if patients are able to walk only slowly they should be even nearer to the toilets.

Mealtimes are a major event in a patient's day. In the dining area the chairs should be at a height which is comfortable for each patient and not so low, or the dining table so high, that plate and mouth are almost at the same level. Furniture equipment manufacturers continue to improve designs for use by disabled people, but often supplies officers, nurses and therapists fail to get together to decide the most appropriate ward furniture to purchase, and money is wasted buying unsuitable items.

At meal times patients should have the opportunity to choose what they would like to eat; where necessary, teeth, whether false or real, should be well looked after to make mastication of a wide variety of different foods possible. The contribution of adequate nutrition to physical and mental well-being is increasingly being recognized, particularly for elderly people. The quality and texture of food is important, and 'sloppy' food is appropriate only for a very limited number of individuals.

Meal times should be relaxed and unhurried. The need for sufficient staff, carers or volunteers to be available to help those with feeding difficulties cannot be over-emphasized, and the role of the dietitian in giving advice on nutrition is increasingly being appreciated in psychiatric hospitals. A recent visit to a psychogeriatric assessment ward at lunch-time showed that every patient had been supplied with a non-slip mat to steady their plates, and a wide range of adapted cutlery was available and in use; very few patients had therefore to be fed or to use feeding cups.

The best time for ward activities to begin is likely to be when breakfast and toileting, and the drug rounds, are complete. Some patients may be able to leave the ward (and every effort should be made to arrange this), and join activities in the social centre, occupational therapy department or, rarely, industrial therapy department. For others however, activities have to be restricted to the ward. It is common to hear staff state that the patients show no interest and just want to be left alone, but for patients who are unable to leave the ward there are many activities which can be introduced.

Occupational therapy

The main aim of the occupational therapist is related to retaining or promoting normal personal relationships, activities and mobility, encouraging self-esteem and confidence, and reducing or preventing confusion. This is attempted through reality orientation programmes and social, creative, domestic and other activities in selected groups with differing needs. Individual work with patients is also used to encourage independence in daily activities and promote use of any remaining abilities. Simple handicraft activities and industrial packing have also been introduced to the wards, and provided there is sufficient staff guidance and enthusiasm these can be successful and enjoyable for a small number of patients. Two factors are important to ensure success. Firstly, correct and continuing assessment and planning; secondly, the involvement of other disciplines, principally the ward staff – close liaison being essential to decide on the best possible methods used in daily activities for habit training and the promotion of normal social conversation and interaction.

Music therapy

Music therapy has been successfully used in both mental handicap and psychiatric long-stay wards, but is most effective when directed by a qualified music therapist.

Speech therapy

The speech therapists are concerned with the patient's total ability to communicate, so that not only are they responsible in the team setting for the speech and language input into therapeutic activities, particularly the reality orientation groups, but they also work to provide an alternative means of communication when verbal language breaks down; this is usually in the form of a symbolic or gestural language, such as Makaton or Amerind. These signing systems can be used to convey simple messages (or indeed, very complicated ones). There is now an increasing awareness of the contribution that speech therapists make to patients not only with communication problems but also with swallowing difficulties. They are also spending more time teaching other staff how to assist patients with speech and swallowing difficulties.

Physiotherapy

A physiotherapy service for long-stay patients can be expected to produce a number of advantages, and many middle-aged and elderly patients with arthritic, neurological and orthopaedic conditions can be helped to regain useful mobility and independence. Dependence on nursing staff can be reduced, and with increasing mobility there is likely to be a reduction in incontinence and avoidance of joint contractures and pressure sores. Chest infections will be resolved more rapidly with physiotherapists assisting patients to remove bronchial secretions. Medical staff can make use of the physiotherapist's ability to assess the patient's physical disabilities and potential. Nurses and other ward personnel can benefit from being taught safe and effective methods of assisting patients – thus avoiding hazards for both patients and themselves. Medical and nursing staff can be advised on the selection and provision of splints and collars and on all disability equipment – such as wheelchairs, crutches and sticks. In close co-operation with nurses and occupational therapists, advice can be given on selection of furniture, such as suitable beds and chairs, and on ways to modify the ward environment to facilitate patients' mobility and function.

Physiotherapy can be most effective if there is a well but simply equipped department easily accessible for all patients and staff, where both acute and long-term patients can be assessed and treated, and where space and quiet facilitate this assessment. Ideally it should be near the wards and other therapy departments so that the therapist's work is closely integrated with the ward practices and time consuming journeys for patients and porters are avoided.

One method of identifying patients, who might benefit from an improved environment and increased activity, is by assessing each one using a very simple functional activity and motivation assessment scale. The assessment scale shown in Figure 15.1 has been used successfully to assess the physical function of long-stay patients in one large psychiatric hospital. The assessment form was devised locally and tested for inter- and intra-observer error on a small pilot study by nurses and therapists. This assessment survey was carried out by two physiotherapists in five long-stay wards. It was found that the best way to ensure effective co-operation from patients and nursing staff was to test the functional activities at a time when the patient was accustomed to carrying them out. This meant visiting the wards in the early morning, about 6.30 a.m., which was the usual time patients got up, or in early evening or in the afternoon to coincide with bed time.

Such a survey can also be used to assess the physical progress or deterioration of patients, and to detect those who would functionally improve if there was some small modification to the environment. It can also be useful for planning realistic teaching programmes for nursing staff on how best to lift and handle patients, whilst avoiding back strain and encouraging active patient participation. It can also give therapists a greater awareness and understanding of the difficulties faced by nurses and patients and is useful as a basis for calculating future staffing needs to provide physiotherapy for those identified as likely to benefit.

The Stow Lodge assessment research project (STARS) developed initially by a multi-disciplinary team at Stow Lodge Hospital, Stowmarket, has created a basis for an ongoing system of patient care planning for continuing-care patients. After multi-disciplinary assessments are completed on individual patients, targets are set, plans made and actions follow. A vital component of the system is the need for multi-disciplinary agreement on the assessment ratings and on all-action plans.

The individual mobility problems the physiotherapist is likely to encounter when assessing and treating elderly patients with dementia are well described by Oddy (1987). Strategies to help overcome communication and behavioural problems using, where applicable, visual, auditory, physical and memory cues to gain a functional response are well described. The strategies provide a framework for therapists to follow in this specialized field of practise.

Exercise sessions held in the wards for groups of patients can help to prevent loss or deterioration of mobility and in some cases re-educate and increase it. Some of the most successful are where ward staff actively co-operate and join in, and there must be extensive consultation between nurses and therapists before the sessions are introduced. They can also improve social awareness and encourage contact with others. Initially it is important to involve only those patients who are interested. At first only two or three people may wish to participate, but one leader will still need two or three helpers to take a group. Careful observation may show one or two other patients who occasionally focus on the group, and occasionally someone who appears to be totally unaware will tap in time to the music. The benefit for patients can begin as part of the day area is cleared for the group; re-arranging the furniture can provide an interest and a reason for moving in an environment in which there is often no incentive to do so. Even patients who cannot walk can be helped to transfer into a different chair for the session. Music has a vital part to play in these sessions, and live music is better than taped music since it can be quickly adapted to the pace of the group. If live music is not available, a tape recorder can be used and efforts made to get the patients to help select the tunes. The types of group activity will vary enormously with the ability of patients and the talent of the group organizer. The book 'Let's Get Moving' (Davies, 1978) is a useful source of ideas. Helpers to the remedial professions often possess a wide range of musical talents. Accordions and violins are portable, and helpers playing them have been able to provide lively, entertaining stimulation. Exercises and the music can be adapted to the patients' pace, and tunes chosen from 1930s or 1940s are usually more appropriate than those composed before the First World War.

Activities must be chosen with great care to suit the patients, and any which could appear childish must be avoided. Activities involving simple equipment, which even the most disabled can handle, provide a sensory stimulus and can improve manipulative skills. Equipment of varying shape, size and surface is important, and activities which involve co-operation with a neighbour in the group and team games help to develop communication between patients. Team games should have a functional purpose and should be designed to encourage trunk and limb mobility – rotation to pass equipment to a neighbour, and lifting a ball from the floor to throw it to a partner. Unexpected speed and agility of movement can be revealed in some of these sessions, and can be regained after repeated practice. It may take weeks of regular sessions before many patients join in, but new admissions to the ward may be happy to participate at once. Patients who have been gazing vacantly into space may begin to make brief eye contact with those taking the sessions, and this may make it possible to begin to establish some form of communication with them. An active, more mobile patient may sit near the group for just a minute or two and then gradually gain confidence and join in for an increasing length of time. It takes a lot of enthusiasm and energy on the part of the organizers to keep the group lively and active, but it is important not to give up too soon and to make every effort to maintain the session at a regular time of day and if possible repeated several times a week. The groups are not a substitute for individual physiotherapy but an adjunct to them, and part of the individual regime which many people need may be able to be combined with the team activities. With increasing activity and participation patients may become more sociable and a little less isolated, and may be willing to join in some suitable activities outside the ward, such as a coach outing.

Gains from a physical activity programme are not likely to be spectacular, but if one or two patients are able to maintain their mobility and, after a few years of being lifted, regain the ability to transfer from bed to chair or manage the lavatory with less help, then these are very real and important achievements. It has been known for patients to make such progress that they have been well enough to be given the opportunity to be transferred back into the community. Many staff will be encouraged and enable other patients to regain some degree of independence.

CASE HISTORIES

The following case histories illustrate the physiotherapists contribution within the team approach.

(i) Mrs A., born in 1892, was admitted to a long-stay psychiatric hospital in 1977 with diagnosis of chronic confusional state, mild senile dementia, and a severe osteoarthritic left knee. She was also partially sighted and had some hearing loss. She was assessed by a physiotherapist soon after admission. The right knee was very painful and had a flexion contracture; the therapist suggested an orthopaedic opinion. The knee gradually deteriorated in spite of ultrasound, exercises and a splint, and walking became increasingly difficult because of pain. The patient was well motivated. In 1978 a manipulation under anaesthetic failed to increase pain-free range, and a caliper was fitted. In 1979 the knee was arthrodesed. The patient was gradually re-mobilized and was able to walk independently with two sticks. In 1980 she was discharged from the long-stay ward and was able to live in a Local Authority old people's home, walking short distances on sticks and using a wheelchair only for longer outings.

(ii) Mrs C., born in 1915, had seven admissions to psychiatric hospital before being admitted to a long-stay ward in 1976. The diagnosis was subnormal schizophrenia with progressive choreo-athetosis with spasticity, right talipes equino varus, and bilateral osteoarthritic knees. On physiotherapy assessment in 1976 it was found that she was unable to stand, walk or transfer. She had not been prescribed her own wheelchair, and she was unable to propel the ward one. Mrs C. was treated daily for over a year; during that time she learnt to transfer from bed to chair, and from chair to toilet, and was able to propel the wheelchair prescribed for her. After serial stretch plasters for her talipes equino varus she was able to stand and walk with some help using a rollator. Her ability varied a great deal, and at times she had very little motivation to independence. The ability to transfer independently was of considerable value for both patient and ward staff after years of immobility and dependence. Occasional reassessment and treatment in physiotherapy maintained this level of achievement for over one year.

(iii) Mr A., born in 1910, was admitted to hospital in 1940 having a history of chronic psychosis and epilepsy. Following a cerebrovascular accident with a right-sided hemiparesis he needed to walk with a rollator. He was referred to physiotherapy in September 1986, as the nurses were concerned about his increasing reluctance to move, leaving him unable to leave an upstairs ward which had been his home for many years. On referral, Mr A's leg was oedematous, and cellulitis had led to skin breakdown. Within a week the therapist had persuaded him to attend the department, and with daily practice he was able to walk to the department. The dressings were carried out on the ward. By gradually increasing the tension of the tubular bandage and by increasing mobility, the swelling was controlled and the skin healed. Within six weeks Mr A. was walking with one stick, and by the end of the year he could discard the tubigrip. One year later he was discharged from hospital to live in a warden-controlled flat.

(iv) A lower limb fracture in an elderly patient who has already been admitted with severe dementia can lead to an assumption that there is little point in trying to regain mobility. The following case history demonstrates that this can be unduly pessimistic. Mrs B., born in 1918, was admitted in 1985 with severe dementia, and although needing help with self-care she was able to feed herself and walked independently until, in April 1987, she sustained a fracture of the left neck of the femur. This was treated by the insertion of an uncemented Thompson's prosthesis. Within a week, with physiotherapy guidance, and with encouragement and assistance from the nurses, she was able to transfer from one chair to another and to walk a few steps with support; however, following a minor urinary infection, and increased pain, she began to hold the affected leg in flexion (X-rays showed no displacement of the prosthesis). By June, Mrs B. was still not weight-bearing, and some flexor muscle tightening had occurred. Daily therapy to stretch the hip and knee flexors, and lying flat for short periods during the day helped to encourage weight-bearing. A temporary back-splint and shoe-raise were fitted and were worn during physiotherapy until the patient was able to walk with a wheeled frame. She progressed to walking with a quadrupod stick, and standby assistance; eventually, with occasional physiotherapy super-vision and guidance to the nurses, the patient again walked unaided fifteen months after the accident.

TEAM APPROACH

Where consultants in elderly patient medicine and psychiatry hold joint multi-disciplinary case conferences, and where social service is well established, then the quality of assessment and management of the elderly people with psychiatric problems is likely to be most successful. There is a psychogeriatric assessment unit in Cornwall where such co-operation occurs. When the team agrees that a patient could live in an elderly people's home in the community, then, through the hospital team, which includes social workers, a place can be obtained in a home which has been purpose-built for elderly mentally ill people. When a resident needs to be admitted to hospital the care staff know that they have the hospital's support. The officers in charge of the home are enthusiastic about the success of this co-ordination of Health and Social Services. The care staff at the home can readily but unobtrusively observe residents, and a pleasant garden hedged with conifers deters the wanderers from venturing further afield.

THE FUTURE

Joint planning endeavours are needed involving senior managers in Health, Local Authority social services, housing, voluntary and private sectors consulting with local staff and carers. To meet future needs for continuing care, small-scale local units should be planned, run by mutual agreement, probably by social services or private or voluntary organisa-tions with adequate Health Service support, these units being provided as near as possible to the patient's own home – perhaps providing day-care for elderly mentally ill people in the community. They could also provide a resource and support centre for carers.

For all the professions, recruitment and low establishments are likely to continue to be a problem and to increase as the number of available young people declines in the 1990s. There must be improvement in facilities provided for staff. This should include not only good residential accommodation, staff rooms and social facilities, but also creches and school holiday clubs to encourage and enable people with young families to return to work. Regular 'back-to-work' courses should be mounted to help to bring people who have had a gap in their careers up to date again.

The gradual improvement in recruitment and staffing levels in the allied health professions has often been achieved by the commitment of district therapists (particularly in physiotherapy) who have assessed the service in their districts and have come to the conclusion that resources are needed for the continuing care of elderly psychiatric patients. Prior to 1974 there were many long-stay psychiatric hospitals where there was no physiotherapy service at all, but since then new departments have been developed, and in some a small number of students are now gaining experience. This trend continues and is expanding into the community service to support clients and staff in elderly people's homes and elderly mentally ill people in their own homes.

Demands on health services continue to grow, and if the needs of the long-stay patients are to be met there must be far greater use of locally trained people. Some elderly patient hospitals already employ remedial therapy helpers – helpers trained by both physiotherapist and occupational therapists and with some nursing involvement. These generic helpers could be trained by nurses, therapists and social workers, and provided a suitable grading and organizational structure can be agreed should be available to work wherever continuing-care elderly mentally ill people are in need of services. This might be in the remaining continuing-care wards, in residential homes, or in patient's own homes and in day-care. The great advantage for elderly people is improved continuity of care while providing helper staff with a satisfying job. For the teachers too, it is an economic use of their teaching time and skills. These helpers can be effectively used to augment physiotherapy and occupational therapy, and can take group activity sessions in the ward as well as assisting patients' mobility with professional guidance. Preferably they should have access to regular in-service training. Youth training scheme recruits can be an imaginative means to augment the corps of helpers without significant financial implications for the Health Service.

If elderly mentally ill patients are transferred to a continuing-care ward, it can be very stressful for some carers who may then welcome the opportunity to join a carers' support group. These are increasingly available for carers in the community but are also valued additions to the work of the continuing-care ward. Such groups provide mutual emotional support for the former carers, and members of the group often assist in many ward activities as well. Volunteers are increasingly working effectively with elderly people but, in long-stay hospitals, they need the support of a full-time paid voluntary service co-ordinator and a planned teaching programme from appropriate staff. At one time there was some resistance from qualified staff to working with volunteers, but this is gradually being overcome – rapidly where voluntary service organizers are carefully selecting and nurturing their volunteers.

Repeated DHSS reports have stressed the need for resources to be used to improve care for elderly mentally ill people, and if these funds can be made available, then the next few years should begin to see more improvements in long-term care. The interest now being shown by recently qualified personnel towards these more deprived patients is encouraging, and if more resources become available to improve community care, then it is to be hoped that there will be a much higher quality of care for fewer people who unfortunately still remain in continuing care wards.

ACKNOWLEDGEMENTS

The helpful suggestions made by Mrs Rosemary Oddy, Superintendent Physiotherapist, Carlton Hayes Hospital, Leicester, have been much appreciated.

REFERENCES

Developing Services for Elderly Mentally Infirm People: Responses to the 'Rising Tide' initiative (1987) Beth Johnson Foundation in association with the Department of Adult and Continuing Education, University of Keele, England.
King's Fund (1986) *Living Well into Old Age: Applying Principles of Good Practice to Services for People with Dementia*, King Edwards Hospital Fund, Project Paper No. 63, London.
Norton, Doreen, Unpublished Report for Scottish Home and Health Department.
The Rising Tide – Developing Services for Mental Illness in Old Age (1982) NHS Health Advisory Service, Sutherland House, 29–37 Brighton Road, Sutton, Surrey.

FURTHER READING

British Geriatrics Society and the Royal College of Nursing (1975) *Improving Geriatric Care*, Royal College of Nursing, London.
Davies, Eira, M. (1978) *Let's Get Moving* Age Concern England, London.
Cowan, Daphne (1976) The assessment of self-care capacity in geriatric psychiatric patients by objective and subjective methods. *Clin. Psychol.* **32**, 59–102.
DHSS (1976) *Priorities for Health and Personal Social Service in England*, HMSO, London.
DHSS (1981) *Care in Action*, HMSO, London.
DHSS (1986) *Health Building Note 40 – Common Activity Spaces Vol. 1*, HMSO, London.
DHSS (1973) *Health Building Note 35 – Department of Psychiatry (mental illness) for a District General Hospital*, HMSO, London.
DHSS (1981) *Identification of Toilet Areas in Psychogeriatric Wards*, a report on colour and sign recognition, HMSO, London.
Diesfeldt, H.F.A. and Diesfeldt-Gronendijk, H. (1977) Improving cognitive performance in psychogeriatric patients: the influence of physical exercise. *Age Ageing*, **6**, 58–64.

Gilleard, C.J. and Pattie, A.H. (1977) The Stockton Geriatric Rating Scale: a shortened version with British normative data. *Brit. J. Psychiat.* **131**, 90–4.

Hare, Mary (1986) *Physiotherapy in Psychiatry*, Heineman, London.

Jacques, Alan (1988) *Understanding Dementia*, Churchill Livingstone, Edinburgh.

Kaplan, J. and Ford, S. (1975) Rehabilitation of the elderly – an eleven year assessment. *Gerontologist*, **15**, 393–7.

Linn, Margaret W. (1976) Studies in rating the physical, mental and social dysfunction of the chronically ill aged. *Med. Care*, **14**, 119–25.

NHS Health Advisory Service. Annual Report 1987. Obtainable from HAS, Sutherland House, 29–37 Brighton Road, Sutton, Surrey.

Oddy, Rosemary (1987) Promoting mobility in patients with dementia: some suggested strategies for physiotherapists. *Physiother. Practice*, **3**, 18–27.

Pelosi, Tony and Gleeson, Margaret (1988) *Illustrated Transfer Techniques for Disabled People*, Churchill Livingstone, Edinburgh.

Powell, R.R. (1974) Psychological effects of exercise therapy upon institutionalised geriatric mental patients. *J. Gerontology*, **29**, 157–61.

Pratt, Rosalie (1971) Prevention of pressure sores and contractures. *Nursing Times*, **67**, 567–9.

Ransome, Helen (1981) Team to keep the elderly active. *Reme. Therapist*, July 10th.

Royal College of Nursing (1988) An instructor's syllabus for handling and moving patients. Royal College of Nursing, London.

Salter, C. de L. and Salter, C.A. (1975) Effects of an individualized activity program on elderly patients. *Gerontologist*, **15**, 404–6.

Stamford, B.A., Hambacher, W. and Fallica, A. (1975) Effects of daily physical exercises on the psychiatric state of institutionalised geriatric mental patients. *Res. Quart.*, **45**, 34–41.

Sykes, Keith (1980) Planning health care for the elderly mentally infirm. *World Hospitals*, **16**, 34–6.

Whitton, James (1977) How to quench the last flame of independence in old age. *Health Soc. Services J.*, **87**, 894–5.

Part Three

IMPROVING QUALITY OF LIFE: CASE-STUDIES

There follow four case-studies or schemes where vigorous attempts have been made to improve the quality of life of patients in long stay hospital accommodation. The first and third case-studies are set in hospital wards while the second and fourth both developed their philosophies of care within accommodation which previously belonged to the local authority. One of these is an NHS Nursing Home Project.

Chapter 16

Roxbourne Hospital

INTRODUCTION

This chapter describes the efforts which have been made to improve the quality of life for continuing-care patients in Roxbourne Hospital, Harrow, Middlesex, England. This hospital, like many other long-stay units for the elderly, was built about 100 years ago and was designed for fever and isolation patients. The buildings are all single-storey, with a number of interconnecting rooms of different sizes. Over the years the accommodation has been adapted to create a number of small wards containing between four to eight beds. Since 1974 there has been a continuing programme of upgrading accommodation and furnishings, providing King's Fund beds, lockers with wardrobe space, brighter and more cheerful curtains and bedcovers.

Day rooms have been created from balconies and previous ward accommodation, each providing a view outside to well-kept gardens and overlooking the arrival of cars and delivery vans, bringing a constant glimpse of the outside world to residents. Individual places in the day rooms are still accepted and kept to. Efforts by well-meaning staff to rearrange the chairs, in order to provide a change of scene or change of company, with a new next-door neighbour from time to time, perhaps with someone who can communicate or is less deaf or confused, are not well-received and only lead to much resentment and unhappiness. After all, this seating space is the resident's own 'home' and as such should be respected. Following the death of a resident, there may well be a bid for their corner in the day room, but certainly not change for change's sake. How often do you resent a visitor sitting in your chair, even for a short stay!

The residents at Roxbourne Hospital, 8 men and 43 women, are all physically dependent and many are confused. All have undergone prolonged intensive rehabilitation for disabilities including cerebral thrombosis, Parkinson's disease, multiple sclerosis, osteoarthritis and rheumatoid arthritis, at one of the two other units in Harrow District. All residents are confined to a chair, only one can walk a few steps with help and one other can stand with the aid of a grab rail for toileting purposes. Approximately one-third of the residents require considerable help with feeding. Their mental test score ranges from 0 to 14 out of 16, with an average of 6 (Denham and Jeffreys, 1972).

Helpers, under the supervision of the visiting physiotherapist, assist in maintaining the limited mobility of the residents. It is noticeable that when the decision is made to stop intensive rehabilitation and to transfer the patient to the continuing-care unit, the resident feels an initial sense of relief that the pressure is 'off', but this can soon be followed by institutionalization where no decisions need to be made and there is acceptance of the daily routine with little choice of any alternative. The future may well hold little pleasure or joy, and expectations are nil.

The residents, unless ill or receiving terminal nursing-care, are dressed daily in their own personal clothing, although when necessary this is supplemented by the hospital wardrobe. The ladies have the benefit of a visiting hairdresser providing the uplifting hair-do, and a manicurist to add the brighter touch of a pretty-coloured nail varnish.

Unfortunately this has left residents still spending much of the day sitting staring into space, with only a few receiving visits from relatives and friends, as they, too, are elderly and often live some distance away. Few can read because of failing sight, and television, a joy to the elderly living alone, tends to become a source of irritation and argument when placed in a day-room or ward, for those who cannot see it, for those who cannot really hear it or for those who want a particular programme. Often the television or radio appears to be switched on during the day for the benefit of the domestic staff, with residents protesting about the constant noise.

IN THE BEGINNING

In 1977, the District occupational therapist, and myself (physiotherapist) were fortunate to be given the opportunity to recruit two part-time helpers for Roxbourne Hospital. We agreed that they should work together to provide a morning programme of activity, which was limited to only four residents at one time by the size of the small room available. We decided to take the residents away from the day rooms to make a change of scene and also to provide a continuing change of company from day to day. Conversation was soon stimulated within this small group, when ideas for daily activities were discussed and residents often found common interests, as many of them came from the local neighbourhood. One session a week was provided by a teacher of drama from the local college of further education. Although there was only room for four residents at any one time, a total of 12 to 16 were given some form of activity during the week, as the choice of activity and decision as to whether to go or not was left to the individual. The original programme provided whist, quizzes and slide shows.

PROGRESS

Following the success of the small activity group, the Regional Health Authority and Past Patients and Friends Committee collaborated to finance the building of an Activity Centre, a prefabricated building to be built within the hospital grounds in close proximity to the wards. The available ground space was 1,582 square feet and within these limits the nursing officer, district occupational therapist and chief speech therapist, two helpers and myself were given the opportunity to plan the rooms. The Centre was to serve a dual purpose: firstly to provide day-time accommodation for the residents and their activity programme, and secondly to act at other times as a Social Centre for the staff at Roxbourne Hospital and for other social activity groups within the District.

The accommodation

The Activity Centre (Figure 16.1) which was completed in October 1978, comprises:

1. *An Entrance Hall.*
2. *The Lounge/Sitting Room.* This is available to residents and their relatives and friends for birthday parties or private conversation. It is papered and furnished, with fitted carpet, a three-piece dralon-covered suite, china display cabinet, nest of tables, and radiogram in order to make it like a room found in many private homes. All the furniture is second-hand and is not ultramodern. As all the residents move around in wheelchairs there is no need for the plastic covered 'geriatric' chair in the lounge.
3. *The Activities Room.* This is light and spacious. The floor is covered in a 'cork'-design vinyl which looks attractive and shows no wheelchair marks. There is a clock on the wall together with pictures made by the residents and photographs of activity centre events. A number of small square tables are provided, each one allowing space for four people in wheelchairs. These tables may be placed together to provide a larger area for some activities, but the smaller more intimate group form makes communication between residents easier. Indoor plants are grown in large moveable pots in the Activities Room and cared for by residents interested in their care. Seedlings and plants are grown and sold at the annual hospital fete.
4. *The Store Room.* This has shelving which provides adequate space for

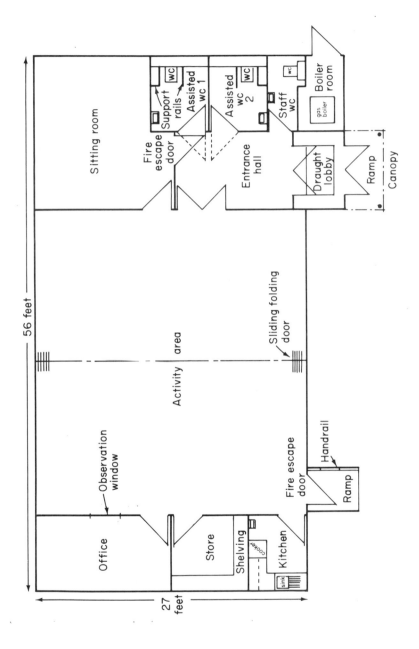

Figure 16.1 Plan of the Activities Centre at Roxbourne Hospital, Harrow, Middlesex.

storing the materials used each day.
5. *The Small Office*. This has a viewing window into the activity room, and contains a desk with telephone which provides an emergency call system to the nearby wards if required.
6. *The Kitchen*. This is equipped with a Baby Belling cooker which is used by a number of residents in the cooking session, to make buns for the morning coffee, provided in the Centre for the residents on arrival from the wards.
7. *The Toilets*. These lead off the entrance hall, and there is one staff toilet and two assisted toilets for patients. It would have been much better to have designed one double-sized assisted toilet for residents who are all unable to stand for transfers. The provision of grab rails is more of a hindrance than a help.

The daily programme

As each day provides a different activity, the residents will move to a different group, possibly two or three times a week. The decision to join an activity every day or just once or twice a week is left to the individual resident to decide. If you have never enjoyed painting, drawing or collage you are certainly not going to change suddenly. Likewise, playing whist is not everybody's choice. Drama and poetry-reading is again an individual interest. New residents are invited and encouraged to join in but never pressurized. Often after looking on for a few visits they will make an active decision as to which day or days they wish to come over.

While each day of the week has a different activity the same programmes are used with minor modifications week by week. The decision to keep to a fairly set pattern makes it easier for the resident to identify the day of the week, as otherwise every day is the same without any means of knowing whether it is Tuesday or Friday. Helpers bring residents across from the wards with the assistance of a porter when available and coffee is provided in the Centre by the domestic help, using the facilities of the small kitchen. The tables are covered with pretty table cloths and often fresh flowers are put on individual tables.

The types of activities undertaken by residents are shown in Table 16.1. The topics used for the quizzes include; identifying well-known buildings, naming animals, birds, trees, towns, famous people etc. 'Twenty Questions' and spelling games are also very popular. Quiz games are competitive with two opposing sides, points being scored by each team, with a reward for the highest scorer. An individual prize for the Brain of Roxbourne is awarded each year, in the form of a silver cup.

Table 16.1 Activities available to residents each week and average numbers attending

Activity	Average Attendance per Session
Drama/Poetry Reading	7
Art/Collage	6
Whist	12
Bingo	20
Cooking	4
Slide-Shows	20
'News' Session	8
Quizzes	14
Sing Song	20

Additional support

Support for the helpers, also comes from the District Speech Therapy Department which provides a member of their staff for two mornings a week, one session being devoted to the Activities Centre where the ideas for the stimulating quiz programme originate. The Occupational Therapy Department also provides qualified support for one session each week.

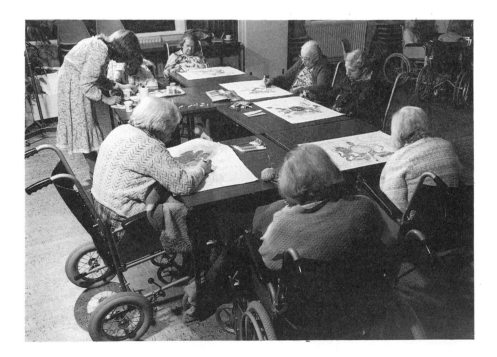

Figure 16.2 Group activity collage.

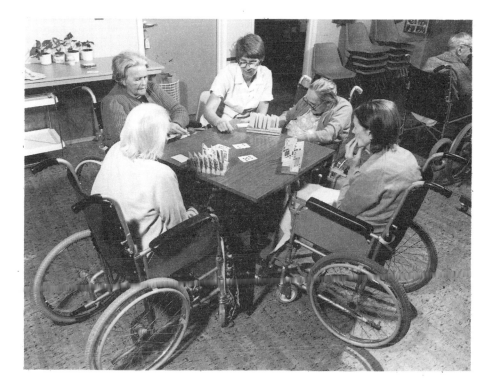

Figure 16.3 Group activity whist.

Two sessions a week, for art/collage and drama are provided by staff from the college of further education funded by the District. These sessions are invaluable. Many 'works of art' are created by the residents including many interesting forms of collage, picture-painting and colouring (Figure 16.2). Easter bonnets have been made and judged at a parade in the Centre. Making Christmas decorations and calendars are of course an annual event, and in 1981 the Royal Wedding provided a wonderful topic for discussion and ideas for decoration-making. Drama includes poetry-reading and simple one-act plays. When a resident finds reading or speaking difficult a helper or volunteer may take their place. The use of volunteers is encouraged so a greater number of residents can be looked after at each session, particularly when the less motivated and more disabled need help. It is essential that the volunteers are totally committed to their involvement and so appear regularly to play their part in the daily programme, otherwise a group activity may have to be cancelled at the last moment, if a volunteer fails to turn up. Our volunteers have become part of the Centre team and are invaluable.

Parties

The Centre has proved very valuable for gathering most of the residents together for a party to celebrate Christmas or Easter. Many of them are active in, and enjoy making decorations. The tables are placed together, covered in party food, with attractive flower arrangements providing a colourful change of scene for everyone. The food is served in small single-mouthful portions, thus making it easier for those having feeding difficulties. At other times groups of local school children visit the Centre to provide dancing displays, drama groups come to produce plays, and old time reviews and musical entertainment are provided by groups from the local church and District Hospital.

Outside visits

These are very popular with a number of the residents and provide a talking point for the following day or days. Details of the visit are discussed over coffee with those who have been left behind. The transport is provided by a converted minibus which accommodates four wheelchairs with safety clamps and belts. Seats for the helpers are placed next to the wheelchairs which gives residents greater confidence during the drive. The most popular visit is to the large shopping centre some ten miles away, where toilets for disabled people are available. Enormous pleasure is gained, not only from the opportunity of deciding what to buy, and being able to choose for themselves, but also for seeing and recognizing known buildings and roads on the way. The hospital provides coffee and sandwiches for the outing; on a longer outing the opportunity for tea or coffee in a cafeteria, with access for wheelchairs, is an added pleasure. Visits to the local parks and nursery gardens are also enjoyed. For outside visits, one helper per wheelchair is necessary. It is worth noting that pushing a chair over a long distance can prove very uncomfortable for the occupant as well as tiring for the helper. Each ward sister is responsible for selecting, in turn, those residents able to go out and the visits most suitable for them.

For the past few years, a few patients have been able to spend a short summer holiday at the seaside, staying in accommodation specially designed for severely disabled people. Because the caring staff in the hotel find it difficult to cope with noisy or very confused patients, we have sent only the more sensible patients. From what they tell us they thoroughly enjoy their time by the sea.

Residents' comments

A number of residents have expressed their opinions about the Activity

Centre and what it has meant to them. 'It makes all the difference to my life – a boon'; 'It is stimulating and makes me think for myself'; 'It keeps me in touch with current affairs'; 'I know what day of the week it is', 'I meet people from other wards and we have something to talk about'; 'I cannot use my hands but my head is alright'; 'It makes such a change', 'It makes the day – I like all the activities', 'I enjoy doing things and watching others do them'; 'It brings back memories – seeing slides of places I remember'; 'I keep up with the world outside'; 'I enjoy having to think'. They also commented on how they felt life would be without the Centre. 'I would go mad'; 'I would switch off'; 'I would sit and stare'; 'I would sleep'; 'There would be nothing to do or think about'; 'I could not live without it'.

Attitudes

The success of the activity centre, from its very small beginnings, has been due largely to the good will and interest of the helpers. Initially there was very little support for the venture from the nursing staff, who felt that any additional resources should go towards supporting an increase in their establishment and for additional equipment. The nurses' task, in a long-stay unit of this kind is hard and may be unrewarding most of the time, with the endless work of bed-pans, toilets, changing bed-linen and bathing. An offer by a physiotherapist to visit each ward, between 8.00 and 9.30 to advise 'on the spot' about getting patients out of bed, into a chair, was readily accepted by the senior nursing staff. The practical advice was welcomed by all grades of nursing staff and was far more relevant than that taught in the school of nursing. Each resident presents with multiple problems not found when teaching lifting and transferring with models. A senior physiotherapist seen working outside her normal working hours has quite an effect on the nurses. It is essential to make these visits regular, either early or late, when the residents are being put back to bed, as both nurses and residents change. It is also valuable to offer advice as and when requested during any working week. However, as the nurses have become more involved with the centre, joining in the parties and taking the residents on outside visits, their enthusiasm and interest has developed.

Another useful move was in the field of in-service training. A regular monthly programme was arranged by the senior nursing officer in the district. These sessions, from 14.00 to 15.15 hours, were attended by all grades of nursing, occupational therapy, physiotheraphy and speech therapy staff involved in caring for the elderly. The programme included: the management of incontinence, the handling of stroke patients, bereavement, drugs, and attitudes between staff, etc. Everyone became interested in these sessions after a rather slow start and the programmes were repeated each month. An amazing amount of free discussion took place and everyone agreed that a greater understanding of each subject talked about was valuable. In the continuing-care units the attitudes of all the senior managers are of utmost importance. Visits from the district heads, district medical staff, and the unit general manager brings support to the unit and simple problems can be solved before they grow into large difficulties.

THE FUTURE

The Activity Centre programme, so far, provides only for the more motivated and less confused residents, a criticism which is often heard. In order to provide an extended programme, we need to increase the establishment of helpers to work on a more individual basis with the more confused and less motivated resident. Additional helpers in turn would require the support from volunteers. Volunteers alone could not fill the role of the helpers, as direction and training is needed to plan suitable programmes for this group of patients.

At present, the Centre is not used all day. A number of residents did stay in the Centre for a longer programme, which included lunch, but after a short trial period found the extra activities too tiring and asked for a morning session only, preferring to rest or read in the afternoon. We hope, in the future, to be able to develop a suitable extended programme to fill the needs of all the residents.

It is still the exception rather than the rule to find regular stimulating activities being organized in continuing-care units; lack of finance is often given as the excuse, though lack of interest is often more apparent. Bingo and sing-song sessions may be held in some units, but no effort is made to find out what the residents are particularly interested in doing. Who should organize these programmes? The answer is the person with the interest, drive and ability to do it, be it a nurse, therapist or someone specifically appointed to do the work. This person should be assisted by the auxillary or nurses and helpers, together with regular volunteers. All these people should be chosen specifically for this work.

REFERENCE

Denham, M.J. and Jeffreys, P.M. (1972) Routine mental testing in the elderly. *Mod. Geriat.*, **2**, 275–9.

Chapter 17

The Anmer Lodge project

The philosophy, and therefore the induction programme, of the Anmer Lodge project grew out of the idea that the elderly in the continuing-care situation should have the choice of increasing their self determination, their freedom of choice and their right to be 'at risk'. At the same time the staff had to consider their own needs and anxieties.

The opportunity for the project came from the need for the Health Authority to expand its number of beds for the long-term care of the elderly. Ideally the chosen site had to be set within the community, be accessible to all by public transport and be in an area where staff could be recruited, i.e., not near a large hospital or other establishment where nurses were employed.

The clients were to be a group of highly dependent elderly people who, in many cases, had been hospitalized for a number of years. Their conceptions of hospital were, in several cases, quite fixed. This might easily have led to a dilemma about whose needs we were meeting. Were we fulfilling *our* needs by changing the life style of some of these elderly residents or were we increasing *their* quality of life? This was a key question we had to consider. On embarking on the project we produced more questions than answers on the way the project should be run. This proved to be an exciting and a motivating factor when it started to get off the ground.

THE BUILDING

Of the various sites considered, Anmer Lodge offered the most promise. It was an Old People's Home of the Part 3 type, built in the 1960s. It offered accommodation on two floors in double and single rooms. The building was constructed on a nucleus basis, that is, a series of sitting rooms with small corridors, each leading to the residents' bedrooms, toilet and bathing facilities. The local borough's policy of providing elderly care on a more community-based model meant that the upper floor of the building could be leased to provide them with further income to expand their community-care programme. After negotiations, the Health Authority took up the lease.

The site was in the northern tip of the Health Authority's boundary, well away from other health care provision. It was within walking distance of an underground railway station and was served by good bus routes. There was good access to local shops, which was seen as an additional major attraction.

The building was on a slight hill which meant that there was access to the grounds at the rear of the upper floor, which had the additional advantage of being self-contained without through traffic. There was a lift and adequate fire exits and, due to the sloping site, ease of access to the outside.

A number of modifications had to be made before the floor could be occupied. These included the installation of a sluice room, an assisted shower, an assisted bathroom with the use of a high/low bath, and modification of the toilet doors to allow wheelchair access. The adjoining matron's flat, which was no longer used, was commandeered and altered to create a large dining room with good access for wheelchairs. In addition there were two nucleus sitting rooms. The kitchen in the matron's flat was modified to take a dishwasher, a large refrigerator/freezer and a microwave oven, in addition to the conventional cooker. This was important if a philosophy and vision of care was to be realized in the way we foresaw.

On completion of the building work we were left with a 20-bedded unit with 12 single rooms, four double rooms, two sitting rooms, a dining room, kitchen, six assisted toilets, one assisted shower, one assisted bathroom, one sluice room, a storage room and a staff room. We also had the use of the personal laundry from the unit downstairs who supplied lunch and dinner for the residents from their main kitchen. There was much co-operation from the local authority staff.

THE INDUCTION PROGRAMME

With the building complete and the recruitment programme started, we now had a vision to be realized.

In the beginning, I felt that the success of the project lay in the induction programme set for the staff prior to the recruiting of residents. This could give us all a grounding of aims and objectives, and ways of realizing them. This would only be a basis, as the major work would be in the follow-up period once we were up and running.

The recruitment of staff proved to be difficult but not impossible. We were looking for trained staff who had a commitment to caring for the elderly and in doing so had a willingness to be creative in delivering the care, and willingness to question all aspects of how they operated and interacted with residents and themselves.

We were also looking for nursing auxiliaries who had no

preconceived ideas of how care should be delivered. We wanted them to use their inborn caring skills and to develop the ability to transfer this from their own home to a more formal caring environment. In fact, none of the auxiliaries who were recruited had any experience in hospital or similar type work, but in their experience of life they had administered care in various forms and in differing situations.

The induction programme had two essential components. Firstly, there had to be an area dealing with policies and procedures, for example, fire drill, administration of medicines etc. Secondly, there had to be time for us all to look at the vision of Anmer Lodge and how that could be realized. It is all too easy to say what should be done when nursing the elderly, but how this is to be put into practice is a very difficult task.

Our vision was to provide care to our elderly residents and their families in an open and loving way, while always maximizing the amount of control the residents had over their lives. The problem we could foresee with this was: was this what the residents actually wanted or was it what we thought they might want? We were envisaging giving choice and maximizing flexibility to people who may have come from a more rigid routine and have been in that routine for many years. We also had to consider their expectation of health care. Many of their conceptions went back to the days of the workhouse, so that expectations might have been very low and they were embroiled in such preconceived ideas as being grateful for whatever was offered. Relatives and friends may also have had such expectations or lack of them.

Our other concern was whether we were so open with our delivery of care that we were leaving ourselves very exposed to criticism for two particular reasons. Firstly, would we be seen as unprofessional by people who were used to seeing health care professionals in a very stereotyped role? Secondly, if we were successful in achieving an openness in our own care, would this give license to relatives to complain excessively, especially if they felt that care in the past had not met their expectations? Would we be dumped upon? This was quite a dilemma for us to face. Taking these factors into account, we set about devising a programme which would hopefully encompass all these issues.

The programme was divided into three sessions per day: 10.00 a.m. to 12.30 p.m., then 2.00 p.m. to 4.30 p.m., and finally 5.30 p.m. to 7.00 p.m. It was based largely on experiential learning, and these components were interspersed with sessions giving factual information. This we felt would cover the issues of overload and give the programme the necessary variety to hold everyone's attention.

On Day one all the new staff arrived and there was an air of anticipation and excitement. This general enthusiasm could be capitalized upon, to give everyone the knowledge that they were all able to contribute to the induction since all had valuable skills to bring to the project.

The first session consisted of practical information and a general tour of the building. This was an informal and gentle introduction to the week. At lunch, medical staff and other heads of department associated with the care of the elderly unit were able to meet the new staff.

In the afternoon there was a session where everyone introduced themselves and gave an account of why they were a nurse and why they chose to work at Anmer Lodge. This gave a general overview of people's experience and perceptions of caring. This also gave everyone a chance to share what they saw were the real issues in caring, such as the needs of both residents and staff. There was a realization that it was not wrong or selfish for nurses to have needs. This, in many cases, was quite a new concept and had gone against a lot of learning that had taken place in the past. In many ways we were re-learning as well as re-educating ourselves.

In the evening session we explored what was working and what was not working in nursing and everyone was able to contribute. Even the nursing auxiliaries who had had no formal caring experience were able to share their experience of nurses through their own hospitalization or through the hospitalization of their children. This was a really useful exercise from the point of view of being able to explore many of the issues in nursing from a personal perspective and from an outsider's point of view. This consequently led on to looking at our personal and professional motivations.

A lively discussion ensued around the real issues of caring and there was an endeavour to define what we really meant by caring. This provided a theme which we were able to touch on throughout the whole week and consequently for months to come in the follow-up sessions.

The first day, although exhausting, gave everyone that opportunity to get to know one another and also to see that they all had something valuable to contribute to the week. This created some safety within the staff group and some general bonding occurred, albeit fragile at this stage of the proceedings.

On the second day we started with drug administration procedure which was very practical and did not involve too much by way of emotional or mental overload.

In the afternoon and evening sessions we returned to the issues of caring, not only looking at caring for residents and meeting their needs, but looking at self-care and care of our colleagues. This we felt was important. Our basis for addressing these issues were around the areas of stress management and 'burn out', which is so often talked about in nursing. Both small and large group exercises were devised, so that the staff could look at what care they needed for themselves to enable them to relate well with residents and to meet their physical, mental, emotional and hopefully spiritual needs. From there we moved on to looking at care of each other.

Many of the staff agreed that nurses are not good at supporting one another. Often to ask for support from a colleague was seen as failure and was something that had not been encouraged in the past. We felt that for us to interact well with residents we must acknowledge this, otherwise the staff might become 'burnt out' very quickly and become emotionally overloaded. This we felt was an important lynch pin in the programme. The balance we had to achieve therefore was firstly, to see that self-care was different from selfishness and, secondly, to get the correct balance between looking after ourselves and not turning inwards on ourselves to the extent that we resented the residents being there. This balance we knew could be quite hard to achieve and proved a very challenging issue for us to address.

On the third day, half-way through the programme, we addressed the issue of the difficult patient. This brought in issues of patients becoming empowered. Nearly everyone could see that quite often the difficult patient was someone who was not prepared to conform or do what we wanted. It was felt important that patients were able to express how they felt since it may be the only way that they could exert their power whilst being ill. This concept was something that everyone seemed to identify with and readily understood. The difficult area was how do we feel when someone is being very critical and possibly being abusive to us? At one level we were able to rationalize it away, saying they need to do this, but we had to combine that with the real fact that staff can still feel very hurt.

For the afternoon session it was felt important to move on to more concrete issues so that staff had a chance to assimilate what they had discussed and experienced. We therefore considered the documentation that we were going to use and how it should be devised to meet the needs of residents and staff. At the end of the session we considered other practical issues such as the serving of meals and dietary factors.

The evening session for that day consisted of looking at what we meant by healing, with particular reference to the caring of elderly residents. We were looking at how they went through phases of being very passive and very dependent, requiring nurses to look after them. This was a phase that everyone could identify with and felt very comfortable with.

We also considered what happened when residents moved away from that phase, and became difficult, non-conformist and challenged what we said to them. This, everyone could see, was where residents were saying, 'I want to take control of what is happening to me'.

We addressed the issue that healing did not necessarily mean getting better, but moving on to another stage of one's life. This was particularly true of the type of client that we would be dealing with. Most, if not the majority, of our residents were going to be with us until they died. We were able to discuss that if they achieved death in a way that left them in control, then that also was healing.

On the fourth day we started by looking at the operational policies of the home. These I had already devised prior to opening but I felt that this was a chance for the staff to comment on them, and since we had been together for three days, we might modify them if they were considered inappropriate or too rigid. There was a lively discussion and all agreed that the policies would certainly have to be reviewed on a three-monthly basis.

In the afternoon we carried on from the third evening session by looking at the resident as a whole person in relation to his/her physical, emotional and spiritual needs so that we were really looking at the resident as a complete person. We continued looking at our perceptions of facing death and what that meant to the resident, what they meant to us and what it meant to the relatives. We looked at video tapes by Elizabeth Kobler Ross which proved to be a useful moving exercise and gave many of us an insight into the various phases that people go through in accepting or not accepting their own death.

On the final day we considered how we could work as a team and bring together all the issues we had discussed in the week. We had already looked at the difficult patient and what we were now going to consider was the difficult colleague. This proved to be a much more difficult problem to address, as all agreed it was much easier to ignore a difficult colleague or hope that his/her behaviour would go away. All admitted that it was difficult to challenge someone's behaviour and it might be a painful experience not only for that person, but also for us. This was felt an important area to talk about, especially if there was to be trust and honesty amongst the staff. This concept was very easy to discuss but difficult to put into practice.

The induction programme had certainly given the staff an insight into themselves and into the way that they were going to work together. It was a start, but the monthly follow-up sessions were considered to be of considerable importance, particularly since policies might need reviewing.

THE FIRST PATIENTS

The next phase was the admission of residents to the unit. It was agreed that we would phase our opening, and start by admitting 10 residents only, since staffing levels were adequate for these numbers only, as opposed to the 20 originally envisaged. Hopefully, any teething problems could be ironed out in the beginning with minimum disruption. The remainder of the staff would be recruited later and steps taken to make sure that they were assimilated and welcomed by the rest of the team. I personally had a fear that there might be a division between old and new staff. In fact, my fears were to be unfounded.

We received our residents over a period of one week, admitting two people each day in order that we got to know them well and that the nurses who were allocated to the residents were able to begin to form a bond between each other and their relatives. We had to acknowledge that fear was felt, not only by ourselves, but also by the residents and their families. In order to allay some of this fear, the residents who were coming from another hospital were visited prior to arrival so that they knew us and could recognize our faces when they arrived.

We also held a meeting at the referring hospital with the relatives of the people who were to come to us. This, as well as giving information to them allowed us to explain our philosophy of care and allowed them to question us. Many of them had fears about their relatives coming out of the present hospital where some had been for a considerable period of time. However, no potential resident was pressurized to come to Anmer Lodge. It was felt most important that they should feel comfortable with the situation and were not unduly distressed by the projected move.

When the first residents arrived at Anmer Lodge, much time and effort was put in to ensuring that they felt welcome. We instituted a system of primary nursing, which meant that each resident had a nurse who was assigned particularly to them to deliver their care. The residents were allocated their rooms and importance was attached to them getting to know each other as a group. In practical terms, the day-to-day routine was worked out to give maximum flexibility for each individual resident. It had been written into the nurses' job descriptions that they would prepare breakfast for the residents. The idea was to maximize the flexibility with which breakfast would be served. In practice, breakfast time varied from 8 a.m. to 11.30 a.m. This was important so that residents could get up at the speed they chose in the morning and were never hurried.

The lunch was set at 1 o'clock. The food came up in a bulk trolley from the unit downstairs. The intention was that the nurses would serve the residents meals in the dining room, paying particular attention to what food they wanted and the amount they wanted. We tried to be sensitive to the amount that each resident would want, bearing in mind that elderly people would rather have small frequent amounts of food rather than large meals.

In the afternoon there was emphasis on diversional activities and socialization between the residents and their visitors. At this time there was a hand-over meeting for the staff, and each day we concentrated on particular resident's needs. The evening meal was a snack served by nursing staff. Its time was very flexible.

Throughout this time individual programmes were developed for each resident and we were keen that routines such as last toileting would not occur and that continence programmes were tailored to each individual's needs.

To maximize the creativity with which care was delivered, regular staff meetings were set up so that we could evaluate the care we were delivering, as well as what we had done and what we had not done so well. Our other emphasis in care was to ensure that if any residents were ill or dying, the other residents were aware that this was going on. We felt it inappropriate to hide anything from the residents, as being a small group they operated very much like an extended family.

CONCLUSION

Within the first months of opening we had achieved a small cohesive resident group with staff who were keen and enthusiastic to meet their needs in a creative and flexible way.

The ongoing process of follow-up to the initial induction will be a key factor in making sure that care continues to be delivered in this way and is a dynamic process, not something that stops when one has achieved certain aims. The real success of the project will be if, in years to come, this type of care can be sustained on a long-term basis.

Chapter 18

The Bolingbroke Hospital long-term care project

INTRODUCTION

The Bolingbroke Hospital long-term care project developed for nine multiple handicapped aged people a standard of accommodation that is beyond our wildest dreams. We do not know whether this is the first time that a home has been created within a hospital; we do know that the furniture and furnishing design is a break through in standards. Suspended from the walls are fabric covered panels, the bedside locker, a wardrobe and a chest of drawers.

The project which took three years to create represents a break-through in standards. Two years after its opening it attracts visitors from home and abroad, and there is no doubt that care of the aged will never be the same again.

Lord Raglan, writing about the spread of civilization, used the analogy of a fish touching the top of the pond to illustrate the spread of ideas. Using that analogy the Bolingbroke project is like a Koy Carp: people ask 'How much did it cost?'; in truth, we do not know. Its design represented the combined efforts of innumerable people from different walks of life.

Major co-operating agencies were the staff of the department of elderly patient medicine attached to St George's Hospital Medical School in Tooting; the Bolingbroke Hospital nursing, therapy, administration, domestic, works and catering departments; the Hotel and Catering Division of the University of Surrey; the London College of Furniture; the Department of Health and Social Security Architect's Department; Charles Den Roche Simple Systems; and a host of others.

During the project we learnt to say 'The cost is not important' and we still hold this to be true. The most important thing was that we decided what we wanted to do, then we raised the money to do it.

If, having read about the project, you wish to visit, then visits are arranged, with the permission of the patients, on Wednesday afternoons between 2.00 and 4.00 p.m. Prior booking is essential. Visitors see less than you would expect to see in a first-class hotel. Our patients do not have private bathrooms, but they have a standard of living that an affluent society could easily afford.

This brief chapter gives no more than a flavour of the project. The chapter starts by just putting the work into its national perspective; then its place within the overall strategy of the department of elderly patient medicine is described. Thereafter the development of the project team is outlined, and established principles are laid down. Finally, the chapter concludes with photographs of the ward which give a glimpse of its splendour.

SOCIAL POLICY SIGNIFICANCE

Underlying the present governmental policies of community care is the notion that care provided out of institutional settings is superior to that provided within. Support for such policies occurs not only among professionals but among the population at large. Consequently long-term care, when provided in institutions such as hospitals, is seen as second best and as incapable of meeting the needs of those for whom it provides. Community care is fostered because it improves choice, but the services provided do not reflect the choice of the sick, they represent the choice of fit professionals.

Multi-handicapped individuals do not choose to be disabled, to have no money, poor housing and no families and friends. It is not they who choose, it is the society in which they live.

Negative attitudes relating to institutions are deep-rooted. On one level the institution is seen as a place of punishment or confinement. Samuel Butler in his book Erehwon used the analogy of punishment for ill-health and treatment for crime; in the care of the aged the crime is to be not rehabilitable, and to have no family or friends.

Closed wards in isolated psychiatric hospitals enhance the view of punishment for sickness. Similarly, the open wards of our long-stay hospitals punish people for being sick; stripped of their possessions, dressed in others' clothes, we punish the elderly for being sick. The concept of punishment is often enhanced, in the minds of the resident by the fact that many departments of elderly patient medicine have allocated beds in old workhouses. Elderly patients remember the workhouse for what it was: a place of confinement and punishment for those who had not learnt the benefit of the work ethic. The image is of dependency, and the stigma is of uselessness. Loss of dignity, and reliance on what is seen as charity, puts the standards of care in long-stay wards way down the list of desirable options.

Couple the inherent defects with the lack of staff training, and it is hardly surprising that community care is perceived as the answer to all problems. Yet the hospital and even the institution is part of the community, and irrespective of how good care at home is there will always be some people who require to be tended within institutions. Hospital care is not always bad, and home care always good, for some the alternative is the truth. For some the hospital and the residential home represent the right choice.

THE DANISH PERSPECTIVE

The Bolingbroke project exists because a King Edward's Hospital Fund for London Working Group went to visit Denmark to see why that country had failed its sick by not introducing rehabilitation. Lack of rehabilitation was the reason for the trip, but the overwhelming impression of the care of older people in Denmark was the quality of the accommodation in which they lived; in nursing homes with single rooms, private lavatories were the norm and residents were encouraged to furnish their rooms with their own possessions. The effect was striking. It is not private care, wherein the standards relate to how much you and your family can afford. It is a compromise between the state and voluntary organizations – private care does not exist. It is not care for profit. The country chooses to tend its aged sick in a dignified way that respects their past contribution to the present society and makes Danes aware that their society will, if the worst comes to the worst, tend them in their old age. It is a society that values its old and does not throw them in the dustbins of the affluent society. However, all is not perfect; the lack of rehabilitation, coupled with the absence of a elderly patient medical service, means that too many are in care. Extra beds are put up in acute hospitals in the bathrooms and corridors, and old wards were being used for people waiting for places in nursing homes.

The British long term care system requires Danish standards of accommodation; the Danish health-care system requires British concepts of rehabilitation. People visiting Denmark without knowledge of rehabilitation may leave with the wrong impression. The quality of long-stay care shows how the society values the aged it cannot rehabilitate. It does not demonstrate that community care, based on rehabilitation, is not the best option for the majority. Personal belongings, single rooms, fabric covered walls, etc. ice the cake of our department of elderly patient medicine, but the project is not the cake; the cake is an effective dedicated medical department specializing in diagnosing, treating and rehabilitating the aged.

REHABILITATION IN PERSPECTIVE

Three health-care legacies of the Second World War were the National Health Service, Rehabilitation and Operational Planning Timm (1967). Pater (1981) describes how the concepts of a National Health Service were rooted in the depression. Means and Smith (1983) place on record that split responsibility between social service departments and hospitals came about because of a combination of complaints and bombing; complaints about patient mismanagement led to the inquiry that recognized that the chronic sick were suffering from lack of medical leadership, non-existent teamwork and lack of rehabilitation; while bombing led to recognition of the fact that the frail elderly could manage in sea-side hotels. Consequently, responsibility for the chronic sick was placed on the Hospital Service whilst responsibility for the frail aged remained with local government. That legislation was the root cause of the emergence of the speciality of elderly patient medicine with specific responsibility for long-stay hospital care.

Now, forty years later, some professional pundits and outside evaluators recommend that the hospitals should cease to have responsibility for long-stay care. Others, including the author of this chapter, champion the cause of introducing the modern principles of elderly patient medicine into pre-admission assessment, rehabilitation and after-care of residents in rest and nursing homes. Ultimately, the decision will not be a medical one. The decision is political. Present regulations represent past political choices. The present emphasis on care in the community mainly in private rest and residential homes represent present political choice. The future arrangements represent future political choices. In evaluating the project and formulating your own ideas as to what is the best way forward, it is important to recognise that the Bolingbroke long-term care project exists in a department which actively champions the case for rehabilitation of the elderly.

THE ROOTS OF THE PROJECT

Responsibility for long-term care was the key. As a senior registrar trained by Professor Exton-Smith, I had learnt the benefit of progressive patient care, and in 1968 on my appointment as a consultant for the Borough of Merton I introduced his principles. The waiting list was 68.

The first priority was the development of a rehabilitative environment; to this end three wards in separate hospitals were re-designed. In my hands progressive patient care did not work, possibly because beds were on more than one site and instead of separate acute, rehabilitation and long-stay wards, the department evolved into combined acute rehabilitation wards and separate long-stay wards. Geography, resource allocation and expedience were responsible for the split. The Merton service then had, and still has, beds on more than one site; some have no on-site investigatory facilities or resident medical staff – clearly beds such as these cannot admit the acutely ill, they have to be used for either rehabilitation or long-stay care. In our case, all off-site beds without on-site radiology were used for long-stay care.

Gradually, in the long-stay ward, my eyes were opened: another dimension arose.

In 1972, following the work of Professor Brocklehurst, an art teacher, Mrs Audrey Huntley, came to Cheam and transformed my views. Soon, visitors were coming to the hospital, not out of pity for the elderly patients, but to admire their work (Figures 17.1 and 17.2).

The next major influence was a film, 'Away from the Workhouse', made in Professor Hall's department in Southampton. In that film the concept of patient committees was introduced; not believing, we took a coach full of staff and one patient to meet the staff and resident of Ashford Hospital. It was true. Thereafter, we too introduced a patient committee which resulted, among other things, in a ward Christmas party, a cheese and wine evening, a summer barbecue and an evening bonfire and fireworks. At that stage, proud of our achievements, Roger Burton, the department's social worker, and I visited Denmark. For the first time in my life I saw in-patients surrounded by possessions. The effect was striking. One felt like a burglar in their room. The belongings showed that more than being just a disease in need of care, the diseased body represented a person who had lived. On my return, Chris Smith, a psychologist doing an MSc course at St George's and I tested the hypothesis that personal belongings had a positive effect.

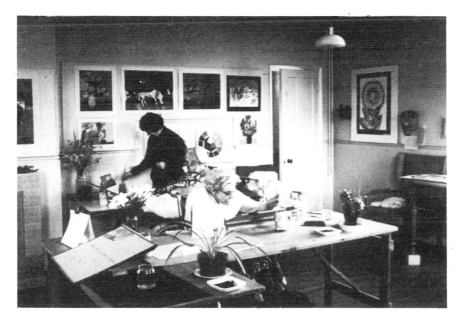

Figure 18.1 Art at Cheam, 1973: The art teacher, Mrs Audrey Huntley, and two artists.

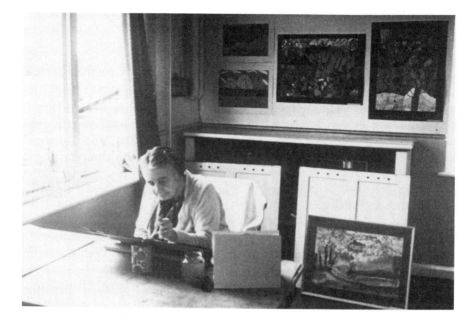

Figure 18.2   An artist at work, 1973.

PERSONAL BELONGINGS: THEIR POSITIVE EFFECT

The test was simple. Second year medical students taking the ageing course were divided into two groups; one group saw a photograph of a patient surrounded by my family photographs, flowers and cards: the other group saw the same patient in bare surroundings. In each room individual students were asked to complete an adjective check list and a semantic differential.

The results, published in the *Gerontologist* (Millard and Smith, 1981), showed that the trend was for the students who saw the possessions to be more positive in their approach to the patient. Thereafter it seemed a simple matter to introduce personal belongings into long-stay care. However, that is far from the case. Impediments abound.

Asset stripping

Long-stay patients undergo social asset stripping. The path to a long-term care ward is not an easy one; few come direct from their own home. Most have passed through other places first – their children's home, or the residential home, often intervene, and at each passage personal belongings are discarded. For many long-stay patients even the simple goal of two photographs is impossible to fulfil, let alone retrieving their cherished possessions.

Institutional rules

Institutional staff resist change. Why put photographs behind her bed when she is blind? Who is to be responsible if they are broken or stolen? What about fire, dust, clutter, infection? At each turn the inertia of the institution has to be overcome.

Unsuitability of the environment

Many long-stay patients are housed in wards designed for infectious diseases. You can't put pictures on curtains. Beds are often under the windows. Equipment attached to the walls gets in the way. Many reasons intervene. In the end at Cheam we compromised with patient identity boards and put up a board on which to pin photographs. Despite the compromise, at the end of two years less than a third of the patients had a few personal mementos.

Belongings damage walls

Picture nails damage the walls. The patients stay for a long time but they are still transient. Others follow. Wards are expensive to decorate. Wilful damage must be avoided.

The first principle taught in schools of hotel and catering is care of the environment. Specifically, if you want to run a nice hospital or residential home make sure that no notices are stuck up with sellotape; sticky tape damages the walls. Walls are expensive to decorate.

THE BOLINGBROKE PROJECT

In 1979, having been appointed Professor of Geriatric Medicine, I gave up working in the London Borough of Merton and moved to be involved with the elderly patient medical services for part of the London Borough of Wandsworth. Prior to my appointment there had been no beds allocated in the District General Hospital. All the beds had been allocated in St Benedicts Hospital, built at the beginning of the century as a boys' school.

Although much good work was being done, the facilities were inadequate for modern diagnosis and treatment, and in 1980 the decision was made to transfer the patients. In 1981 the Bolingbroke Hospital, a 100-bed acute hospital, received on transfer from St Benedict's Hospital

95 long-stay patients. To capitalize on the forced marriage of acute and long-stay it was decided that all six wards should become acute; within one year all bar one had succeeded. The failure of that ward to succeed led to the project.

THE BOLINGBROKE WARDS

Five of the six wards were of the traditional Nightingale design; most were small, containing between 15 and 21 beds. One ward, with 13 beds, previously used as the private patients' ward, was badly in need of redecorating, replumbing and rewiring. The staff in the single room ward had achieved its goal and developed a first class rehabilitative environment. Their reward was the transfer of the long-stay patients from the ward that had failed to develop a rehabilitative approach.

APPOINT A PROJECT CO-ORDINATOR

Key to the success of any innovative project is the employment of an individual who shares the dream. In our case we were able to use the salary of a technician's post in the Medical School supplemented by the St George's Hospital Endowment funds to employ Ms Rosemary Horsfall as a research assistant. Trained as a nurse, she had for several years been case-work co-ordinator with Counsel and Care for the Elderly. She brought knowledge of the statutory and voluntary sector residential and nursing homes and shared our desire to develop a model unit. Her contribution was the root cause of our success.

SELECTING THE WARD-BASED STAFF

Our next approach was to choose the correct staff. To this end all the nurses, trained and untrained, on day and night duty working in Charles Ryall Ward were interviewed individually by the project co-ordinator, myself and a senior nurse manager. All wanted to move – so all stayed.

People visiting now will be surprised to find that many of the present nurses who run the ward so well were in the original group. The reason for their desire to move is retrospectively clear. People dislike change. In the case of the staff of the project ward they had already had one major upheaval. In addition, they had succeeded in the primary task of developing a rehabilitative environment, and the reward for their success was to be punished; from the glamour of acute and rehabilitation they were to become long-stay.

FREEDOM OF CHOICE

People talk of the rights of staff and patients to choose. In reality there is little choice. Managers choose what happens to wards, staff and patients have to accept. The managerial team who decide the operational policy must then sell that policy to the staff whom they employ.

If children are failing at school you should look at the teachers and not the taught. In like manner, if patients are not being well managed one should look at the managers and not at the staff they employ.

BUILD THE TEAM

It is tempting to try, at any cost, to avoid the traumas associated with the building of a team, for inherent in teamwork is conflict. Yet, without teams, nothing can be achieved. The knowledge required to develop a new style of patient management is not contained in any individual, and teams therefore have to be built.

INVOLVE THE PATIENTS

The patients, too, are part of the team. Changing their world involves them more intimately than it involves us. They, too, will probably not like the idea of change, yet if life is to advance they realise that change must occur. During any project regular meetings with the patients are essential. At these meetings it is important that the patients should be aware of the reasoning behind the project and the object that you wish to achieve. Listen to them; they have much wisdom.

Some may not understand, but it was not our practice to exclude them. The motto of the project was 'The best for the worst' and if that is your philosophy there is little to be gained by exclusion. Some did not live to see the finished project, but both they and their relatives willingly accepted that to achieve our final goal they had to be inconvenienced. How much, they, nor we, realised.

To achieve our goal we actually allowed the contractors to knock part of the wall down in the ward in which they were housed. At that stage we had ten patients in a ward designed for six. The patients and staff were overcrowded, cramped and uncomfortable. Yet no-one complained because they were willing participators in the dream.

INVOLVE THE ANCILLARY STAFF

In addition to telling the patients, ensure that the ancillary staff know what is happening. Call the porters, the cleaners, the domestics and the works staff together and tell them what you are doing and why you are doing it. They, too, have ideas and they can contribute to the success of the whole. They take pride in their work and have justifiable pride in the achievement. That our project succeeded was to a large extent due to their willingness to help. Without them we could have achieved nothing; ignore them and you too will achieve nothing, for you can design the finest environment but unless they look after it you achieve nothing. Overlook ancillary staff training and involvement and you overlook the very building blocks of your new ward.

INVOLVE THE PROFESSIONALS ALLIED TO MEDICINE

A third essential group were the therapists, the social workers, the dietitians, and the nurses. They have much of the expertise that we required; as such, they needed to be consulted and involved throughout the project. Without them we could not have developed the idea, formulated and discussed the principles, and developed the teaching.

Each profession has its own skills. Do not expect a ward sister to be an expert in colour co-ordination, nor a therapist to design a bathroom. Each profession has its own knowledge base.

Involved as well were representatives of the hospital administration, the hospital engineers, and the works department. Each group has its own skills, but they, too, need be complemented by others. Hospital works departments have considerable expertise in upgrading hospitals but they have little skills in designing hotels. If you are to design a hotel within the hospital turn outwards and involve others. However, before you can involve others you must begin.

DEVELOP A DEMONSTRATION ROOM

The key to the successful completion of our project was decorating one room. The cost involved was minimal. We solely wallpapered one room, put up a picture rail, attached a few pictures and carpeted the floor.

One patient and their family were involved in the selection of the colour scheme. Sadly the patient died three weeks after the room was completed, and the next patient therefore entered an already decorated room. However, it was the co-operation of this patient and her son that ensured our success.

The principle that we wished to demonstrate was that the patients had their room with their possessions and that visitors and staff could enter only with the resident's permission. The willingness of our first resident, and subsequently of other residents, to allow strangers into their rooms has ensured that the concepts spread.

Retrospectively it seems surprising that all the visitors came to see was a wallpapered and carpeted room. However, from that room the whole project grew, and it was in that room that we identified the basic principles of care.

Public and private space

Separate the public and the private space. The reason that we decided to do this was that visitors were entering the patient's room space without her permission. Then the day room was at the far end of the ward. The solution was to move the day room to the other end. Now the day room is the first room that the visitor enters, and the room is separated from the general hustle and bustle of the hospital by a door with a knocker.

The day room is public space – the bedrooms are private space. No visitors are allowed into this space without permission. Separating public and private space identifies territory and also has the advantage that you can restrict access and prevent casual theft of personal belongings.

Personalized accommodation

The room is the patient's: their room, their name on the door; their chosen colour scheme; their belongings; their pictures on the wall. At first we put up the names on card, but now each patient has his or her name and title picked out in vinyl letters on a sweet chestnut panel; that final touch was by the young men who built the furniture.

Prior to that we recognize that personalization damages the walls. Wallpaper gets torn adjusting the bed; wheelchairs knock the walls. Picture nails, too, mark the walls, and pictures leave fade marks. In addition, when the patient died it was difficult to justify re-wallpapering a room which has only just been decorated. Redecoration, too, takes time, and time is limited. Hospital beds must be kept in use.

Eventually, everything was suspended from the walls. The bedside locker, the chest of drawers, the wardrobe and decorative fabric panels were all suspended from a hanging rail.

Money is not the problem

Share the dream. Speak to the League of Friends. Talk to pensioners' groups. Mention it in public lectures. Welcome visitors.

In our case we were fortunate. The League of Friends paid for the first room to be upgraded. The King Edward's Hospital fund for London gave £ 25 000. The Hotel and Catering Division of the University of Surrey advised us on the room arrangement. The London College of Furniture staff and students designed the newstyle of furniture and furnishing. The DHSS Architect's Department re-designed the layout. The project eventually cost over £ 250 000, yet it would never have begun if we had not learnt to say 'Money is not the problem'. Decide what you want to do. When you know what you want to do, look for the money to pay for it.

Build a model

Our dream nearly failed because we did not build a model. Architects can understand lines on plans, I cannot. The demonstration room showed what we wanted to do, and from that room we learnt the first two principles, but we were not knowledgeable enough to develop a comprehensive plan. Fortunately, Mr Brian Hitchcox of the DHSS Architect's Department was, and half-way through the project he built a model. That model, which still hangs from the wall in the Education Centre, showed our mistakes. We had totally overlooked the necessity of re-designing the bathrooms and sluices. We had failed to make proper use of the balcony. We had failed to make a proper bridge between the project ward and the next door ward, and we had failed even to consider the design of the six-bed bay. Following examination of that model we all realized that we were out of our depth. Mock-up rooms and model layouts are an essential prerequisite of planning.

Recognize your own limitations

The Bolingbroke project stands as witness to the skills of others. The day it was completed I realized that, alone, I could never have even begun to design the finished project. My training skills are medical. I hope that I understand the basic principles of running a department of elderly patient medicine. I know something about the reasons why patients fall, become immobile or confused, for they are the common problems of my professional trade. I now recognize that I know nothing about the manufacture and design of furniture; or the way to lay out a hotel room; or how to plan a hospital ward; or colour co-ordinate, or a host of other tasks. My part was to have a dream, but the fulfilment of that dream rested on the creation of an environment in which others could bring their professional skills to play.

Build on the people that you have

No dreams will ever materialize if one spends one's time bemoaning the material with which you have to work. Start where you are with the staff, the patients and the buildings that you have. Take an inventory of the good things that you have. Recognize what people can do, and don't continue to harp on what they cannot. Take pride in providing the best service for the worst people; surprisingly, then you will find that the worst people become the best, for they truly require the professional skills that you have developed.

Visit other wards and departments within your own hospital. Have an open day in your own ward. Ask others to visit you. Apply for grants to travel elsewhere. Arrange if you can, a visit by staff of your hospital to another hospital. Make it an annual event. On those visits you will see that, although you do some things better than others, others do some things better than you.

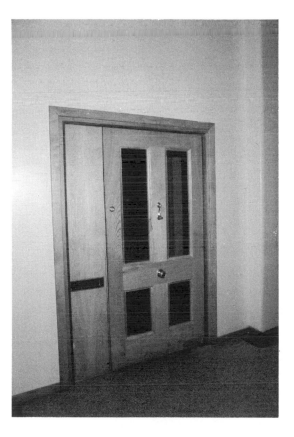

Figure 18.3 Front door and knocker.

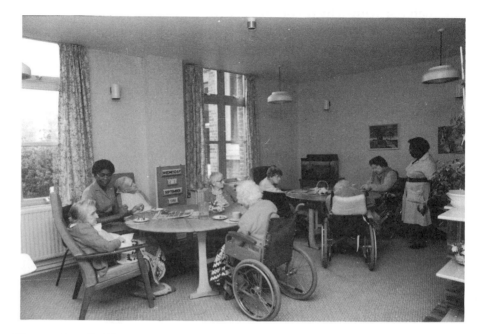

Figure 18.4 Public space.

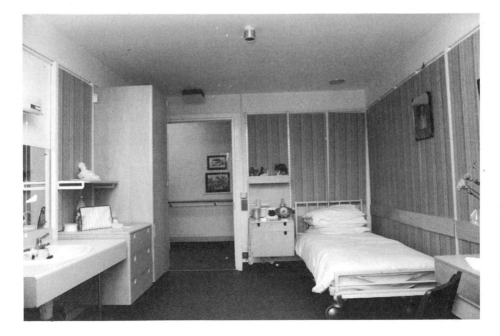

Figure 18.5 The hanging furniture and decorative panels.

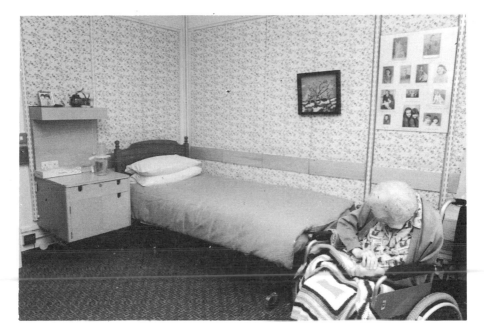

Figure 18.6 Miss Chapman in her room.

CONCLUSION

The Bolingbroke project stands as silent witness to the way that a civilized society could choose to tend its sick and frail dependents. The decorative standards seem to many visitors to be too high. Only time will tell whether the concept of hanging furniture and fabric panels from the walls is the correct one. Universal usage requires the project to be marketed and sold, and that requires the skills of others. However, what is certain is that the care of the long-stay elderly patient in the United Kingdom will never be the same again, for the project shows that a better world is possible.

Figures 18.3 to 18.6 show a view of the front door with its knocker, the space of the dayroom, and the decorative design of two rooms. The chosen pictures do not illustrate the carpets on the floors, the names on the doors, or the blue and pink bathrooms which contain special baths and equipment necessary for the staff to do their work. Hopefully, however, they may give the reader in this country and abroad some insight into the project and perhaps, who knows, encourage them to try to do the same thing where they are.

ACKNOWLEDGEMENTS

I thank Mrs Elizabeth Mosby for preparing the manuscript; the multi-disciplinary laboratory staff at St George's Hospital Medical School for taking the photographs; Ms Charlotte Walden for an early draft of this article, and Dr Paul Higgs for his assistance. In addition, I acknowledge with gratitude the debt I owe to countless people, both living and dead, for the assistance which they gave in making a dream reality.

REFERENCES

Means, R. and Smith, R. (1983) From public assistance institutions to 'Sunshine Hotels': changing state perceptions about residential care for older people 1939–1948. *Ageing Society*, **3**, 157–81.

Millard, P.H. and Smith, C.S. (1981) Personal belongings – a positive effect? *Gerontologist*, **21**, 85–90.

Pater, J.E. (1981) The Makings of the National Health Service. King Edward's Hospital Fund for London.

Timm, O.K. (1967) Rehabilitation; to what? *J. Am. Geriat. Soc.* **15**, 709–16.

Chapter 19

Jubilee House

INTRODUCTION

Jubilee House is one of three experimental homes which were set up, on the initiative of the DHSS (1983) to test the feasibility of providing nursing home care for the elderly people within the National Health Service. The homes, situated in Portsmouth, Sheffield and Fleetwood, were designed to cater for those people who require 'continuous non-psychiatric nursing to a degree which cannot be provided through the community health services, but who do not need the full range of hospital services or active medical treatment'. The residents are people who would normally live on a long-stay hospital ward.

The nursing homes are intended to be the residents' permanent home. If admission to hospital is necessary, residents return to the home as soon as the acute phase of treatment is completed. Whilst the homes were not specifically intended to provide terminal care, residents who become terminally ill will be supported at the home.

The experimental schemes were initially jointly financed by the Department of Health and Social security and the three participating district health authorities on a roughly 50–50 basis. Some funding from the DHSS continued during the evaluation period of three to four years. After this time funding became the sole responsibility of the health authority.

The project was intended to start in 1983 but the opening of both the Fleetwood and Portsmouth homes was delayed until the autumn of 1984. All the homes were existing buildings which were converted for the project. The Fleetwood and Sheffield homes had been respectively a hotel and a maternity unit, whilst Jubilee House in Portsmouth had previously been a local authority home for the blind. The homes provide between 24 and 30 places. Most residents have single rooms but double rooms were provided in anticipation of their use by married couples or friends.

Referrals for admission to the home can be made only by a consultant geriatrician. The advantage of this is that all potential residents will have a full assessment by the geriatric team and will be admitted only if they are judged to be unable to benefit from further active medical treatment or rehabilitation. The result of this careful vetting is that dependency levels have been shown to be similar to those of long-stay wards, and greater, on average, that those privately-run nursing homes (Health Care Research Unit, 1986). Once admitted to the home the residents' medical cover is provided by a general practitioner, and consultants are involved only if requested to make a domicilary visit. The general practitioner who cares for residents at Jubilee House is paid on the basis of one clinical session per week, although he prefers to divide this into two shorter regular visits each week. Between planned visits he, or his deputizing service, provides emergency cover. Residents have the option to keep their own general practitioner, but only one resident has ever expressed a wish to do so.

EVALUATION OF NHS NURSING HOME PROJECTS

The evaluation of the three homes is being undertaken by the Health Care Research Unit at Newcastle University. Their study compares existing long-stay accommodation for the elderly with the NHS nursing home in each of the three authorities. There are three components to the experimental design. The first is a randomized controlled trial which forms the major part of the research. It aims to compare the residents in the experimental homes with patients in associated long-stay wards. The objectives of this are to compare clinical effectiveness, patient satisfaction, staff satisfaction and the cost of the two modes of care, and so to provide a sound basis for judging the social efficiency of the two modes of care (Bond, 1984).

Patients referred to the project, who must all be over 65 and from a defined catchment area, have been randomly allocated to Jubilee House or to a control group. Those allocated to the Jubilee House group were offered a place in the nursing home, whilst the control group were accommodated in existing NHS facilities. Patients on the waiting list for private homes were not included in the study. Data have been collected from both groups using a variety of questionnaires given by a local field worker to residents, staff and relatives. Data have also been obtained from medical and nursing notes, and from details provided by the health authority's finance department.

The second part of the evaluation is a descriptive study of the alternative modes of care in the experimental and non-experimental settings. The final component to the evaluation is a baseline and follow-up survey of all the institutions used by elderly people within the catchment area. This describes facilities available and dependency characteristics of patients and residents.

Detailed results were not available at the time of writing, but it appears that clinical care equates with the best in hospital provision, and that quality of life is enhanced both by the homely environment and the greater individual freedom which can be attained in a small unit. Jubilee House costs, assuming 100% occupancy, are £282 per resident week (March, 1990) and this compares favourably with other NHS facilities.

JUBILEE HOUSE

Jubilee House has 25 residents in 21 single and two double rooms. The home also boasts: two dining rooms; a kitchen (all food is cooked on site); one large sitting room and several smaller sitting areas; an activity room including cooking facilities; a small gym; a visitors' bedroom and two visitors' tea bars.

The bedrooms are furnished but residents can bring their own furniture if they wish. Each resident has a commode which is disguised and which doubles as a comfortable chair. All residents use a commode at night, and some prefer them during the day. The saving in staff time having this facility always available easily justifies the expense of their purchase. Bedside cupboards include a lockable drawer to which the resident alone has access. All rooms have a TV aerial point and, one resident has had a private telephone installed. Bedrooms, corridors and sitting rooms are fully carpeted. People able to propel their own wheelchairs might find carpets a slight disadvantage as they can move more easily on a hard surface but, for most residents, the contribution made by the carpets to the homely environment is far more important.

There was some concern as to how single rooms would be accepted by residents who have, almost invariably, experienced ward accommodation for some time before admission. These fears have proved unfounded. Expecting a male admission and having only a bed in a double room where the other occupant was female, we asked every resident if they would like to share. Even those people who appeared to take little notice of their surroundings gave a distinct 'no'. They were not going to give up their private rooms. With very few exceptions the double rooms have been occupied by new residents waiting for a room of their own. Once settled in a room residents are encouraged to think of it as their own. They can arrange the furniture as they like, bring as many of their own possessions as they like and even decorate it to their own taste. No changes are made without the resident's agreement.

An anticipated disadvantage of single rooms was that residents would be reluctant to use the communal areas and would risk becoming isolated. Contrary to expectations, the main sitting room which, because of its position acts as a throughfare, is the place where most residents choose to spend the major part of their day. Although some residents prefer to eat in their rooms, dining rooms are well used. Both are furnished with round tables seating four people. The height of two of these tables has been raised as the optimum table-top position varies from person to person. Finding the correct level can be critical for those who are struggling to eat independently despite physical disabilities. A pleasant ambiance to the dining room has been seen as a priority, and a measure of success is that staff choose to eat with the residents rather than using their own dining room.

The gym was not an original part of the plan but treatment from the physiotherapist, employed for four hours a week, has proved important as much for morale as for actual physical improvement. The physiotherapist felt that there was a need for large pieces of equipment such as parallel bars which could not be housed in sitting areas without compromising the homely character.

Management

The head of home in each of the experimental units is a nurse who is responsible for the care of the residents as well as management of the home and all its staff.

Jubilee House is part of the district health authority community unit but is managerially largely self-contained. The head of home's role included the management of a budget of £376 000 which includes all staff and non-staff costs. The budget may be analysed as follows:

	£
Trained nurses	133 335
Care assistants	125 564
Bank staff (all grades)	5 314
Occupational therapy and physiotherapy	2 463
Medical officer	2 051
Catering staff	22 442
Domestic staff	16 180
Clerical	2 683
Total staff costs	310 032
Catering provisions and equipment	12 826
Domestic equipment	3 093
Drugs, dressings and medical equipment	10 231
Gas and electricity	11 568
Rates	6 881
Laundry	1 222
Disposable linen	1 334
Maintenance	6 857
Telephone and stationary	2 029
Other non-staff costs	917
Total non-staff costs	56 968

(All costs are based on figures available for the year ending March 1990.)

The head of home is also responsible for a petty cash float of £300 and for administering the finances of those residents who prefer not to handle their own affairs.

There is no direct charge for care or accomodation but, as for prolonged hospitalization, pensions are reduced to minimal levels, currently £9.40 per week.

Domestic and catering services, including the purchase of provisions, are the responsibility of the head of home. Her remit also includes administrative responsibility for the occupational therapist and physiotherapist although they relate to their respective district heads for professional matters.

Numbers of care staff employed are determined by the health authorities' criteria for registering nursing homes. Although actual registration is unnecessary, Jubilee House is inspected in the same way as private nursing homes. It is mandatory to have an RGN on duty at all times and a minimum of five care staff during the day. Whole-time equivalents for 24-hour cover are: RGN 8.67 and care assistant 14.76. The majority of these staff, including the head of home, work on a part-time basis. Student nurses based at Jubilee House for 6–7 weeks as part of their care of the elderly experience, are supernumerary. Whole-time equivalents for other staff are as follows:

Domestic assistants	2.30
Cook and catering assistants	2.51
Clerical officer	0.54
Porter/handyman	0.38
Occupational therapist	0.03
Physiotherapist	0.11
Physio helper	0.11

To remain cost effective, Jubilee House has always depended on maintaining a 'bank' of qualified staff who were willing to cover holidays of regular night staff. The bank system has now been successfully extended to include care assistants and domestic and catering staff.

Philosophy of care

Jubilee House was chosen as part of the research from about 50 proposals (Hooper, 1983) from different health authorities partly because of the suitability of the available building and partly by the ideologies of care described by the local champions of the scheme. The nurses who head the three homes were given a common training designed to help them make the most of their nursing knowledge and skills without compromising the residents' right to run their own lives. In view of the lack, at that time, of a coherent body of knowledge relating to nursing care in the long-stay elderly units, the three were encouraged to become self-sufficient as regards their own educational needs. Equipped with this training, the heads of homes were in a good position to realise the initial aspirations of their local projects. The running of Jubilee House has been firmly based on the following philosophy which formed part of the original submission to the DHSS.

> The rights of the resident to independence, individuality and dignity will be respected at all times as will their right to exercise choice and make decisions. Residents will be consulted, either directly or, if this is not feasible, through a friendly 'other', in all matters affecting their health and welfare. They will have control over their daily life, including times of awakening and taking meals with recognition of their need for privacy, fellowship and entertainment at appropriate times.

This philosophical principal is prominently displayed and frequently referred to in Jubilee House. It acts as a yardstick against which all decisions should be measured. It is important that all staff are aware of the ideals of the home because the nature of long-stay care means that different needs may conflict. Health requirements and personal choice are often at odds. Optimum mobility, for instance, is encouraged but never demanded. That may be the principal aim of a rehabilitation ward but our goals are different. A resident may be advised to stop smoking, but the decision is his, no matter what the medical implications.

Breakfast is served between 8 a.m. and 11 a.m. with one member of care staff based in the dining room to give assistance as necessary. The relaxed atmosphere and lack of time constraint means that this is the largest daily intake of both food and drink for some of the more severely disabled residents. As the kitchen is next to the dining room the catering staff are able to get to know the individual likes and dislikes of all the residents. Cooked breakfasts are prepared on demand, and choice is virtually limitless. The desire of one resident for cheese and biscuits and another for a breakfast of ice cream causes no problem. Routine is not discouraged provided it is structured by the individual resident and not the institution. Cleaning schedules can be arranged to suit the residents so the residents feel no pressure to be up at a particular time. Such a requirement is written into the tendering document for domestic services. Baths can be taken at any time, and as frequently or infrequently as the resident chooses.

A variety of diversional and social events are organized, but there is no compulsion to attend. Regular sessions are arranged for the differing needs of residents. As the residents change so does the popularity of different forms of entertainment. Quiz games such as 'Trivial Pursuits' seem to be a constant favourite. An unusually large number of mentally alert residents at present has led us to set up the very successful weekly coffee mornings. These are hosted, in the main office, by the clerical officer. The aim is to give an opportunity to people who may have similar interests to get to know each other and also to emphasize that there is no part of the home which is outside the residents' sphere. We have an activities nurse who organizes outings and events. Equally important are the small touches which are the responsibility of all staff. Newspapers must find their way to the person who has ordered them. Television and music must be an active choice rather than a background drone. Magazines must be continually renewed and always available. Thought needs to be given to where people sit and who they sit with.

Recognition of the importance of personal territory was one of the original reasons for testing the nursing home style as an alternative to the long-stay ward. Nobody enters a resident's room without knocking and waiting for a reply where this is possible, or allowing a reasonable pause where it is not. Staff have no right of entry. Most residents like the security of occasional visits from staff during the night but those who prefer to remain undisturbed have the right to do so.

All residents have a lockable drawer to which staff have no access. This can be used for valuables, drugs for those few residents who are physically and mentally capable of administering their own medicines, or simply for private belongings. On one occasion a resident forceably demonstrated his right to refuse treatment by locking away his speech therapy excercises and refusing to relinquish the key. Many residents have extended their desire for personal territory beyond the confines of their own room. There is a pattern of people claiming their own spot in the sitting room and their own place in the dining room. A trial of having place names at dining tables was warmly accepted.

One of the reasons for the choice of Jubilee House for the nursing home project was its reasonable proximity to shops and post office. It was never envisaged that residents would walk to the shops, indeed most cannot walk at all, but the hope was that they could be taken by their visitors. Unfortunately the half-mile distance is further than all but the most energetic relatives can push a wheelchair. Care assistants are willing but pressures on their time mean that these excursions are not as frequent as had been hoped. There has been little interest in the local pub but this is presumable because local culture dictates that public houses are male domains while the residents of Jubilee House are, of course, predominantly female. The most important local facility has proved to be the church, situated immediately opposite the home, which has always numbered several Jubilee House residents amongst its regular congregation.

Keeping in touch with their local community was an important part of the concept. To this end the League of Friends provided a Mini Metro converted to take one wheelchair. A major advantage of this over a larger minibus is that ease of loading and driving means that it can be used by relatives with a minimum of instruction. Ownership of the car remains with the League of Friends and they are responsible for insurance which covers any driver. Residents can tour the local town and sea front or visit friends rather than waiting for larger excursions which are complicated to organize and not to everybody's taste. Contributions to the cost of petrol are voluntary, but most residents prefer to pay their expenses. The emphasis on smaller outings does not, of course, preclude the more organized trip for which a minibus is hired.

The residents' committee is a major influence in shaping the pattern of life. Our hope that it could function with no staff input has proved unrealistic, but the care assistant who convenes meetings was nominated and elected by the residents. The few necessary communal structures to daily life are decided by the residents committee. Lunch and supper times have been changed more than once according to their instruction.

As residents realise that the committee gives them a genuine role in the management of the home they become more vocal, more likely to express any dissatisfactions, and more likely to raise matters not prompted by staff (Miller, 1986). For instance, one grievance was that residents did not like the way death was handled in the home. We had been devoting our energies to comforting the relatives and the body was removed with a minimum of fuss to avoid upsetting the other residents. The residents felt excluded. They wanted to take a much larger part in the process. At the instigation of the committee regular bulletins are now given to all residents if one of their number is ill, and a garden of remembrance has a named rose for each person who has died at Jubilee House. Far from wanting death to be handled discreetly residents wanted to be able to discuss their grief for the death of a friend and their wishes and fears concerning their own death. It is salutory to note that nurses have been banned from the meetings because of their tendency to answer for residents without giving them time to voice their own opinions.

The vital role played by relatives and friends is not forgotten. Tea bars provide the means for visitors to make themselves a drink. A spare bedroom is available for overnight accommodation. Residents can invite friends to join them for meals, and there is an open invitation to a buffet tea held every Sunday. A cupboard full of toys and a garden slide make Jubilee House popular with young visitors.

Although the physical environment was carefully planned it was always recognized that attitudes of staff were likely to have an even greater influence on the residents' quality of life.

Before opening in 1984 all staff took part in a two-week study programme principally to discuss the extent to which residents could exercise the freedom to structure their own lives and to take risks. Participants were asked to consider their own position as future residents of such a home and all agreed that, provided safety of others was not jeopardized, there was no justification for imposing any restrictions on a mentally able person. A mentally infirm resident may require some guidance but this should still be minimal. The effectiveness of this course became clear as the staff who had benefitted from it were gradually replaced by new recruits who were sometimes more authoritarian in their approach. It became obvious that attitudes of all staff should be continually challenged. Whilst reinforcing the philosophy with other staff, the senior staff themselves are challenged by the constructive criticism of a professional suppport group. This group, consisting of a consultant geriatrician, the Director of Nurse Education and four other senior nurses, meets quarterly to review progress and developments.

With a care staff consisting predominantly of unqualified assistants it is important that the expertise and skill of the trained nurse is used to its best advantage. Staff nurse and care assistant work side by side meeting the residents' needs but the plans for care are drawn up by qualifed staff working as primary nurses. These primary nurses have up to six residents for whom they are responsible. Any task they perform for the resident is an opportunity to make an assessment of their needs: is the integrity of their skin threatened; are they taking sufficient fluid; is their pain control adequate?

Student nurses spend six or seven weeks at Jubilee House as part of their experience of geriatric nursing. To direct the students' awareness towards areas specific to long-stay care, and to encourage confidence in the choice of equipment, learning objectives have been drawn up. These include: to understand the importance to residents of privacy, dignity, choice and control; to understand the need for personal territory and possessions; to understand the role of the resident's family and ways in which this may be influenced by staff; and to compare the available pressure relief mattresses and cushions in terms of effectiveness, comfort and cost.

One of the intentions of the experimental home project, as highlighted in the training programme for the heads of home, was that appropriate use of the nursing process and nursing models in long-stay elderly care would be clarified.

The fundamental structure of the nursing process, that there should be a continual cycle of assessment, planning, implementation and evaluation of care is based on a widely used problem-solving tool. The logic of this cycle is hard to dispute but the application of the process has seen a plethora of documents which are, in the main, more appropriate for the use in acute areas than long-stay areas. The result has been that many long-stay nurses have shied away from using the process. At Jubilee House the nursing process has been accepted enthusiastically, but the structure has been adapted to meet the needs of an area where changes are slow but time is always in short supply and where the majority of the care givers are unqualified and work part-time. Our written plans are unconventional but they are tailor-made to help the long-stay expert nurse to collect information, organize her ideas and communicate her decisions to the rest of the team.

The trained nurses have skills and knowledge which they should share with their residents rather than impose on them. Their expertise is needed to prevent complications arising from underlying disabilities. Jubilee House staff have been asked why they need trained nurses when they have no dressings and no catheters. The answer is, of course, that there are no dressings and no catheters because it employs trained nurses.

Nurses at Jubilee House should have a broad knowledge base but there are several areas in which they must be expert. These include:

Psychology of institutional living
Psychological and physical effects of loss of body function
Supporting those who have suffered bereavement, including loss of
    health and home
Maintenance of healthy skin
Control of chronic pain
Changing sleep patterns and altered sensory perceptions in the elderly
Nutrition and aids to independent eating
Comfort in seating, and safety in moving disabled people
Dignified control of elimination

Goffman (1960) describes the potential problems of living in an institution where leisure, work and family activities are all under the control of one authority. Awareness of the tendency for staff in these circumstances to control and standardize residents' lives in order to simplify the running of the organization is vital if senior staff are to be alert to and so avoid such developments within the home.

The most common disabilities suffered by residents are those resulting from residual damage caused by strokes. The nurse must be aware of the extent to which functional and sensory capacities may be altered beyond that which is immediately apparent. She must be knowledgable about equipment which can help the resident make the most of their remaining abilities and she must be able to empathize with somebody who may be struggling to come to terms with the loss of their healthy self-image. As well as understanding the effects of topical application, including soap, to elderly skin the nurse in long-stay care must be expert at preventing the development of pressure sores. Jubilee House residents all fall into a high-risk category and, as frequent turning is impractical as well as unpopular with residents, we make extensive use of mechanical aids. With the help of trust funds we have acquired nine water mattresses and ten silicore mattresses. An additional purchase of a Pegasus airwave mattress is anticipated by the League of Friends. Similarly, for chairs, we have three Roho cushions and various gel– and water-cushions. If it were not for these aids we could not function adequately without increasing staffing levels and so increasing revenue costs.

Jubilee House was initially furnished with four different easy-chair designs, but this did not give sufficient diversity to suit all residents. Over the last four years the range has been gradually increased. Those chairs described as 'geriatric' (high with a straight back and lumber support) have, in practice, proved to be the least popular. Domestic style recliner chairs are favoured by several people but, in hind sight, a design with 'wings' would have been more suitable than the hospital contract design we were offered. It is not possible to have only chairs designed for domestic use mainly because they usually have low seats which cause difficulties for staff transferring the heavier residents from one chair to another.

Despite having two hoists available, a fair amount of lifting cannot be avoided. This was taken into account when furniture was chosen. All beds purchased had a 'high–low' facility and were recommended for nursing home use. Unfortunately they required subsequent alteration as the lowest point (19 inches) was still higher than desirable. Principles of safe lifting come high on the list of educational objectives.

The majority of residents have either occasional or regular urinary incontinence despite efforts to regain control wherever possible. Catheters are used occasionally, so that nurses must know about recent developments in catheter care and selection. Residents are offered a choice of pads so that they can select whichever is most comfortable and effective for them. At night they may choose either pad and pants or Kylie sheet.

Faecal incontinence is largely preventable, but constipation remains a problem despite high levels of roughage in the diet. An individual bowel chart prescribes bowel care worked out between the primary nurse and her resident. Most people are content to use suppositories but, as one resident who objected pointed out, 'we do not give away our bottom halves when we come to live in a home'. Some residents use their own tried-and-tested remedies from 'ex-lax' chocolate to sitting over a commode pot full of hot water. The importance of a soft toilet seat and a variety of padded commode seats should not be underestimated.

CONCLUSION

The role of the nurse is not to control and order the lives of the residents but rather to offer a wealth of expertise which can help them to make the most of the years remaining to them.

Care at home remains the ideal, but there will always be those for whom it is impractical. For these, the most disabled of our elderly population, we must continue to seek the best that our financial resources can supply.

However political changes influence the care of elderly people, this experimental project has shown that health authorities can afford to look for alternatives to the traditional long-stay ward. With the right attitudes, the right education, and the right environment our last few years can be a dignified and enjoyable end to a long life.

REFERENCES

Bond, J. (1984) Evaluation of long-stay accommodation of elderly people, in *Gerontology – Social and Behavioural Perspectives* (ed. D.B. Bromley), Croom Helm, London.

DHSS (1983) The Experimental National Health Service Nursing Home – an Outline

Goffman, E. (1960) Characteristics of total institution, in *Identity and Anxiety* (eds M.R. Stein, A.J. Vidick and D.M. White), Free Press of Glencoe, Illinois.

Health Care Research Unit (1986) University of Newcastle-upon-Tyne, Report No. 29, vol. 2.

Hooper, J. (1983) An NHS home of their own. *Health Soc. Service J.* July 21.

Miller, L. (1986) The making of a home. *Nursing Times*, June 11.

Sander, R. (1987) The nursing process in long stay care. *Geriat. Nursing Home Care*, February.

Sander, R. (1988) Longterm Support. *Geriat. Nursing Home Care*, March.

Index